ISSN 1536-5255

# NUTRITION
## A KEY TO GOOD HEALTH

**INFORMATION PLUS® REFERENCE SERIES**
Formerly published by Information Plus, Wylie, Texas

GALE®

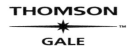

THOMSON

GALE

Detroit • New York • San Diego • San Francisco • Cleveland • New Haven, Conn. • Waterville, Maine • London • Munich

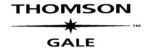

## Nutrition: A Key to Good Health
Helen S. Fisher

**Project Editor**
Ellice Engdahl

**Editorial**
Andrew Claps, Paula Cutcher-Jackson, Kathleen J. Edgar, Dana Ferguson, Debra Kirby, Prindle LaBarge, Elizabeth Manar, Sharon McGilvray, Charles B. Montney, Heather Price

**Permissions**
Ann Taylor

**Product Design**
Cynthia Baldwin

**Composition and Electronic Prepress**
Evi Seoud

**Manufacturing**
Keith Helmling

**LIBRARY OF CONGRESS CATALOGING-IN-PUBLICATION DATA**

ISBN 0-7876-5103-6 (set)
ISBN 0-7876-7343-9
ISSN 1536-5255

Printed in the United States of America
10 9 8 7 6 5 4 3 2 1

# NUTRITION
## A KEY TO GOOD HEALTH

# TABLE OF CONTENTS

# PREFACE

*Nutrition: A Key to Good Health* is one of the latest volumes in the Information Plus Reference Series. The purpose of each volume of the series is to present the latest facts on a topic of pressing concern in modern American life. These topics include today's most controversial and most studied social issues: abortion, capital punishment, care for the elderly, crime, health care, the environment, immigration, minorities, social welfare, women, youth, and many more. Although written especially for the high school and undergraduate student, this series is an excellent resource for anyone in need of factual information on current affairs.

By presenting the facts, it is Gale's intention to provide its readers with everything they need to reach an informed opinion on current issues. To that end, there is a particular emphasis in this series on the presentation of scientific studies, surveys, and statistics. These data are generally presented in the form of tables, charts, and other graphics placed within the text of each book. Every graphic is directly referred to and carefully explained in the text. The source of each graphic is presented within the graphic itself. The data used in these graphics are drawn from the most reputable and reliable sources, in particular from the various branches of the U.S. government and from major independent polling organizations. Every effort has been made to secure the most recent information available. The reader should bear in mind that many major studies take years to conduct, and that additional years often pass before the data from these studies are made available to the public. Therefore, in many cases the most recent information available in 2003 dated from 2000 or 2001. Older statistics are sometimes presented as well if they are of particular interest and no more recent information exists.

Although statistics are a major focus of the Information Plus Reference Series, they are by no means its only content. Each book also presents the widely held positions and important ideas that shape how the book's subject is discussed in the United States. These positions are explained in detail and, where possible, in the words of their proponents. Some of the other material to be found in these books includes: historical background; descriptions of major events related to the subject; relevant laws and court cases; and examples of how these issues play out in American life. Some books also feature primary documents or have pro and con debate sections giving the words and opinions of prominent Americans on both sides of a controversial topic. All material is presented in an even-handed and unbiased manner; the reader will never be encouraged to accept one view of an issue over another.

## HOW TO USE THIS BOOK

Food and nutrition are subjects of vital importance to everyone. Nutritionists, doctors, and psychologists are constantly studying the effects of diet on a person's body and mind, while economists and business people study the food purchasing habits of consumers. As a result of this research, our understanding of what Americans should eat, what they actually eat, and why, is constantly changing. This book presents the most recent research on major nutrition and nutrition-related topics, with a particular emphasis on controversial or rapidly changing areas, such as obesity among Americans, food safety, eating disorders, and the ever-changing definition of a healthful diet.

*Nutrition: A Key to Good Health* consists of ten chapters and three appendices. Each of the chapters is devoted to a particular aspect of nutrition in the United States. For a summary of the information covered in each chapter, please see the synopses provided in the Table of Contents at the front of the book. Chapters generally begin with an overview of the basic facts and background information on the chapter's topic, then proceed to examine subtopics of particular interest. For example, Chapter 6, Food

Labeling, begins with a history of government involvement in food labeling and health claims, explaining how the current regulatory system came about. It then describes the government's nutrition label, what it is for, and what its various parts mean. From there, the chapter moves on to describe how the government regulates health claims on food packaging, as well as other common claims such as "light," or "healthy." Then the chapter describes exceptions to the normal labeling rules, and concludes with statistics on whether or not people actually pay attention to nutritional labeling. Readers can find their way through a chapter by looking for the section and sub-section headings, which are clearly set off from the text. They can also refer to the book's extensive index if they already know what they are looking for.

**Statistical Information**

The tables and figures featured throughout *Nutrition: A Key to Good Health* will be of particular use to the reader in learning about this issue. These tables and figures represent an extensive collection of the most recent and important statistics on nutrition and related issues—for example, graphics in the book cover the amount of fat in a typical American's diet, the recommended calorie intake for men and women of different ages and activity levels, the percentage of Americans who say they would avoid purchasing bioengineered foods, and the number of Americans who receive government food assistance. Gale believes that making this information available to the reader is the most important way in which we fulfill the goal of this book: to help readers to understand the issues and controversies surrounding nutrition in the United States and to reach their own conclusions.

Each table or figure has a unique identifier appearing above it for ease of identification and reference. Titles for the tables and figures explain their purpose. At the end of each table or figure, the original source of the data is provided.

In order to help readers understand these often complicated statistics, all tables and figures are explained in the text. References in the text direct the reader to the relevant statistics. Furthermore, the contents of all tables and figures are fully indexed. Please see the opening section of the index at the back of this volume for a description of how to find tables and figures within it.

**Appendices**

In addition to the main body text and images, *Nutrition: A Key to Good Health* has three appendices. The first is the Important Names and Addresses directory. Here the reader will find contact information for a number of government and private organizations that can provide further information on food and nutrition. The second appendix is the Resources section, which can also assist the reader in conducting his or her own research. In this section, the author and editors of *Nutrition: A Key to Good Health* describe some of the sources that were most useful during the compilation of this book. The final appendix is the detailed Index, which facilitates reader access to specific topics in this book.

**ADVISORY BOARD CONTRIBUTIONS**

The staff of Information Plus would like to extend their heartfelt appreciation to the Information Plus Advisory Board. This dedicated group of media professionals provides feedback on the series on an ongoing basis. Their comments allow the editorial staff who work on the project to make the series better and more user-friendly. Our top priorities are to produce the highest-quality and most useful books possible, and the Advisory Board's contributions to this process are invaluable.

The members of the Information Plus Advisory Board are:

- Kathleen R. Bonn, Librarian, Newbury Park High School, Newbury Park, California

- Madelyn Garner, Librarian, San Jacinto College—North Campus, Houston, Texas

- Anne Oxenrider, Media Specialist, Dundee High School, Dundee, Michigan

- Charles R. Rodgers, Director of Libraries, Pasco-Hernando Community College, Dade City, Florida

- James N. Zitzelsberger, Library Media Department Chairman, Oshkosh West High School, Oshkosh, Wisconsin

**COMMENTS AND SUGGESTIONS**

The editors of the Information Plus Reference Series welcome your feedback on *Nutrition: A Key to Good Health*. Please direct all correspondence to:

Editors

Information Plus Reference Series

27500 Drake Rd.

Farmington Hills, MI 48331-3535

# ACKNOWLEDGMENTS

*The editors wish to thank the copyright holders of material included in this volume and the permissions managers of many book and magazine publishing companies for assisting us in securing reproduction rights. We are also grateful to the staffs of the Detroit Public Library, the Library of Congress, the University of Detroit Mercy Library, Wayne State University Purdy/ Kresge Library Complex, and the University of Michigan Libraries for making their resources available to us.*

*Following is a list of the copyright holders who have granted us permission to reproduce material in* Information Plus: Nutrition. *Every effort has been made to trace copyright, but if omissions have been made, please let us know.*

*For more detailed source citations, please see the sources listed under each individual table and figure.*

**Agricultural Research Service:** Figure 2.12, Table 2.1, Table 2.2, Table 2.3, Table 2.4, Table 2.5, Table 2.6, Table 2.7, Table 2.8, Table 2.11, Table 2.12, Table 2.13, Table 2.14, Table 2.15

**Calorie Control Council:** Figure 9.5

**Centers for Disease Control and Prevention:** Table 3.12, Table 3.13, Table 7.5, Figure 9.9, Table 9.7, Figure 7.4, Figure 7.5, Figure 7.6, Figure 7.7, Table 7.1, Table 7.6, Table 7.7, Figure 7.9, Table 9.6

**Centers for Disease Control and Prevention, National Center for Chronic Disease Prevention and Health Promotion:** Figure 3.3, Figure 3.6, Table 8.1, Figure 8.1

**Centers for Disease Control and Prevention, National Center for Health Statistics:** Figure 9.1, Table 9.1, Table 9.2, Figure 9.2, Figure 9.4

**Food Marketing Institute:** Table 5.1, Table 5.2, Table 5.3, Table 5.4, Table 5.5, Table 5.6, Table 5.7, Figure 7.15, Figure 7.16, Table 8.9, Table 8.10, Table 8.11

**Gallup Organization:** Figure 9.6

**National Academy of Sciences:** Table 3.7, Table 6.3

**National Institutes of Health, Clinical Nutrition Service:** Table 3.11

**National Institutes of Health, National Heart, Lung, and Blood Institute:** Table 3.17, Table 9.4

**National Institutes of Health, National Institute of Diabetes and Digestive and Kidney Diseases, Weight Control Information Network:** Table 9.5

**Oklahoma State University:** Table 3.14

**Oxford University Press:** Table 7.8

**U.S. Census Bureau:** Table 2.10, Table 4.6

**U.S. Department of Agriculture:** Table 3.1, Figure 3.1, Table 3.2, Figure 3.2, Table 3.10, Table 3.15, Table 3.18, Figure 4.9, Figure 7.13, Figure 9.3, Table 9.3, Figure 10.3, Table 10.4

**U.S. Department of Agriculture, Agricultural Research Service, Beltsville Human Nutrition Research Center:** Table 8.6, Table 8.7, Table 8.8

**U.S. Department of Agriculture, Center for Nutrition Policy and Promotion:** Table 3.3, Table 3.4, Table 3.5, Figure 3.8, Table 3.19, Table 8.2, Figure 8.2, Figure 8.3, Figure 8.4, Table 8.4, Table 8.5

**U.S. Department of Agriculture, Economic Research Service:** Table 1.5, Table 1.6, Figure 1.7, Figure 2.1, Figure 2.2, Figure 2.3, Figure 2.4, Figure 2.5, Figure 2.6, Figure 2.7, Figure 2.8, Figure 2.9, Figure 2.10, Figure 2.11, Table 2.9, Table 3.16, Figure 3.7, Table 4.1, Figure 4.1, Table 4.3, Figure 4.2, Figure 4.5, Table 4.5, Table 4.7, Table 4.8, Table 7.3, Table 7.4, Figure 7.1, Figure 7.8, Table 7.10, Table 7.11, Table 8.3, Figure 8.5, Table 8.12, Figure 8.6, Figure 8.7, Table 8.13, Figure 8.8, Figure 8.9, Figure 8.10, Figure 8.11, Figure 8.12, Table 10.1, Table 10.2, Figure 10.1, Figure 10.2, Table 10.3, Figure 10.5, Figure 10.6, Figure 10.7, Figure 10.8, Figure 10.9

**U.S. Department of Agriculture, Food and Nutrition Service:** Figure 4.6, Figure 4.7, Figure 4.8, Figure 10.4

**U.S. Department of Agriculture, National Agricultural Statistics Service:** Table 1.1, Figure 1.1, Figure 1.2, Table 1.2, Figure 1.3, Table 1.3, Figure 1.4, Figure 1.5, Table 1.4, Figure 1.6

**U.S. Department of Agriculture, World Agricultural Outlook Board, Interagency Agricultural Projections Committee:** Table 1.7, Table 1.8, Table 1.9, Figure 1.8

**U.S. Department of Labor:** Table 4.2, Figure 4.3, Table 4.4, Figure 4.4

**U.S. Environmental Protection Agency, National Center for Environmental Economics:** Figure 7.12

**U.S. Food and Drug Administration:** Table 3.6, Table 3.8, Table 3.9, Figure 3.4, Figure 3.5, Table 6.1, Figure 6.4, Figure 6.5, Table 6.5, Table 6.6, Figure 7.10, Table 7.12, Figure 7.11, Table 7.13, Figure 7.14, Table 7.14

**U.S. Food and Drug Administration, Center for Devices and Radiological Health:** Table 6.4

**U.S. Food and Drug Administration, Center for Food Safety and Applied Nutrition:** Figure 6.1, Figure 6.2, Figure 6.3, Table 6.2, Figure 7.2, Figure 7.3

**U.S. General Accounting Office:** Table 7.2, Table 7.9

**Wheat Foods Council & American Bakers Association:** Figure 9.7, Figure 9.8

CHAPTER 1

# AGRICULTURE

The farm has long held a cherished place in American tradition. The wholesome, hard-working family raising corn or cattle has often been mythically portrayed as the backbone of the "heartland of America." Americans have frequently looked upon the farmer and rancher as the creators of this country's bounty. Today farming is undergoing a major transformation as fewer, larger farms produce food with the help of high-technology mechanization, not family members.

## THE *CENSUS OF AGRICULTURE*

The Bureau of the Census of the U.S. Department of Commerce conducted the first agriculture census in 1840 as part of the fifth decennial (occurring every ten years) population census. Other agriculture censuses were taken as Congress saw fit. Beginning in 1982 the agricultural census has been taken every five years. In 1997 the Bureau of the Census turned over the responsibility of conducting the *Census of Agriculture* to the National Agricultural Statistics Service (NASS) of the U.S. Department of Agriculture (USDA). Some of the data presented here come from the *1997 Census of Agriculture.* The *2002 Census of Agriculture* will be available in spring 2004.

## PORTRAIT OF FARMS

### Farm Numbers in 2002

The USDA defines a farm as "any place from which $1,000 or more of agricultural products were produced and sold, or normally would have been produced and sold, during the census year." According to *Farms and Land in Farms,* a February 2003 report of the NASS, in 2002 there were 2.16 million farms in the United States. This figure is up very slightly (0.1 percent) from the number of farms in 2001, but is the first significant increase in the number of farms in the United States since 1998–99. (See Table 1.1.) The size of the average farm in 2002 was 436

**TABLE 1.1**

**Number of farms, land in farms, and average size farm, 1992–2002**

| Year | Number of farms | Land in farms | Average farm size |
|---|---|---|---|
| | *Number* | *1,000 Acres* | *Acres* |
| 1992 | 2,107,840 | 978,503 | 464 |
| 1993 | 2,201,590 | 968,845 | 440 |
| 1994 | 2,197,690 | 965,935 | 440 |
| 1995 | 2,196,400 | 962,515 | 438 |
| 1996 | 2,190,500 | 958,675 | 438 |
| 1997 | 2,190,510 | 956,010 | 436 |
| 1998 | 2,191,360 | 953,500 | 435 |
| 1999 | 2,192,070 | 947,440 | 432 |
| 2000 | 2,172,280 | 943,090 | 434 |
| 2001 | 2,155,680 | 941,310 | 437 |
| 2002 | 2,158,090 | 941,480 | 436 |

Note: A farm is any establishment from which $1,000 or more of agricultural products were sold or would normally be sold during the year.

SOURCE: "Number of Farms, Land in Farms, and Average Size Farm: United States, 1992–2002," in *Farms and Land in Farms,* U.S. Department of Agriculture, National Agricultural Statistics Service, Washington, DC, February 2003

acres. Average farm size dropped quite a bit (5.1 percent) in the one-year period from 1992 to 1993, from 464 acres to 440 acres, but decreases in farm size were small thereafter. Figure 1.1 shows the distribution of farms and farmland by geographic region. Figure 1.2 shows farmland acreage by state.

The largest increase in the number of farms in the one-year period between 2001 and 2002 occurred in the Southern region of the United States. The region added 5,700 farms, or 0.6 percent. In comparison, the largest loss of farms occurred in the North Central region, which saw a decrease of 3,300 farms, or 0.4 percent.

Between 2000 and 2002, California, Delaware, Iowa, Missouri, Nebraska, and New York experienced a steady

FIGURE 1.1

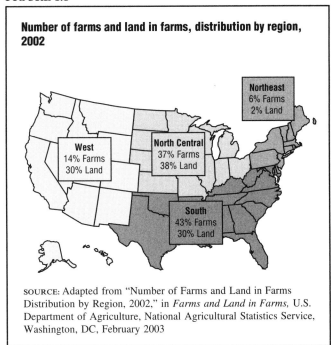

**Number of farms and land in farms, distribution by region, 2002**

Northeast
6% Farms
2% Land

West
14% Farms
30% Land

North Central
37% Farms
38% Land

South
43% Farms
30% Land

SOURCE: Adapted from "Number of Farms and Land in Farms Distribution by Region, 2002," in *Farms and Land in Farms,* U.S. Department of Agriculture, National Agricultural Statistics Service, Washington, DC, February 2003

decline in the number of farms, with the largest decrease (7.6 percent) in Delaware. (See Table 1.2.) During the same period, Alaska, Arkansas, Montana, Oklahoma, Oregon, South Carolina, and Texas experienced small increases.

Overall, the number of farms by state increased slightly between 2001 and 2002. (See Figure 1.3.) Thirty-two states retained the same number of farms from 2001 to 2002, nine states added farms, and nine states lost farms. The largest gain in farms during the one-year period occurred in Texas (3,000 farms).

**Land Use**

According to the *1997 Census of Agriculture* (the latest data available), of the 932 million acres of farmlands in 1997, 46.3 percent accounted for cropland and 42.5 percent for pastureland and rangeland. Of the 431 million acres of cropland, 71.8 percent was used for harvested crops, and 8.8 percent was used for cover crops, had failed crops, or was summer-fallowed (plowed and tilled but left unseeded). About 4.4 percent remained idle, and 15 percent was used for pasture.

**Farm Real Estate Values**

Farm real estate values, including land and buildings, have been increasing steadily since 1998. (See Table 1.3.) An August 2002 announcement from the NASS states that in January 2002, farm real estate value was $1,210 per acre, an increase of 5.2 percent from the previous year. Every state except Delaware, Nevada, New Mexico, and Washington showed gains from the previous year. The Northeast region had the highest average value of farm

real estate ($2,810 per acre). The Mountain region, at $507 per acre, had the lowest farm real estate value as of January 2002.

In 1997, 60.5 percent of all farms in the United States were small—between 1 and 179 acres in size. Half (50.3 percent), however, sold less than $10,000 and accounted for only 1.5 percent of total farm sales. Conversely, farms with sales of $500,000 or more made up only 3.6 percent of all farms, but accounted for more than half (56.6 percent) of all sales. The total market value of agricultural products (crops as well as livestock, poultry, and their products) sold in 1997 reached $196.9 billion, up 45 percent since 1987 ($136 billion). The average sales per farm were $102,970, up 58 percent from $65,165 in 1987.

According to *Farms and Land in Farms,* dry weather, below-normal yields, and lower commodity prices contributed to the shifting of farms among economic sales classes between 2000 and 2002. The number of farms with sales in the range of $1,000–$9,999 increased by 1.0 percent, to 1,172,770 in 2002. Farms with the smallest amount in sales—less than $10,000—accounted for the only increase (1.0 percent) in the number of farms between 2000 and 2002. (See Figure 1.4.) Farms with the highest amount in sales—over $100,000—had the largest decrease (1.1 percent) in their numbers between 2000 and 2002. Figure 1.5 shows the distribution of farms by size among sales classes in 2002.

Small farm operations (those with less than $10,000 in sales) accounted for 54.4 percent of all farms in 2002, but had the smallest amount of land—13.2 percent. (See Figure 1.6.) Farm operations earning more than $100,000 in sales in 2002 had 57.7 percent of all land, but only 16.1 percent of all farms.

The very smallest farms—those that have enough crops and livestock to have sales of at least $1,000—reported sales of under $1,000 from 1999 to 2002. (See Table 1.4.) These smaller farms are growing, however: their numbers increased by 16.1 percent and their acreage increased by 50 percent between 1999 and 2002.

**WHO GROWS AMERICA'S FOOD?**

**Fewer Farmers**

Until the Industrial Revolution, the U.S. economy was mainly agricultural. In 1810, 84 percent of the labor force worked in farming. By 1950, 12.2 percent of the labor force worked in farming. In 2000 farmers accounted for only 2.4 percent of the workforce.

In 1998 (the latest data available) family workers, including farm operators and unpaid workers, made up 69 percent of farm labor. Hired farm workers accounted for the remaining 31 percent. Service workers, including crew leaders and custom crews (workers who provided skilled

**FIGURE 1.2**

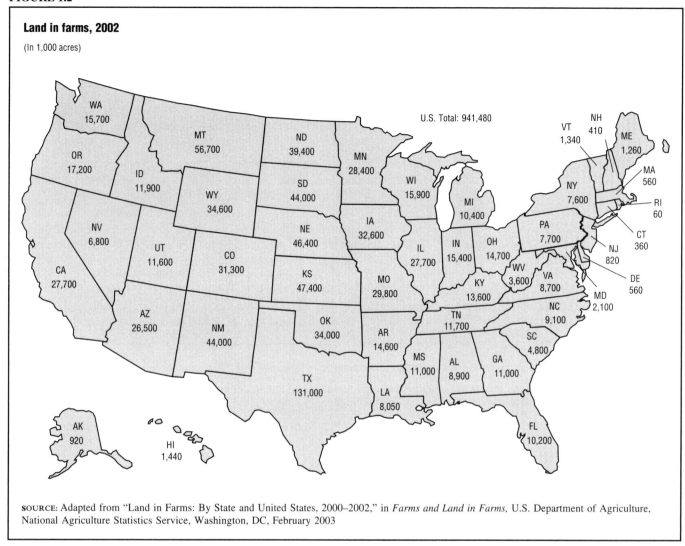

**Land in farms, 2002**

(In 1,000 acres)

U.S. Total: 941,480

WA 15,700
OR 17,200
ID 11,900
MT 56,700
ND 39,400
MN 28,400
WI 15,900
MI 10,400
NY 7,600
VT 1,340
NH 410
ME 1,260
MA 560
RI 60
CT 360
PA 7,700
NJ 820
DE 560
MD 2,100
NV 6,800
UT 11,600
WY 34,600
SD 44,000
IA 32,600
IL 27,700
IN 15,400
OH 14,700
WV 3,600
VA 8,700
CA 27,700
CO 31,300
NE 46,400
KS 47,400
MO 29,800
KY 13,600
NC 9,100
AZ 26,500
NM 44,000
OK 34,000
AR 14,600
TN 11,700
SC 4,800
MS 11,000
AL 8,900
GA 11,000
TX 131,000
LA 8,050
FL 10,200
AK 920
HI 1,440

SOURCE: Adapted from "Land in Farms: By State and United States, 2000–2002," in *Farms and Land in Farms,* U.S. Department of Agriculture, National Agriculture Statistics Service, Washington, DC, February 2003

labor and their own equipment), made up 9 percent of all workers on farms.

Several key factors have driven workers out of farming. Technological advances, such as the increased use of fertilization, improved irrigation, and larger tractor equipment, have led to dramatic increases in productivity and reductions in employment. Relatively high costs of land and equipment have restricted access to farming for many and forced others to abandon farming. The expansion of the service sector created a demand for labor in nonfarm industries, and higher earnings attracted many workers away from agriculture. On the other hand, Hispanic immigration, largely from Mexico, has provided a large pool of low-wage agricultural labor.

Since the 1970s dramatic changes have been seen in farming—from the use of black farm workers to Hispanic workers, from smaller to larger farms, from lower to higher levels of educational attainment, and, to some extent, from male to female ownership. Finally, unpaid work by family members, which was once typical in farms, has declined substantially.

## WHAT AMERICA GROWS

### Crops

America's beautiful "amber waves of grain" are most likely to be cornfields and soybean fields. Corn is not only the largest crop produced, but it is also the nation's largest export. According to the NASS, in its *Statistical Highlights of U.S. Agriculture for 2001 and 2002: Bulletin 976,* farmers harvested 68.8 million acres of corn for grain, 73.0 million acres of soybeans, and 48.7 million acres of wheat in 2001. Another 26.6 million acres were harvested of cotton, sorghum, and barley.

### Livestock and Poultry

According to *Agricultural Statistics 2002* (USDA, Washington, D.C., 2002), in 2000 U.S. cash receipts from farm marketings totaled $194 billion, up 2.9 percent from $188.1 billion in 1999. Livestock receipts totaled $99.5

**TABLE 1.2**

**Number of farms, by state, 2000–02**

| State | 2000 | 2001 | 2002 |
|---|---|---|---|
| | *Number* | *Number* | *Number* |
| Alabama | 47,000 | 47,000 | 47,000 |
| Alaska | 580 | 580 | 590 |
| Arizona | 7,500 | 7,300 | 7,300 |
| Arkansas | 48,000 | 48,000 | 48,500 |
| California | 87,500 | 85,000 | 84,000 |
| Colorado | 29,500 | 30,000 | 30,000 |
| Connecticut | 3,900 | 3,900 | 3,900 |
| Delaware | 2,600 | 2,500 | 2,400 |
| Florida | 44,000 | 44,000 | 44,000 |
| Georgia | 50,000 | 50,000 | 50,000 |
| Hawaii | 5,500 | 5,300 | 5,300 |
| Idaho | 24,500 | 24,000 | 24,000 |
| Illinois | 78,000 | 76,000 | 76,000 |
| Indiana | 64,000 | 63,000 | 63,000 |
| Iowa | 95,000 | 93,500 | 92,500 |
| Kansas | 64,000 | 63,000 | 63,000 |
| Kentucky | 90,000 | 88,000 | 89,000 |
| Louisiana | 29,500 | 29,000 | 29,000 |
| Maine | 6,800 | 6,700 | 6,700 |
| Maryland | 12,400 | 12,400 | 12,200 |
| Massachusetts | 6,100 | 6,000 | 6,000 |
| Michigan | 52,000 | 52,000 | 52,000 |
| Minnesota | 79,000 | 79,000 | 79,000 |
| Mississippi | 43,000 | 42,000 | 43,000 |
| Missouri | 109,000 | 108,000 | 107,000 |
| Montana | 27,600 | 27,500 | 28,000 |
| Nebraska | 54,000 | 53,000 | 52,000 |
| Nevada | 3,000 | 3,000 | 3,000 |
| New Hampshire | 3,100 | 3,100 | 3,100 |
| New Jersey | 9,600 | 9,600 | 9,600 |
| New Mexico | 15,200 | 15,000 | 15,000 |
| New York | 38,000 | 37,500 | 37,000 |
| North Carolina | 57,000 | 56,000 | 56,000 |
| North Dakota | 30,300 | 30,300 | 30,000 |
| Ohio | 80,000 | 78,000 | 78,000 |
| Oklahoma | 85,000 | 86,000 | 87,000 |
| Oregon | 40,000 | 40,000 | 41,000 |
| Pennsylvania | 59,000 | 59,000 | 59,000 |
| Rhode Island | 700 | 700 | 700 |
| South Carolina | 24,000 | 24,000 | 24,500 |
| South Dakota | 32,500 | 32,500 | 32,500 |
| Tennessee | 90,000 | 91,000 | 90,000 |
| Texas | 226,000 | 227,000 | 230,000 |
| Utah | 15,500 | 15,000 | 15,000 |
| Vermont | 6,700 | 6,600 | 6,600 |
| Virginia | 49,000 | 49,000 | 49,000 |
| Washington | 40,000 | 39,000 | 39,000 |
| West Virginia | 20,500 | 20,500 | 20,500 |
| Wisconsin | 77,000 | 77,000 | 77,000 |
| Wyoming | 9,200 | 9,200 | 9,200 |
| United States | 2,172,280 | 2,155,680 | 2,158,090 |

SOURCE: "Number of Farms: By State and United States, 2000–2002," in *Farms and Land in Farms*, U.S. Department of Agriculture, National Agricultural Statistics Service, Washington, DC, February 2003

**FIGURE 1.3**

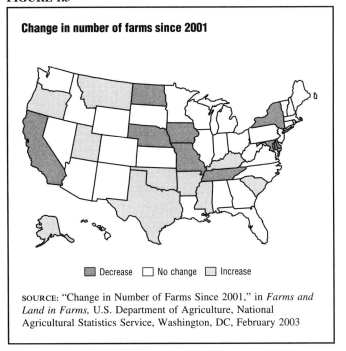

**Change in number of farms since 2001**

Decrease ☐ No change ☐ Increase

SOURCE: "Change in Number of Farms Since 2001," in *Farms and Land in Farms*, U.S. Department of Agriculture, National Agricultural Statistics Service, Washington, DC, February 2003

billion, an increase of 4.2 percent from 1999. More than half ($57.1 billion) of the livestock value consisted of meat animals and miscellaneous livestock. Poultry and eggs cash receipts totaled $21.7 billion, and dairy products, $20 billion.

As incomes have risen over the years, the need for a higher-quality diet has also increased, and animal products have often filled that need. Years ago chickens were raised mainly for egg production. The meat from chickens was only a by-product of egg production. Chickens were often scavengers, eating feed and other things that could be found around the farmyard, such as insects. Because chickens were used mainly for egg laying, chicken meat was expensive relative to the price of pork and beef.

Eventually, however, growers changed the way chickens were raised, putting them in environmentally controlled conditions. This was called confinement production. The growers kept the newly developed hybrid chickens in small areas and fed them high-quality grains. Drugs reduced losses from disease, making confinement possible. This resulted in lower prices for chicken meat, so more people could afford it. Close control of all production stages, from feed preparation to slaughter, further reduced costs. Chicken has become one of the least expensive meats a person can buy, with the price declining by about two-thirds from the mid-1950s to the end of the century.

Raising swine (hogs) for pork production has also changed. As with chickens, confining the hogs in small areas, using medicines to control disease, feeding them better food, and managing farms more efficiently have increased pork production not just in the United States but around the world. In fact, more pork is sold on the world market than beef, while chicken is gaining in popularity.

**Organic Agriculture**

The National Organic Standards Board of the USDA defines organic agriculture in this manner:

**TABLE 1.3**

**Farm real estate: average value per acre of land and buildings, by state, March 1, 1970, and January 1, 1998–2002**

| State | March 1, 1970 | January 1, 1998 | January 1, 1999 | January 1, 2000 | January 1, 2001 | January 1, 2002 |
|---|---|---|---|---|---|---|
| | Dollars | Dollars | Dollars | Dollars | Dollars | Dollars |
| Alabama | 200 | 1,440 | 1,520 | 1,680 | 1,800 | 1,900 |
| Arizona[1] | 70 | 987 | 1,070 | 1,180 | 1,360 | 1,520 |
| Arkansas | 260 | 1,150 | 1,220 | 1,250 | 1,300 | 1,370 |
| California | 479 | 2,610 | 2,770 | 2,850 | 3,000 | 3,100 |
| Colorado | 95 | 618 | 630 | 670 | 695 | 710 |
| Connecticut | 921 | 5,950 | 6,300 | 6,600 | 6,900 | 7,300 |
| Delaware | 499 | 2,660 | 2,750 | 2,800 | 2,950 | 2,950 |
| Florida | 355 | 2,240 | 2,260 | 2,400 | 2,600 | 2,800 |
| Georgia | 234 | 1,510 | 1,630 | 1,880 | 2,100 | 2,300 |
| Idaho | 177 | 1,020 | 1,090 | 1,170 | 1,200 | 1,250 |
| Illinois | 490 | 2,130 | 2,250 | 2,380 | 2,530 | 2,640 |
| Indiana | 406 | 2,060 | 2,220 | 2,350 | 2,500 | 2,590 |
| Iowa | 392 | 1,700 | 1,770 | 1,820 | 1,900 | 1,980 |
| Kansas | 159 | 577 | 580 | 590 | *610 | 620 |
| Kentucky | 253 | 1,450 | 1,530 | 1,600 | 1,770 | 1,850 |
| Louisiana | 321 | 1,210 | 1,210 | 1,250 | 1,270 | 1,310 |
| Maine | 161 | 1,190 | 1,200 | 1,250 | 1,300 | 1,400 |
| Maryland | 640 | 3,180 | 3,300 | 3,600 | 3,800 | 4,000 |
| Massachusetts | 565 | 5,210 | 5,500 | 5,900 | 6,500 | 7,200 |
| Michigan | 326 | 1,670 | 1,850 | 2,150 | 2,300 | 2,500 |
| Minnesota | 226 | 1,160 | 1,230 | 1,320 | 1,360 | 1,450 |
| Mississippi | 234 | 1,050 | 1,100 | 1,180 | 1,250 | 1,300 |
| Missouri | 224 | 1,070 | 1,130 | 1,250 | 1,380 | 1,520 |
| Montana | 60 | 294 | 296 | 350 | 375 | 384 |
| Nebraska | 154 | 645 | 670 | 695 | 730 | 755 |
| Nevada[1] | 53 | 392 | 420 | 440 | 460 | 460 |
| New Hampshire | 239 | 2,250 | 2,250 | 2,300 | 2,400 | 2,600 |
| New Jersey | 1,092 | 7,000 | 7,000 | 7,100 | 7,400 | 8,000 |
| New Mexico[1] | 42 | 217 | 217 | 217 | 220 | 220 |
| New York | 273 | 1,280 | 1,340 | 1,410 | 1,500 | 1,600 |
| North Carolina | 333 | 2,080 | 2,250 | 2,500 | 2,800 | 2,900 |
| North Dakota | 94 | 401 | 406 | 415 | 425 | 440 |
| Ohio | 399 | 2,040 | 2,220 | 2,300 | 2,480 | 2,700 |
| Oklahoma | 173 | 610 | 625 | 634 | 670 | 710 |
| Oregon | 150 | 960 | 1,000 | 1,020 | 1,050 | 1,100 |
| Pennsylvania | 373 | 2,390 | 2,500 | 2,720 | 2,840 | 2,950 |
| Rhode Island | 734 | 6,500 | 6,500 | 6,600 | 6,900 | 7,300 |
| South Carolina | 261 | 1,480 | 1,520 | 1,600 | 1,650 | 1,700 |
| South Dakota | 84 | 348 | 360 | 380 | 405 | 440 |
| Tennessee | 268 | 1,810 | 1,950 | 2,150 | 2,240 | 2,310 |
| Texas | 148 | 593 | 610 | 630 | 680 | 720 |
| Utah[1] | 92 | 807 | 855 | 900 | 975 | 1,050 |
| Vermont | 224 | 1,520 | 1,570 | 1,650 | 1,750 | 1,900 |
| Virginia | 286 | 1,920 | 2,040 | 2,200 | 2,350 | 2,490 |
| Washington | 224 | 1,190 | 1,190 | 1,200 | 1,190 | 1,190 |
| West Virginia | 136 | 1,090 | 1,070 | 1,150 | 1,280 | 1,370 |
| Wisconsin | 232 | 1,240 | 1,370 | 1,700 | 2,000 | 2,200 |
| Wyoming | 41 | 222 | 220 | 240 | 260 | 285 |
| 48 States | 196 | 974 | 1,020 | 1,080 | 1,150 | 1,210 |

[1] Excludes Native American Reservation Land.

SOURCE: "Table 9-14.—Farm real estate: Average value per acre of land and buildings, by State, Mar. 1, 1970, and Jan. 1, 1998–2002," in *Agricultural Statistics 2003*, U.S. Department of Agriculture, National Agricultural Statistics Service, Washington, DC, 2003

Organic agriculture is an ecological production management system that promotes and enhances biodiversity, biological cycles and soil biological activity. It is based on minimal use of off-farm inputs and on management practices that restore, maintain and enhance ecological

**FIGURE 1.4**

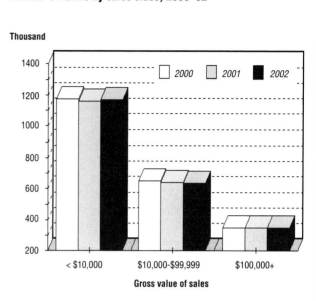

**Number of farms by sales class, 2000–02**

SOURCE: "U.S. Number of Farms by Sales Class, 2000–2002," in *Farms and Land in Farms,* U.S. Department of Agriculture, National Agricultural Statistics Service, Washington, DC, February 2003

harmony. 'Organic' is a labeling term that denotes products produced under the authority of the Organic Foods Production Act. The principal guidelines for organic production are to use materials and practices that enhance the ecological balance of natural systems and that integrate the parts of the farming system into an ecological whole. Organic agriculture practices cannot ensure that products are completely free of residues; organic growing methods are used to minimize pollution from air, soil and water. Organic food handlers, processors and retailers adhere to standards that maintain the integrity of organic agriculture products. The primary goal of organic agriculture is to optimize the health and productivity of interdependent communities of soil life, plants, animals and people.

Organic farming, which became one of the fastest growing segments of U.S. agriculture during the 1990s, continued its momentum into 2001. According to "U.S. Organic Farming: A Decade of Expansion," in the November 2002 issue of *Agricultural Outlook,* the rapid increase was spurred by consumer demand for organically produced food—a demand that grew by 20 percent or more annually. In fact, by 2001 U.S. organics sales exceeded $9 billion and accounted for approximately 2 percent of total food sales, according to industry data.

Certified organic cropland more than doubled in the United States during the 1990s, and several livestock sectors—dairy, eggs, and chicken—grew even faster. Farmers and ranchers in 49 states dedicated 1.3 million acres of farmland to organic production by 1997. Between 1997 and 2001 they added 1 million more acres, bringing the total to 2.3 million acres. (See Table 1.5.)

**FIGURE 1.5**

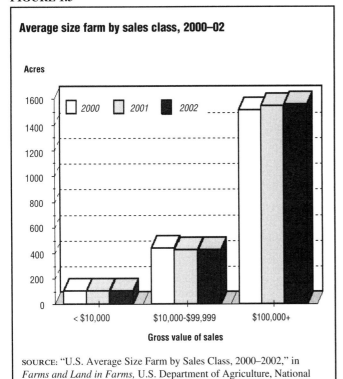

Average size farm by sales class, 2000–02

SOURCE: "U.S. Average Size Farm by Sales Class, 2000–2002," in *Farms and Land in Farms,* U.S. Department of Agriculture, National Agricultural Statistics Service, Washington, DC, February 2003

**TABLE 1.4**

Percent of farms and land in farms for places with less than $1,000 of reported sales, but with sufficient crops and livestock to normally have sales of at least $1,000, 1999–2002

| | Percent of total | |
| Year | Farms | Land |
| --- | --- | --- |
| 1999 | 15.5 | 2.0 |
| 2000 | 15.0 | 2.0 |
| 2001 | 16.0 | 2.0 |
| 2002 | 18.0 | 3.0 |

SOURCE: "Percent of Farms and Land in Farms for Places With Less Than $1,000 of Reported Sales, but with Sufficient Crops and Livestock to Normally Have Sales of at Least $1,000, United States, 1999–2002," in *Farms and Land in Farms,* U.S. Department of Agriculture, National Agricultural Statistics Service, Washington, DC, February 2003

According to *U.S. Organic Farming in 2000–2001: Adoption of Certified Systems,* a February 2003 report of the Economic Research Service of the USDA, every state except Mississippi and Delaware had some certified cropland, and nearly nine-tenths had certified pastureland. Organic animal production systems were certified in 37 states in 2001, compared with 23 states in 1997. In addition, certified organic cropland more than doubled in 12 states between 1997 and 2001, and certified organic pasture more than doubled in nearly two dozen states. (See Table 1.5.)

**FIGURE 1.6**

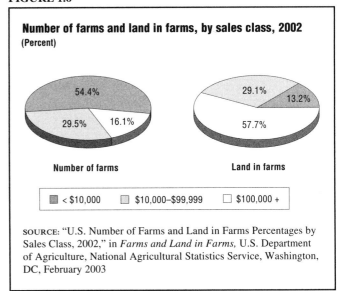

Number of farms and land in farms, by sales class, 2002
(Percent)

SOURCE: "U.S. Number of Farms and Land in Farms Percentages by Sales Class, 2002," in *Farms and Land in Farms,* U.S. Department of Agriculture, National Agricultural Statistics Service, Washington, DC, February 2003

California ranked first in certified organic cropland acreage in 2001, with nearly 150,000 acres. (See Figure 1.7) California's organic cropland acreage was mostly used for fruit and vegetable production. North Dakota took second place, with nearly 145,000 acres, mostly used for wheat, soybeans, and other field crops. Table 1.6 shows all states with their corresponding certified organic acreage in 2001. These acres include both land on which crops are grown and land used primarily in ranching.

The increasing popularity of organic farming has led to the inclusion of new initiatives in the Farm Security and Rural Investment Act of 2002 (Farm Act), designed to provide research and technical assistance for organic food farmers. The initiatives include authorization of $5 million for a national cost-share assistance program to help organic farmers with small operations cover a large portion of the costs of certification.

## THE 1996 AND 2002 FARM ACTS

The Federal Agriculture Improvement and Reform Act of 1996 (PL 104-127; also called the 1996 Farm Act) removes much of the former government control over what crops farmers are required to grow and how much is grown. Between 1973 and 1995, farmers were paid not to plant certain crops if there was a surplus of these crops. If crop prices dropped below specified levels, the federal government would make up the difference through "deficiency payments" to farmers.

The 1996 Farm Act changed income supports for eight major field crops—corn, sorghum, barley, oats, wheat, rice, upland cotton, and soybeans—by replacing the deficiency payments with a seven-year program of payments (production flexibility contract payments) to ease farmers out of their reliance on price supports. These payments are fixed amounts that decrease over time until 2002.

**TABLE 1.5**

## Organic farming, 1992–2001

| Item | 1992 | 1993 | 1994 | 1995 | 1996 | 1997 | 2000 | 2001 | Change 1992-1997 | Change 1997-2001 | Change 2000-2001 |
|---|---|---|---|---|---|---|---|---|---|---|---|
| | | | | *1,000 acres* | | | | | | *Percent* | |
| **Certified organic farmland** | | | | | | | | | | | |
| Pasture/rangeland | 532 | 491 | 435 | 279 | – | 496 | 810 | 1,040 | 7 | 109 | 28 |
| Cropland | 403 | 465 | 557 | 639 | – | 850 | 1,219 | 1,305 | 111 | 53 | 7 |
| Total farmland | 935 | 956 | 991 | 918 | – | 1,357 | 2,029 | 2,344 | 44 | 74 | 16 |
| | | | | | *Number* | | | | | | |
| **Certified organic livestock** | | | | | | | | | | | |
| Cattle | 6,796 | 9,222 | 3,300 | – | – | 4,429 | 13,829 | 15,197 | -35 | 243 | 10 |
| Milk cows | 2,265 | 2,846 | 6,100 | – | – | 12,897 | 38,196 | 48,677 | 469 | 277 | 27 |
| Hogs and pigs | 1,365 | 1,499 | 2,100 | – | – | 482 | 1,724 | 3,135 | -65 | 550 | 82 |
| Sheep and lambs | 1,221 | 1,186 | 1,600 | – | – | 705 | 2,279 | 4,207 | -42 | 497 | 85 |
| Total livestock[1] | 11,647 | 14,753 | 13,100 | – | – | 18,513 | 56,028 | 71,216 | 59 | 285 | 27 |
| **Certified organic poultry** | | | | | | | | | | | |
| Layer hens | 43,981 | 20,625 | 47,700 | – | – | 537,826 | 1,113,746 | 1,611,662 | 1,123 | 200 | 45 |
| Broilers | 17,382 | 26,331 | 110,500 | – | – | 38,285 | 1,924,807 | 3,286,456 | 120 | 8,484 | 71 |
| Turkeys | – | – | – | – | – | 750 | 9,138 | 98,653 | | 13,054 | 980 |
| Total poultry[2] | 61,363 | 46,956 | 158,200 | – | – | 798,250 | 3,047,691 | 4,996,771 | 1,201 | 2,110 | 64 |
| **Certified organic operations[3]** | 3,587 | 3,536 | 4,060 | 4,856 | – | 5,021 | 6,592 | 6,949 | 40 | 38 | 5 |

– Indicates data not available. Numbers may not add to total due to rounding.
[1] Total livestock includes other and unclassified animals.
[2] Total poultry includes other and unclassified animals.
[3] Does not include subcontracted organic farm operations.

SOURCE: "U.S. Organic Farming Continues to Expand," in *Agricultural Outlook,* U.S. Department of Agriculture, Economic Research Service, Washington, DC, November 2002

Under the Farm Security and Rural Investment Act of 2002 (also called the 2002 Farm Act), the production flexibility contract payments were replaced by direct payments. According to information on the Economic Research Service (ERS) Web site (http://ers.usda.gov/Features/farmbill) production flexibility contract payments have been replaced by fixed direct payments for eligible producers of wheat, corn, barley, sorghum, oats, upland cotton, and rice. In order to receive payments on these covered crops a producer must enter into annual agreements for crop years 2002–2007.

Producers of soybeans, peanuts, and other oilseeds are eligible for direct payments if they establish oil crop plantings as part of their base acreage and participate in the initial program enrollment. Farm owners have a one-time opportunity to select from two options for determining base acreage used to calculate these payments. Program payment yields also must be established for newly designated oil crop base acres.

## BASELINE PROJECTIONS TO 2012

The *USDA Agricultural Baseline Projections to 2012* (USDA, Washington, D.C., 2003) presents projections for the agricultural sector from 2001 to 2012. The projections assume that the 2002 Farm Act will continue to be in force.

## Crops, Livestock, and Poultry

The USDA predicts that, overall, total acreage planted with the eight major field crops will rise from 248 million acres in 2001 to 251.6 million acres in 2012, an increase of 1.5 percent. Corn and wheat are expected to account for much of the increase—6.2 percent and 3.2 percent, respectively. (See Table 1.7.)

The USDA predicts that red meat consumption in the United States will gradually decrease from 118.1 pounds per person in 2001 to 111.6 in 2012 (a decrease of 5.5 percent). Poultry consumption, on the other hand, is expected to increase substantially (9.7 percent) over the same period, from 95.2 pounds to 104.5 pounds. (See Table 1.8.)

In 2001 consumers spent 45 percent of their meat expenditures on beef; by 2012 this is expected to drop to 42 percent. (See Table 1.9.) The per capita expenditure, however, will increase, from about $224 to $232. On the other hand, the percentage of expenditures on chicken (broilers) is expected to rise from 24.2 percent to 28.5 percent over the same period, while per capita dollars will rise sharply, from $121 to $158. The USDA attributes the increase in poultry expenditures to lower production costs and prices relative to those of other meats, but consumer interest in lower-fat diets might also play a role.

**FIGURE 1.7**

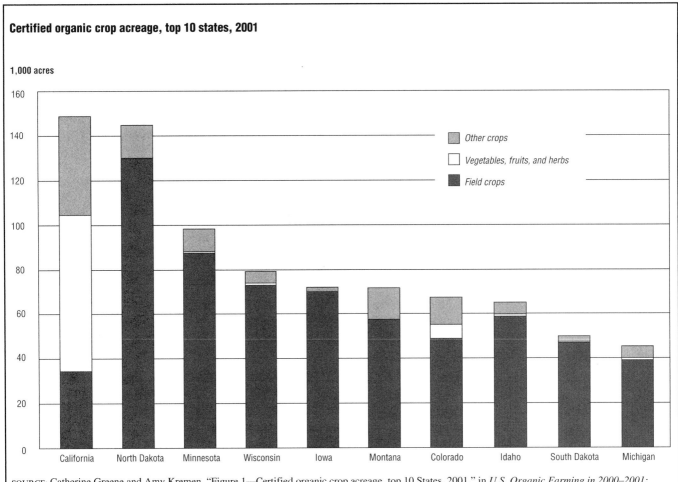

**Certified organic crop acreage, top 10 states, 2001**

1,000 acres

SOURCE: Catherine Greene and Amy Kremen, "Figure 1—Certified organic crop acreage, top 10 States, 2001," in *U.S. Organic Farming in 2000–2001: Adoption of Certified Systems,* Agriculture Information Bulletin No. 780, U.S. Department of Agriculture, Economic Research Service, Resource Economics Division, Washington, DC, February 2003

## Farm Income

The USDA projects regarding farm income over the period 2001–12 show that farm income will rise to more than $40 billion by 2005, and to over $50 billion in 2012 and beyond. (See Figure 1.8.) This is an apparently positive forcast. Nonetheless, the gains that are projected for farm incomes (2 percent annually) will not keep pace with inflation, which is expected to increase at a faster rate (2.7 percent annually). This means that in real terms (adjusted for inflation) farm income will decline over the period.

TABLE 1.6

## Certified organic acreage by state, 1997, 2000, and 2001

| State | Certifiers active by state | | | Total certified acreage | | |
|---|---|---|---|---|---|---|
| | 1997 | 2000 | 2001 | 1997 | 2000 | 2001 |
| | | Number | | | Acres | |
| **U.S. Total** | 40 | 53 | 53 | 1,346,558 | 2,029,073 | 2,343,924 |
| Alabama | 1 | 3 | 1 | 1 | 495 | 35 |
| Alaska | 1 | 1 | 1 | 174,190 | 168 | 168 |
| Arizona | 3 | 5 | 5 | 9,861 | 7,849 | 8,933 |
| Arkansas | 3 | 5 | 5 | 997 | 20,107 | 24,848 |
| California | 6 | 9 | 11 | 102,819 | 157,804 | 163,158 |
| Colorado | 3 | 6 | 7 | 258,873 | 602,463 | 581,614 |
| Connecticut | 2 | 3 | 3 | 1,066 | 1,190 | 1,430 |
| Delaware | 1 | 0 | 0 | 165 | - | - |
| Florida[1] | 4 | 5 | 6 | 32,745 | 5,136 | 12,059 |
| Georgia | 1 | 2 | 3 | 572 | 633 | 546 |
| Hawaii | 4 | 6 | 7 | 595 | 699 | 736 |
| Idaho[1] | 3 | 2 | 3 | 111,430 | 108,609 | 84,048 |
| Illinois | 2 | 8 | 8 | 10,699 | 19,467 | 21,324 |
| Indiana | 3 | 7 | 8 | 1,994 | 5,617 | 4,175 |
| Iowa | 4 | 9 | 8 | 35,769 | 68,939 | 80,354 |
| Kansas | 3 | 5 | 5 | 24,314 | 34,867 | 29,480 |
| Kentucky | 1 | 1 | 1 | 5,666 | 6,291 | 6,552 |
| Louisiana | 1 | 2 | 1 | 371 | 161 | 96 |
| Maine | 3 | 2 | 1 | 6,761 | 9,363 | 9,785 |
| Maryland | 2 | 3 | 3 | 1,645 | 3,009 | 3,590 |
| Massachusetts | 3 | 5 | 5 | 1,134 | 1,265 | 1,269 |
| Michigan | 2 | 8 | 9 | 16,762 | 31,348 | 46,485 |
| Minnesota | 5 | 8 | 8 | 63,685 | 81,953 | 103,297 |
| Mississippi | 0 | 0 | 0 | - | - | - |
| Missouri | 3 | 8 | 9 | 8,300 | 11,748 | 13,310 |
| Montana | 4 | 5 | 6 | 80,112 | 121,175 | 209,025 |
| Nebraska | 3 | 5 | 5 | 29,208 | 47,615 | 47,003 |
| Nevada | 1 | 3 | 3 | 255 | 3,032 | 1,954 |
| New Hampshire | 1 | 3 | 1 | 265 | 495 | 510 |
| New Jersey | 1 | 2 | 4 | 1,334 | 2,094 | 6,982 |
| New Mexico | 4 | 4 | 4 | 26,455 | 40,826 | 42,113 |
| New York | 4 | 7 | 9 | 27,718 | 46,089 | 45,086 |
| North Carolina | 4 | 2 | 2 | 980 | 1,474 | 1,377 |
| North Dakota | 2 | 4 | 5 | 90,790 | 153,737 | 159,300 |
| Ohio | 3 | 4 | 5 | 12,015 | 40,213 | 41,460 |
| Oklahoma | 3 | 4 | 2 | 3,992 | 3,206 | 3,922 |
| Oregon[1] | 1 | 3 | 7 | 16,984 | 26,958 | 27,501 |
| Pennsylvania | 5 | 9 | 8 | 6,511 | 18,873 | 20,984 |
| Rhode Island | 1 | 1 | 1 | 132 | 156 | 210 |
| South Carolina | 2 | 1 | 1 | 41 | 168 | 14 |
| South Dakota | 3 | 6 | 6 | 32,319 | 46,532 | 57,417 |
| Tennessee | 1 | 1 | 2 | 1,351 | 1,434 | 300 |
| Texas | 2 | 4 | 6 | 30,880 | 100,726 | 266,320 |
| Utah | 3 | 5 | 6 | 20,215 | 30,891 | 33,530 |
| Vermont | 2 | 2 | 2 | 21,146 | 29,170 | 30,659 |
| Virginia | 4 | 4 | 3 | 4,416 | 9,520 | 7,428 |
| Washington | 3 | 5 | 5 | 11,459 | 37,731 | 34,238 |
| West Virginia | 3 | 2 | 2 | 733 | 565 | 540 |
| Wisconsin | 3 | 7 | 9 | 47,622 | 80,285 | 91,619 |
| Wyoming | 1 | 3 | 3 | 75 | 6,927 | 17,138 |

[1] Three states reported significant wild-crafted acreage in 1997: Florida (25,000 acres), Idaho (52,388 acres), and Oregon (6,000 acres).

SOURCE: Catherine Greene and Amy Kremen, "Table 3—Certified organic acreage by State, 1997, 2000, and 2001," in *U.S. Organic Farming in 2000–2001: Adoption of Certified Systems,* Agriculture Information Bulletin No. 780, U.S. Department of Agriculture, Economic Research Service, Resource Economics Division, Washington, DC, February 2003

## TABLE 1.7

**Planted and harvested acreage for major field crops, baseline projections, 2001–12**

|  | 2001 | 2002 | 2003 | 2004 | 2005 | 2006 | 2007 | 2008 | 2009 | 2010 | 2011 | 2012 |
|---|---|---|---|---|---|---|---|---|---|---|---|---|
|  |  |  |  |  |  | *Million acres* |  |  |  |  |  |  |
| **Planted area**, 8 major crops |  |  |  |  |  |  |  |  |  |  |  |  |
| Corn | 75.8 | 78.8 | 80.5 | 80.0 | 79.0 | 79.0 | 79.0 | 79.5 | 80.0 | 80.0 | 80.0 | 80.5 |
| Sorghum | 10.3 | 9.3 | 9.0 | 9.1 | 9.2 | 9.2 | 9.3 | 9.3 | 9.4 | 9.5 | 9.5 | 9.6 |
| Barley | 5.0 | 5.1 | 5.0 | 5.0 | 5.1 | 5.1 | 5.1 | 5.1 | 5.1 | 5.1 | 5.1 | 5.1 |
| Oats | 4.4 | 5.0 | 5.0 | 4.7 | 4.5 | 4.5 | 4.5 | 4.5 | 4.5 | 4.5 | 4.5 | 4.5 |
| Wheat | 59.6 | 60.4 | 65.0 | 62.0 | 60.5 | 60.5 | 60.5 | 60.5 | 60.5 | 60.5 | 61.0 | 61.5 |
| Rice | 3.3 | 3.2 | 3.3 | 3.3 | 3.2 | 3.2 | 3.2 | 3.2 | 3.2 | 3.2 | 3.2 | 3.2 |
| Upland cotton | 15.5 | 14.1 | 13.8 | 14.1 | 14.2 | 14.2 | 14.1 | 14.1 | 14.0 | 14.0 | 13.9 | 13.9 |
| Soy beans | 74.1 | 73.0 | 71.5 | 72.5 | 72.5 | 72.8 | 72.8 | 72.8 | 73.0 | 73.0 | 73.0 | 73.3 |
| Total | 248.0 | 248.9 | 253.1 | 250.7 | 248.2 | 248.5 | 248.5 | 249.0 | 249.7 | 249.8 | 250.2 | 251.6 |
| **Harvested area**, 8 major crops |  |  |  |  |  |  |  |  |  |  |  |  |
| Corn | 68.8 | 70.5 | 73.5 | 73.0 | 72.0 | 72.0 | 72.0 | 72.5 | 73.0 | 73.0 | 73.0 | 73.5 |
| Sorghum | 8.6 | 7.5 | 7.7 | 7.8 | 7.9 | 7.9 | 8.0 | 8.0 | 8.1 | 8.2 | 8.2 | 8.3 |
| Barley | 4.3 | 4.1 | 4.4 | 4.4 | 4.5 | 4.5 | 4.5 | 4.5 | 4.5 | 4.5 | 4.5 | 4.5 |
| Oats | 1.9 | 2.1 | 2.5 | 2.2 | 2.0 | 2.0 | 2.0 | 2.0 | 2.0 | 2.0 | 2.0 | 2.0 |
| Wheat | 48.6 | 45.8 | 54.2 | 51.8 | 50.5 | 50.5 | 50.5 | 50.5 | 50.5 | 50.5 | 50.9 | 51.4 |
| Rice | 3.3 | 3.2 | 3.2 | 3.2 | 3.2 | 3.2 | 3.2 | 3.2 | 3.2 | 3.2 | 3.2 | 3.2 |
| Upland cotton | 13.6 | 12.6 | 12.4 | 12.7 | 12.8 | 12.8 | 12.7 | 12.7 | 12.6 | 12.6 | 12.5 | 12.5 |
| Soy beans | 73.0 | 71.8 | 70.2 | 71.2 | 71.2 | 71.4 | 71.4 | 71.4 | 71.7 | 71.7 | 71.7 | 71.9 |
| Total | 222.1 | 217.6 | 228.1 | 226.3 | 224.1 | 224.3 | 224.3 | 224.8 | 225.6 | 225.7 | 226.0 | 227.3 |

SOURCE: "Table 6. Planted and harvested acreage for major field crops, baseline projections," in *USDA Agricultural Baseline Projections to 2012*, Staff Report WAOB-2003-1, U.S. Department of Agriculture, Office of the Chief Economist, Interagency Agricultural Projections Committee, Washington, DC, February 2003

## TABLE 1.8

**Per capita meat consumption, retail and boneless weight, 2001–12**

| Item | Units | 2001 | 2002 | 2003 | 2004 | 2005 | 2006 | 2007 | 2008 | 2009 | 2010 | 2011 | 2012 |
|---|---|---|---|---|---|---|---|---|---|---|---|---|---|
| **Retail weight:** |  |  |  |  |  |  |  |  |  |  |  |  |  |
| Total beef | Pounds | 66.2 | 67.7 | 64.3 | 62.9 | 61.7 | 60.8 | 60.0 | 59.6 | 59.4 | 59.5 | 59.8 | 60.0 |
| Total veal | Pounds | 0.6 | 0.6 | 0.6 | 0.5 | 0.5 | 0.5 | 0.5 | 0.4 | 0.4 | 0.4 | 0.4 | 0.4 |
| Total pork | Pounds | 50.2 | 51.6 | 50.1 | 50.0 | 50.4 | 50.4 | 50.4 | 50.5 | 50.3 | 50.3 | 50.2 | 50.3 |
| Lamb and mutton | Pounds | 1.1 | 1.2 | 1.2 | 1.1 | 1.1 | 1.1 | 1.1 | 1.1 | 1.0 | 1.0 | 1.0 | 1.0 |
| Total red meat | Pounds | 118.1 | 121.0 | 116.2 | 114.6 | 113.7 | 112.8 | 111.9 | 111.6 | 111.2 | 111.2 | 111.4 | 111.6 |
| Broilers | Pounds | 76.5 | 79.5 | 80.1 | 79.7 | 80.5 | 81.1 | 81.6 | 82.4 | 83.0 | 83.6 | 84.1 | 84.5 |
| Other chicken | Pounds | 1.2 | 1.4 | 1.2 | 1.2 | 1.3 | 1.3 | 1.3 | 1.3 | 1.3 | 1.3 | 1.3 | 1.3 |
| Turkeys | Pounds | 17.5 | 17.5 | 17.5 | 17.6 | 17.8 | 18.0 | 18.1 | 18.3 | 18.4 | 18.5 | 18.6 | 18.7 |
| Total poultry | Pounds | 95.2 | 98.4 | 98.8 | 98.6 | 99.6 | 100.4 | 101.0 | 101.9 | 102.7 | 103.4 | 104.0 | 104.5 |
| Red meat & poultry | Pounds | 213.3 | 219.4 | 215.0 | 213.1 | 213.3 | 213.2 | 213.0 | 213.5 | 213.8 | 214.5 | 215.4 | 216.1 |
| **Boneless weight:** |  |  |  |  |  |  |  |  |  |  |  |  |  |
| Total beef | Pounds | 62.7 | 64.1 | 60.9 | 59.6 | 58.4 | 57.6 | 56.8 | 56.5 | 56.3 | 56.4 | 56.6 | 56.8 |
| Total veal | Pounds | 0.5 | 0.5 | 0.5 | 0.4 | 0.4 | 0.4 | 0.4 | 0.4 | 0.3 | 0.3 | 0.3 | 0.3 |
| Total pork | Pounds | 47.2 | 48.4 | 47.1 | 47.0 | 47.4 | 47.4 | 47.4 | 47.4 | 47.3 | 47.2 | 47.2 | 47.2 |
| Lamb & mutton | Pounds | 0.8 | 0.9 | 0.9 | 0.8 | 0.8 | 0.8 | 0.8 | 0.8 | 0.8 | 0.8 | 0.7 | 0.7 |
| Total red meat | Pounds | 11.1 | 113.9 | 109.3 | 107.8 | 107.0 | 106.2 | 105.4 | 105.0 | 104.7 | 104.7 | 104.9 | 105.1 |
| Broilers | Pounds | 54.8 | 56.9 | 57.4 | 57.1 | 57.6 | 58.1 | 58.4 | 59.0 | 59.4 | 59.8 | 60.2 | 60.5 |
| Other chicken | Pounds | 0.7 | 0.9 | 0.7 | 0.7 | 0.8 | 0.8 | 0.8 | 0.8 | 0.8 | 0.8 | 0.8 | 0.8 |
| Turkeys | Pounds | 13.8 | 13.8 | 13.8 | 13.9 | 14.1 | 14.2 | 14.3 | 14.4 | 14.5 | 14.6 | 14.7 | 14.8 |
| Total poultry | Pounds | 69.4 | 71.6 | 71.9 | 71.8 | 72.5 | 73.1 | 73.5 | 74.2 | 74.7 | 75.2 | 75.7 | 76.1 |
| Red meat and poultry | Pounds | 180.5 | 185.5 | 181.3 | 179.6 | 179.5 | 179.3 | 178.9 | 179.2 | 179.4 | 179.9 | 180.6 | 181.2 |

SOURCE: "Table 21. Per capita meat consumption, retail and boneless weight," in *USDA Agricultural Baseline Projections to 2012*, Staff Report WAOB-2003-1, U.S. Department of Agriculture, Office of the Chief Economist, Interagency Agricultural Projections Committee, Washington, DC, February 2003

Nutrition: A Key to Good Health

**TABLE 1.9**

## Consumer expenditures for meats, 2001–12

| Item | 2001 | 2002 | 2003 | 2004 | 2005 | 2006 | 2007 | 2008 | 2009 | 2010 | 2011 | 2012 |
|---|---|---|---|---|---|---|---|---|---|---|---|---|
| Beef, dollars per person | 223.59 | 224.73 | 220.01 | 223.08 | 223.72 | 225.09 | 226.35 | 227.45 | 228.77 | 229.86 | 230.80 | 231.99 |
| Percent of income | 0.86 | 0.84 | 0.79 | 0.77 | 0.74 | 0.71 | 0.69 | 0.66 | 0.64 | 0.61 | 0.59 | 0.57 |
| Percent of meat expenditures | 44.85 | 44.25 | 43.86 | 43.76 | 43.51 | 43.16 | 42.80 | 42.52 | 42.27 | 42.11 | 41.95 | 41.75 |
| Pork, dollars per person | 135.02 | 137.13 | 134.84 | 135.25 | 137.35 | 138.56 | 139.91 | 141.13 | 142.72 | 143.45 | 144.44 | 145.92 |
| Percent of income | 0.52 | 0.51 | 0.49 | 0.47 | 0.46 | 0.44 | 0.43 | 0.41 | 0.40 | 0.38 | 0.37 | 0.36 |
| Percent of meat expenditures | 27.08 | 27.00 | 26.88 | 26.53 | 26.71 | 26.57 | 26.45 | 26.38 | 26.37 | 26.28 | 26.26 | 26.26 |
| Broilers, dollars per person | 120.70 | 127.67 | 128.47 | 132.84 | 134.15 | 138.63 | 143.06 | 146.68 | 150.03 | 152.93 | 155.38 | 158.29 |
| Percent of income | 0.47 | 0.47 | 0.46 | 0.46 | 0.44 | 0.44 | 0.43 | 0.43 | 0.42 | 0.41 | 0.40 | 0.39 |
| Percent of meat expenditures | 24.21 | 25.14 | 25.61 | 26.06 | 26.09 | 26.58 | 27.05 | 27.42 | 27.72 | 28.02 | 28.24 | 28.49 |
| Turkeys, dollars per person | 19.20 | 18.30 | 18.28 | 18.63 | 18.98 | 19.28 | 19.56 | 19.65 | 19.69 | 19.64 | 19.52 | 19.43 |
| Percent of income | 0.07 | 0.07 | 0.07 | 0.06 | 0.06 | 0.06 | 0.06 | 0.06 | 0.05 | 0.05 | 0.05 | 0.05 |
| Percent of meat expenditures | 3.85 | 3.60 | 3.64 | 3.65 | 3.69 | 3.70 | 3.70 | 3.67 | 3.64 | 3.60 | 3.55 | 3.50 |
| Total meat, dollars per person | 498.50 | 507.83 | 501.60 | 509.80 | 514.19 | 521.56 | 528.88 | 534.90 | 541.22 | 545.88 | 550.14 | 555.64 |
| Percent of income | 1.93 | 1.89 | 1.81 | 1.76 | 1.70 | 1.66 | 1.61 | 1.55 | 1.50 | 1.45 | 1.40 | 1.36 |

SOURCE: "Table 22. Consumer expenditures for meats," in *USDA Agricultural Baseline Projections to 2012,* U.S. Department of Agriculture, Office of the Chief Economist, Interagency Agricultural Projections Committee, Washington, DC, February 2003

**FIGURE 1.8**

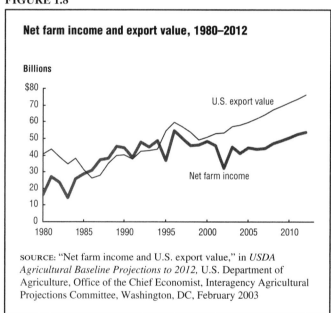

## Net farm income and export value, 1980–2012

Billions

SOURCE: "Net farm income and U.S. export value," in *USDA Agricultural Baseline Projections to 2012,* U.S. Department of Agriculture, Office of the Chief Economist, Interagency Agricultural Projections Committee, Washington, DC, February 2003

# CHAPTER 2

# WHAT DO AMERICANS EAT?

Over the past 20 years Americans have slowly changed their eating habits. While earlier generations grew up eating meat, potatoes, and apple pie, food purchasers today are often choosing convenience foods and foods away from home. Many Americans are aware that there is a direct link between diet and disease. Cholesterol can clog arteries, causing cardiovascular disease and eventual heart attack, the number one killer in America. Americans consumed less red meat and more poultry and fish in the 1990s than in the 1980s. And while Americans are eating more grains, they still do not eat as many whole-grain products, legumes, vegetables, or fruits as recommended by the federal *Dietary Guidelines for Americans.* In addition Americans are eating more foods with large amounts of refined sugars.

## SOURCES OF DATA

The title of this chapter, more precisely stated, should be "What Did Americans Eat?"—because comprehensive data of U.S. food consumption come from three surveys conducted by the Agricultural Research Service (ARS), an element of the U.S. Department of Agriculture. These studies have been completed over the course of two or more years and, by the time they have issued, the data have become relatively outdated. Currently available comprehensive data look back some seven years and are from the ARS's three-year survey that extended from 1994 through 1996, supplemented by a 1998 survey of food intake by children. Data on the ARS's 1999–2002 survey have not yet been published.

The 1994–96 study, part of the *Continuing Survey of Food Intakes by Individuals* (CSFII), also known as the *What We Eat in America Survey* (ARS, Beltsville, MD, 1997), surveyed 5,100 individuals across the nation and is the most recent "snapshot" of food intake for the United States. Earlier surveys in the CSFII series took place in 1985–86 and 1989–91. In the 1994–96 survey, participants

tracked their food intake for two nonconsecutive days, and 1,920 of those 20 years old and older also answered questions on their attitudes and knowledge about dietary guidance and health. The responses of the latter group were recorded in the *Diet and Health Knowledge Survey* (ARS, Beltsville, MD, 1997).

## FOOD INTAKE
### Red Meat, Poultry, and Fish

The CSFII found that most Americans (85.7 percent) ate meat, poultry, or fish on a given day. Frankfurters, sausages, and luncheon meats, as well as mixtures of meat, poultry, and fish (for example, casserole, meat loaf, corn dogs, tuna salad, chicken soup, and sandwiches such as cheeseburgers) were the most popular forms of meat. An almost equal proportion of participants reported eating beef (19.7 percent) and poultry (21.7 percent). (See Table 2.1.)

Meat becomes part of the American diet at an early age. While almost 30 percent of babies under one year old ate some kind of meat as part of their meals, by the time they reached the age of 1–2 years, 80 percent (4 out of 5 children) were consuming meat regularly. Among adults, young women between the ages of 12 and 29 were less likely to eat meat, although 4 out of 5 still did so. (See Table 2.1. Note: The data tables for percentages of individuals who ate particular foods were based on day one of the survey.)

### Grain Products

Nearly everyone (96.7 percent) had eaten some grain products during day one of the survey. Yeast breads and rolls were the most popular grain products, consumed by two-thirds (65.9 percent) of all individuals, followed by cereals and pasta, eaten by nearly half (46.8 percent) of all survey participants. Cakes, cookies, and other pastries

TABLE 2.1

**Percent of individuals consuming various types of meat over the course of one day, by sex and age, 1996**

| Sex and age (years) | Percentage of population | Total | Beef | Pork | Lamb, veal, game | Organ meats | Frankfurters, sausages, luncheon meats | Poultry Total | Poultry Chicken | Fish and shellfish | Mixtures mainly meat, poultry, fish |
|---|---|---|---|---|---|---|---|---|---|---|---|
| | Percent | | | | | | Percent | | | | |
| **Males and females:** | | | | | | | | | | | |
| Under 1 | 1.1 | 29.9 | 1.7† | 1.7† | 0.0† | 0.0† | 3.2† | 6.2† | 5.4† | 2.6† | 18.6 |
| 1–2 | 3.0 | 80.2 | 12.5 | 7.4 | .9† | 0.0† | 27.1 | 24.5 | 22.1 | 5.1 | 37.2 |
| 3–5 | 4.7 | 85.5 | 15.8 | 13.0 | 1.2† | .1† | 33.5 | 26.5 | 24.9 | 6.9 | 30.1 |
| 5 and under | 8.8 | 76.5 | 12.8 | 9.6 | 1.0† | .1† | 27.4 | 23.2 | 21.5 | 5.7 | 31.0 |
| **Males:** | | | | | | | | | | | |
| 6–11 | 4.6 | 84.3 | 21.5 | 12.6 | .6† | 0.0† | 28.5 | 20.0 | 18.9 | 3.0† | 40.0 |
| 12–19 | 5.9 | 87.8 | 25.9 | 15.5 | .6† | 0.0† | 39.9 | 19.6 | 18.6 | 4.5 | 38.0 |
| 20–29 | 7.2 | 89.6 | 23.4 | 16.1 | .9† | 0.0† | 27.9 | 23.4 | 17.9 | 7.6 | 39.8 |
| 30–39 | 8.1 | 90.6 | 26.1 | 17.2 | 1.3† | .1† | 32.3 | 18.1 | 15.4 | 10.1 | 42.9 |
| 40–49 | 7.0 | 88.9 | 28.7 | 16.3 | .4† | .3† | 33.7 | 22.5 | 19.4 | 10.1 | 39.4 |
| 50–59 | 4.7 | 91.3 | 24.1 | 20.8 | 1.1† | .7† | 33.6 | 17.7 | 13.0 | 16.3 | 34.7 |
| 60–69 | 3.4 | 90.8 | 23.0 | 18.3 | 1.6† | .4† | 34.6 | 19.6 | 15.3 | 12.9 | 37.7 |
| 70 and over | 3.4 | 92.1 | 20.8 | 27.1 | 1.6† | .4† | 34.1 | 18.2 | 16.7 | 11.5 | 34.0 |
| 20 and over | 33.9 | 90.3 | 25.0 | 18.4 | 1.0† | .3† | 32.3 | 20.2 | 16.6 | 10.9 | 39.0 |
| **Females:** | | | | | | | | | | | |
| 6–11 | 4.4 | 84.3 | 14.8 | 9.3 | .2† | .3† | 27.2 | 26.5 | 23.8 | 5.9 | 37.1 |
| 12–19 | 5.6 | 81.1 | 19.4 | 11.0 | 0.0† | 0.0† | 26.4 | 25.0 | 22.8 | 5.0 | 34.5 |
| 20–29 | 6.9 | 77.7 | 14.8 | 11.2 | .3† | .3† | 22.7 | 18.7 | 17.8 | 6.5 | 39.7 |
| 30–39 | 8.6 | 83.9 | 15.6 | 15.9 | .4† | 0.0† | 29.8 | 22.3 | 19.5 | 6.7 | 38.1 |
| 40–49 | 7.2 | 86.4 | 15.9 | 19.8 | 1.1† | 0.0† | 23.1 | 22.6 | 17.9 | 10.1 | 34.7 |
| 50–59 | 5.1 | 86.1 | 14.6 | 17.8 | 1.2† | .9† | 20.7 | 25.9 | 19.5 | 12.3 | 39.2 |
| 60–69 | 3.9 | 87.1 | 16.7 | 14.3 | 1.8† | 0.0† | 29.0 | 20.7 | 18.5 | 11.0 | 34.9 |
| 70 and over | 5.1 | 87.9 | 18.6 | 26.4 | .5† | .9† | 20.6 | 23.2 | 21.4 | 11.1 | 27.8 |
| 20 and over | 36.8 | 84.4 | 15.9 | 17.3 | .8 | .3† | 24.6 | 22.1 | 19.0 | 9.2 | 36.1 |
| All individuals | 100.0 | 85.7 | 19.7 | 16.0 | .8 | .2 | 28.7 | 21.7 | 18.8 | 8.5 | 36.9 |

†Estimates based on small cell sizes may tend to be less statistically reliable than estimates based on larger cell sizes. Cell size refers to the unweighted number of individuals in a given sex-age group or demographic group.
Note: Excludes breast-fed children.

SOURCE: "Meat, poultry, and fish: Percentages of individuals consuming foods from various food groups, by sex and age, 1 day, 1996," in *Results From USDA's 1996 Continuing Survey of Food Intakes by Individuals and 1996 Diet and Health Knowledge Survey*, U.S. Agricultural Research Service, Beltsville, MD, 1997

were nearly as popular, indulged in by 41.9 percent of participants. (See Table 2.2.)

### Fruits and Vegetables

Although nutritionists encourage people to eat fruits for a healthy diet, the survey revealed that many people did not follow this advice. Overall little more than half the participants (52.6 percent) reported eating fruits. About one-fifth (20.1 percent) consumed their citrus fruits in the forms of juices, and about 13 percent had eaten an apple or a banana. Young children and those over 60 were more likely to have eaten apples and bananas. (See Table 2.3.)

While 82.7 percent of individuals ate vegetables, the primary choice was potatoes (45.6 percent), with 28.5 percent choosing fried potatoes, usually French fries. The next most popular vegetables were tomatoes (eaten by 39.9 percent), which, in addition to the fresh variety, were ingested in various prepared forms, including tomato juice; ketchup, salsa, chili sauce, and other tomato sauces; and other mixtures with tomatoes as a main ingredient, such as tomato-based soup. (See Table 2.4.)

### Milk and Milk Products

Whole milk has a high fat content that is generally not considered desirable; experts advise drinking skim (fat-free) milk instead. The survey found that many consumers had switched to low-fat milk (25.4 percent, which included both reduced-fat and low-fat milk) but were not as enthusiastic about skim milk (11.5 percent). One-third (33 percent) ate cheese, and 16.1 percent ate milk desserts, primarily ice cream. (See Table 2.5.)

### Beverages and Miscellaneous Foods

Carbonated soft drinks were the most popular beverage, consumed by half (50.3 percent) of the participants, although coffee was more popular with those 20 and older (54.2 percent). Over one-fifth (22.5 percent) of men 20 and older drank an alcoholic beverage, compared with 12.1 percent of women in the same age group. Twice as many children (40.4 percent) ages 3–5 consumed fruit drinks and "-ades," compared with 21.2 percent (Table 2.3) of the same age group who consumed citrus fruit juices. Overall, about one-third of children ages 1–11 drank fruit drinks and -ades. (See Table 2.6.)

TABLE 2.2

**Percent of individuals consuming various types of grain products over the course of one day, by sex and age, 1996**

| Sex and age (years) | Percentage of population | Total | Yeast breads and rolls | Cereals and pasta | | | | Quick breads, pancakes, french toast | Cakes, cookies, pastries, pies | Crackers, popcorn, pretzels, corn chips | Mixtures mainly grain |
| | | | | Total | Ready-to-eat cereals | Rice | Pasta | | | | |
| | Percent | | | | Percent | | | | | | |
| **Males and females:** | | | | | | | | | | | |
| Under 1 | 1.1 | 74.4 | 10.3† | 65.5 | 6.0† | .9† | 2.0† | 6.2† | 16.5 | 8.0† | 13.7 |
| 1–2 | 3.0 | 98.7† | 53.5 | 70.5 | 46.5 | 13.5 | 11.7 | 27.3 | 44.9 | 32.8 | 41.8 |
| 3–5 | 4.7 | 99.4† | 63.4 | 66.5 | 50.1 | 10.5 | 9.8 | 27.1 | 46.5 | 39.0 | 48.1 |
| 5 and under | 8.8 | 95.9 | 53.2 | 67.7 | 43.2 | 10.3 | 9.4 | 24.4 | 42.1 | 32.9 | 41.5 |
| **Males:** | | | | | | | | | | | |
| 6–11 | 4.6 | 98.2† | 57.9 | 56.1 | 46.8 | 8.0 | 7.0 | 27.4 | 51.7 | 32.1 | 41.6 |
| 12–19 | 5.9 | 97.8† | 64.5 | 49.8 | 34.8 | 11.7 | 9.3 | 23.3 | 44.3 | 29.1 | 51.8 |
| 20–29 | 7.2 | 93.7 | 57.9 | 35.4 | 15.9 | 11.5 | 9.1 | 22.4 | 30.0 | 27.3 | 40.1 |
| 30–39 | 8.1 | 93.7 | 65.9 | 37.2 | 22.3 | 11.5 | 7.3 | 23.9 | 37.9 | 26.1 | 35.8 |
| 40–49 | 7.0 | 96.3† | 70.0 | 45.3 | 21.1 | 13.9 | 11.1 | 21.6 | 45.7 | 22.5 | 34.5 |
| 50–59 | 4.7 | 97.8† | 72.0 | 39.1 | 21.7 | 12.2 | 7.2 | 25.7 | 40.5 | 29.3 | 31.1 |
| 60–69 | 3.4 | 97.9† | 79.7 | 51.7 | 29.6 | 11.2 | 7.5 | 23.6 | 38.1 | 23.3 | 24.1 |
| 70 and over | 3.4 | 97.6† | 79.1 | 58.8 | 38.9 | 4.8† | 4.7† | 20.7 | 52.9 | 25.6 | 20.2 |
| 20 and over | 33.9 | 95.6 | 68.6 | 42.4 | 23.0 | 11.4 | 8.2 | 23.0 | 39.7 | 25.7 | 33.1 |
| **Females:** | | | | | | | | | | | |
| 6–11 | 4.4 | 99.4† | 65.8 | 59.5 | 43.6 | 8.6 | 9.2 | 26.9 | 51.7 | 35.8 | 43.7 |
| 12–19 | 5.6 | 97.4† | 62.8 | 47.4 | 30.1 | 8.4 | 10.1 | 19.1 | 40.7 | 25.6 | 44.3 |
| 20–29 | 6.9 | 97.3† | 62.8 | 41.6 | 25.1 | 10.5 | 6.8 | 19.5 | 39.6 | 26.8 | 42.5 |
| 30–39 | 8.6 | 95.4 | 64.1 | 38.2 | 23.1 | 8.2 | 9.4 | 23.4 | 37.8 | 31.1 | 38.6 |
| 40–49 | 7.2 | 97.0† | 69.4 | 43.3 | 21.0 | 15.1 | 8.3 | 20.4 | 40.6 | 26.7 | 32.4 |
| 50–59 | 5.1 | 98.3† | 70.7 | 39.7 | 18.6 | 11.6 | 6.9 | 26.6 | 37.6 | 24.5 | 28.9 |
| 60–69 | 3.9 | 97.2† | 73.0 | 42.5 | 24.6 | 8.3 | 8.5 | 20.1 | 42.8 | 27.2 | 20.2 |
| 70 and over | 5.1 | 98.3† | 75.2 | 52.6 | 31.8 | 4.5† | 3.0† | 25.9 | 52.9 | 20.4 | 17.4 |
| 20 and over | 36.8 | 97.1 | 68.3 | 42.5 | 23.8 | 10.0 | 7.4 | 22.5 | 41.3 | 26.6 | 31.9 |
| All individuals | 100.0 | 96.7 | 65.9 | 46.8 | 28.2 | 10.3 | 8.2 | 23.1 | 41.9 | 27.6 | 36.0 |

†Estimates based on small cell sizes may tend to be less statistically reliable than estimates based on larger cell sizes. Cell size refers to the unweighted number of individuals in a given sex-age group or demographic group.

Note: Excludes breast-fed children.

SOURCE: "Grain products: Percentages of individuals consuming foods from various food groups, by sex and age, 1 day, 1996," in *Results From USDA's 1996 Continuing Survey of Food Intakes by Individuals and 1996 Diet and Health Knowledge Survey,* U.S. Agricultural Research Service, Beltsville, MD, 1997

More than half of those who were surveyed (54.1 percent) reported consuming fats and oils, including vegetable oils, table and cooking fats, salad dressings, nondairy cream substitutes, tartar sauce, and other sauces that were mainly fat or oil. A similar proportion of the respondents (52.3 percent) consumed sugars and sweets, which included sweet sauces, gelatin desserts, jellies, jams, preserves, and candies. Eggs were eaten by about one-fifth (19.1 percent of those surveyed. (See Table 2.7.)

## FOOD AND NUTRIENT INTAKE BY CHILDREN

*The Supplemental Children's Survey* (ARS, Beltsville, MD, December 1999), part of the *Continuing Survey of Food Intakes by Individuals* (*CSFII 1998),* added intake data from 5,559 children from birth to 9 years of age to the data collected from 4,235 children of the same age who participated in *CSFII 1994–96.* The 1994–96 survey included the collection of data from persons of all ages. The results of the supplemental survey were based on all four years of the last CSFII (1994–96 and 1998) for children 9 and under, and on *CSFII 1994–96* only for individuals 10 and older.

## Red Meat, Poultry, and Fish

The supplemental survey found that most people age 19 and younger (82.8 percent) had eaten meat, poultry, or fish on a given day. (See Table 2.8.) Frankfurters, sausages, and luncheon meats were the most popular forms of meat (30.9 percent), but were especially popular with children age 9 and younger (32.4 percent). (See Table 2.8.) Poultry and beef were about equally popular with respondents 19 and younger—22.7 percent of individuals had eaten poultry and 19.6 percent had eaten beef on one day of the survey.

## Grain Products

Almost all respondents (97.6 percent) had eaten some grain products on one day of the survey. (See Table 2.8.) Yeast breads and rolls were the most popular choices, consumed by 62.4 percent of individuals age 19 or younger, followed by cereals and pasta, eaten by more than half (57.6 percent) of all respondents. Cakes, cookies, pastries, and pies were popular with nearly half (46.1 percent) of respondents, as were crackers, popcorn, pretzels, and corn chips, consumed by about one-third (32.5 percent).

**TABLE 2.3**

**Percent of individuals consuming various types of fruit over the course of one day, by sex and age, 1996**

| Sex and age (years) | Percentage of population | Total | Citrus fruits and juices | | Dried fruits | Other fruits, mixtures, and juices | | | | | |
|---|---|---|---|---|---|---|---|---|---|---|---|
| | | | Total | Juices | | Total | Apples | Bananas | Melons and berries | Other fruits and mixtures mainly fruit | Noncitrus juices and nectars |
| | Percent | | | | | Percent | | | | | |
| Males and females: | | | | | | | | | | | |
| Under 1 | 1.1 | 63.4 | 1.9† | .5† | 0.0† | 62.9 | 19.5 | 11.8 | 1.6† | 39.7 | 32.2 |
| 1–2 | 3.0 | 79.4 | 28.8 | 21.8 | 5.4 | 68.0 | 23.2 | 22.8 | 7.8 | 23.4 | 40.3 |
| 3–5 | 4.7 | 65.7 | 26.3 | 21.2 | 3.9 | 54.8 | 17.7 | 13.7 | 6.3 | 16.9 | 26.2 |
| 5 and under | 8.8 | 70.1 | 24.0 | 18.7 | 3.9 | 60.3 | 19.8 | 16.6 | 6.2 | 22.0 | 31.7 |
| Males: | | | | | | | | | | | |
| 6–11 | 4.6 | 47.5 | 18.5 | 16.1 | .4† | 39.8 | 18.0 | 7.0 | 6.5 | 11.8 | 9.5 |
| 12–19 | 5.9 | 42.1 | 23.6 | 18.3 | 1.1† | 26.3 | 7.6 | 5.6 | 5.0 | 8.9 | 7.4 |
| 20–29 | 7.2 | 39.0 | 21.2 | 19.4 | .5† | 25.1 | 6.4 | 7.9 | 4.7 | 9.0 | 3.0† |
| 30–39 | 8.1 | 36.9 | 20.3 | 16.9 | 1.2† | 21.9 | 5.1 | 8.8 | 4.9 | 7.5 | 3.7 |
| 40-49 | 7.0 | 47.6 | 25.3 | 19.4 | 1.8† | 31.9 | 10.4 | 12.0 | 6.0 | 11.5 | 5.6 |
| 50–59 | 4.7 | 56.5 | 31.2 | 23.6 | 2.3† | 42.5 | 13.7 | 20.5 | 7.3 | 13.2 | 5.9 |
| 60–69 | 3.4 | 64.8 | 34.1 | 25.7 | 4.7 | 49.6 | 15.1 | 25.8 | 11.0 | 14.5 | 4.6 |
| 70 and over | 3.4 | 67.3 | 34.7 | 28.5 | 6.9 | 53.5 | 19.9 | 28.2 | 13.3 | 20.8 | 5.5 |
| 20 and over | 33.9 | 48.2 | 25.9 | 20.9 | 2.2 | 33.5 | 10.2 | 14.6 | 6.9 | 11.5 | 4.5 |
| Females: | | | | | | | | | | | |
| 6–11 | 4.4 | 62.0 | 25.5 | 18.2 | 1.2† | 47.5 | 15.7 | 7.2 | 6.6 | 19.5 | 14.7 |
| 12–19 | 5.6 | 44.6 | 23.6 | 19.5 | 1.3† | 29.9 | 11.3 | 6.0 | 5.5 | 9.2 | 9.3 |
| 20–29 | 6.9 | 47.6 | 28.5 | 21.6 | .8† | 31.6 | 10.1 | 11.5 | 4.5 | 10.0 | 6.2 |
| 30–39 | 8.6 | 47.6 | 20.9 | 16.2 | 3.5† | 34.2 | 9.1 | 13.7 | 10.5 | 11.7 | 4.2 |
| 40–49 | 7.2 | 49.6 | 22.6 | 16.2 | 1.2† | 37.8 | 12.3 | 13.1 | 9.7 | 12.6 | 5.4 |
| 50–59 | 5.1 | 61.5 | 33.5 | 23.5 | 3.1† | 48.4 | 14.9 | 20.6 | 11.5 | 13.9 | 3.2† |
| 60–69 | 3.9 | 66.1 | 32.7 | 22.5 | 4.3† | 52.2 | 15.5 | 24.4 | 14.8 | 18.1 | 5.3 |
| 70 and over | 5.1 | 69.9 | 36.7 | 29.3 | 5.8† | 56.6 | 12.7 | 25.6 | 9.0 | 22.3 | 5.6† |
| 20 and over | 36.8 | 55.0 | 27.8 | 20.7 | 2.9 | 41.4 | 11.9 | 16.9 | 9.6 | 14.0 | 5.0 |
| All individuals | 100.0 | 52.6 | 25.8 | 20.1 | 2.4 | 39.1 | 12.2 | 13.9 | 7.6 | 13.4 | 8.2 |

†Estimates based on small cell sizes may tend to be less statistically reliable than estimates based on larger cell sizes. Cell size refers to the unweighted number of individuals in a given sex-age group or demographic group.

Note: Excludes breast-fed children.

SOURCE: "Fruits: Percentages of individuals consuming foods from various food groups, by sex and age, 1 day, 1996," in *Results From USDA's 1996 Continuing Survey of Food Intakes by Individuals and 1996 Diet and Health Knowledge Survey,* U.S. Agricultural Research Service, Beltsville, MD, 1997

## Fruits and Vegetables

Despite the emphasis by nutritionists and other health professionals on the importance of fruit in a well-rounded, healthy diet, the survey found that only 57.8 percent of people age 19 and younger ate fruits on a given day. (See Table 2.8.) Twenty-five percent of respondents consumed citrus fruits, 15.2 percent had eaten apples, and 9.7 percent had eaten bananas.

While 78.3 percent of individuals had eaten vegetables on one day of the survey, nearly half (46.8 percent) preferred potatoes. (See Table 2.8.) Tomatoes (consumed by 34.6 percent) and lettuce and lettuce-based salads (consumed by 16.6 percent) were the next most popular choices of vegetables.

## Milk and Milk Products

The survey found that 86.7 percent of respondents had consumed dairy products on one day of the survey, and 68.1 percent had consumed milk (See Table 2.8.). Low-fat milk consumption (reported by 33.1 percent of respondents) surpassed whole-milk consumption (reported by

30.1 percent of respondents). Skim milk, having the lowest amount of fat and therefore considered by nutritionists and other health professionals to be the healthiest type of milk, was only consumed by 7.5 percent of those participating in the survey. More than one-third (34 percent) of respondents ate cheese, and 18.6 percent consumed milk desserts.

## Beverages and Miscellaneous Foods

Carbonated soft drinks were the most popular beverage, consumed by nearly half (47.8 percent) of children age 19 and younger (See Table 2.8.). Nearly one-third of children 9 and under had consumed carbonated soft drinks on one day of the survey. Fruit drinks and fruit -ades were the next most popular beverages, consumed by 32.3 percent of all individuals age 19 and younger. People 19 and younger also preferred tea (consumed by 11.9 percent) to coffee (consumed by 2.4 percent).

Half (50.8 percent) of respondents age 19 years and younger had consumed sugars and sweets on one day of the survey. (See Table 2.8.) The percentage of children

TABLE 2.4

**Percent of individuals consuming various types of vegetables over the course of one day, by sex and age, 1996**

| Sex and age (years) | Percentage of population | Total | White potatoes Total | White potatoes Fried | Dark-green vegetables | Deep-yellow vegetables | Tomatoes | Lettuce, lettuce-based salads | Green beans | Corn, green peas, lima beans | Other vegetables |
|---|---|---|---|---|---|---|---|---|---|---|---|
| | Percent | | | | | | Percent | | | | |
| Males and females: | | | | | | | | | | | |
| Under 1 | 1.1 | 52.7 | 13.9 | 5.2† | 3.6† | 20.8 | .6† | 0.0† | 15.5 | 9.4† | 14.4 |
| 1–2 | 3.0 | 74.4 | 40.5 | 25.1 | 7.0 | 11.7 | 26.2 | 5.8 | 11.0 | 17.6 | 20.1 |
| 3–5 | 4.7 | 73.3 | 46.5 | 34.2 | 6.2 | 9.9 | 33.2 | 9.2 | 7.5 | 14.2 | 22.4 |
| 5 and under | 8.8 | 71.0 | 40.3 | 27.4 | 6.2 | 11.9 | 26.6 | 6.9 | 9.7 | 14.7 | 20.6 |
| Males: | | | | | | | | | | | |
| 6–11 | 4.6 | 76.8 | 51.6 | 38.7 | 8.2 | 7.9 | 34.2 | 15.2 | 7.6 | 16.4 | 26.6 |
| 12–19 | 5.9 | 80.8 | 48.9 | 35.8 | 2.1† | 9.4 | 45.7 | 27.9 | 3.7† | 6.1 | 33.2 |
| 20–29 | 7.2 | 82.6 | 50.4 | 36.8 | 7.0 | 6.8 | 47.3 | 24.0 | 3.4† | 7.0 | 38.1 |
| 30–39 | 8.1 | 87.9 | 50.1 | 34.2 | 9.9 | 10.7 | 42.7 | 26.4 | 6.3 | 10.9 | 52.7 |
| 40–49 | 7.0 | 86.9 | 46.2 | 29.1 | 8.6 | 13.9 | 39.7 | 27.5 | 7.5 | 15.5 | 52.1 |
| 50–59 | 4.7 | 90.8 | 47.5 | 25.2 | 11.6 | 15.9 | 46.6 | 32.3 | 6.7 | 17.3 | 48.9 |
| 60–69 | 3.4 | 85.1 | 43.0 | 18.9 | 16.2 | 20.3 | 43.9 | 29.4 | 8.8 | 12.3 | 52.8 |
| 70 and over | 3.4 | 83.8 | 46.9 | 13.8 | 13.1 | 18.6 | 36.1 | 27.3 | 12.3 | 16.6 | 50.1 |
| 20 and over | 33.9 | 86.3 | 48.0 | 28.8 | 10.2 | 13.0 | 43.0 | 27.3 | 6.8 | 12.6 | 48.7 |
| Females: | | | | | | | | | | | |
| 6–11 | 4.4 | 83.7 | 54.5 | 43.6 | 3.9† | 14.1 | 35.6 | 17.7 | 6.5 | 16.9 | 30.5 |
| 12–19 | 5.6 | 84.0 | 49.6 | 41.7 | 14.1 | 13.1 | 41.6 | 30.6 | 3.2† | 5.4 | 38.4 |
| 20–29 | 6.9 | 79.6 | 41.4 | 25.8 | 8.0 | 11.3 | 42.7 | 25.3 | 5.9 | 5.3 | 41.3 |
| 30–39 | 8.6 | 85.3 | 47.1 | 26.6 | 13.4 | 15.7 | 39.7 | 31.0 | 4.5 | 12.3 | 46.3 |
| 40–49 | 7.2 | 82.1 | 40.1 | 23.1 | 12.0 | 16.7 | 37.7 | 33.5 | 6.2 | 10.7 | 43.3 |
| 50–59 | 5.1 | 82.5 | 40.3 | 20.1 | 14.9 | 15.6 | 42.9 | 32.2 | 8.2 | 10.1 | 48.1 |
| 60–69 | 3.9 | 82.3 | 36.8 | 14.9 | 13.9 | 14.4 | 41.0 | 29.7 | 9.8 | 9.2 | 50.0 |
| 70 and over | 5.1 | 85.7 | 41.7 | 15.5 | 11.8 | 10.7 | 38.8 | 25.0 | 8.7 | 15.5 | 51.6 |
| 20 and over | 36.8 | 82.9 | 41.9 | 22.1 | 12.2 | 14.2 | 40.3 | 29.6 | 6.8 | 10.5 | 46.2 |
| All individuals | 100.0 | 82.7 | 45.6 | 28.5 | 9.9 | 13.0 | 39.9 | 25.6 | 6.7 | 11.6 | 42.0 |

†Estimates based on small cell sizes may tend to be less statistically reliable than estimates based on larger cell sizes. Cell size refers to the unweighted number of individuals in a given sex-age group or demographic group.

Note: Excludes breast-fed children.

SOURCE: "Vegetables: Percentages of individuals consuming foods from various food groups, by sex and age, 1 day, 1996," in *Results From USDA's 1996 Continuing Survey of Food Intakes by Individuals and 1996 Diet and Health Knowledge Survey,* U.S. Agricultural Research Service, Beltsville, MD, 1997

19 and younger who consumed fats and oils was almost as high (43.2 percent) as that for those consuming sugars and sweets. Eggs were consumed by 16.4 percent of respondents.

## PER CAPITA FOOD CONSUMPTION

The USDA Economic Research Service (ERS) tracks the annual per capita food consumption by Americans in its food supply series *Food Consumption, Prices, and Expenditures.* The ERS calculates the amount of food available for human consumption by subtracting measurable uses (exports; seed, feed, and industrial use; and end-of-year inventories) from the total food supply (food produced, imports, and beginning inventories). (See Figure 2.1.) Consumption per person is then calculated by dividing the food available for human consumption (also referred to as "food disappearance") by the U.S. total population, including the armed forces overseas.

Food disappearance is not an accurate measure of how much food is eaten, but an indicator of trends in consumption over time. ERS data do not reflect how much food is purchased and then wasted, how much is fed to pets, or how much fish and game are obtained by consumers without purchasing them. The data also include unknown amounts of foods used as ingredients in processed foods that are exported.

In the last 30 years the consumption patterns of Americans have undergone some changes. Factors responsible for these changes include:

- The introduction of convenience foods and the growth of the away-from-home food market.

- Advances in food enrichment and fortification.

- Improved nutrition labeling.

- Continuing public education on the correlation of diet and health.

- Sociodemographic trends, such as the rise in single-parent and two-earner households, the growing numbers of working women, an aging population, and increased racial and ethnic diversity.

### Red Meat, Poultry, and Fish

Meat traditionally has been part of the diet of many Americans. Despite advice from nutritionists and other

TABLE 2.5

**Percent of individuals consuming various types of milk and milk products over the course of one day, by sex and age, 1996**

| Sex and age (years) | Percentage of population | Total | Milk, milk drinks, yogurt | | | | | | | Milk desserts | Cheese |
|---|---|---|---|---|---|---|---|---|---|---|---|
| | | | Total | Fluid milk | | | | | Yogurt | | |
| | | | | Total | Whole | Low fat | Skim | | | | |
| | Percent | | | | | | | Percent | | | |
| Males and females: | | | | | | | | | | | |
| Under 1 | 1.1 | 82.9 | 82.9 | 8.6† | 4.8† | 1.3† | 0.0† | 1.0† | 13.7 | 4.8† |
| 1–2 | 3.0 | 95.3 | 91.6 | 87.3 | 54.8 | 32.0 | 2.6† | 8.8 | 13.0 | 32.0 |
| 3–5 | 4.7 | 92.9 | 85.6 | 82.5 | 40.8 | 39.4 | 6.8 | 5.4 | 21.8 | 35.4 |
| 5 and under | 8.8 | 92.4 | 87.3 | 74.6 | 40.9 | 32.0 | 4.5 | 6.0 | 17.8 | 30.3 |
| Males: | | | | | | | | | | | |
| 6–11 | 4.6 | 90.1 | 80.6 | 75.5 | 28.5 | 43.4 | 8.0 | 2.6† | 29.1 | 28.0 |
| 12–19 | 5.9 | 82.1 | 67.4 | 61.0 | 20.9 | 30.5 | 10.7 | 2.2† | 12.8 | 40.8 |
| 20–29 | 7.2 | 70.1 | 44.0 | 40.0 | 12.9 | 19.5 | 8.4 | 3.8 | 10.3 | 36.8 |
| 30–39 | 8.1 | 73.8 | 50.7 | 46.7 | 18.7 | 20.3 | 7.7 | 3.3 | 14.0 | 40.8 |
| 40–49 | 7.0 | 71.7 | 50.4 | 47.4 | 14.8 | 20.2 | 12.5 | 4.2 | 12.2 | 30.9 |
| 50–59 | 4.7 | 73.0 | 52.6 | 50.3 | 11.0 | 26.7 | 12.6 | 2.0† | 18.8 | 28.5 |
| 60–69 | 3.4 | 79.6 | 64.9 | 61.7 | 16.5 | 28.0 | 17.2 | 2.3† | 20.9 | 29.9 |
| 70 and over | 3.4 | 84.1 | 69.0 | 66.9 | 21.3 | 29.4 | 20.2 | .8† | 27.3 | 28.0 |
| 20 and over | 33.9 | 74.1 | 52.7 | 49.5 | 15.6 | 22.7 | 11.7 | 3.1 | 15.5 | 33.8 |
| Females: | | | | | | | | | | | |
| 6–11 | 4.4 | 89.4 | 84.1 | 78.3 | 37.5 | 37.5 | 6.5 | .9† | 20.3 | 23.8 |
| 12–19 | 5.6 | 74.9 | 49.8 | 45.5 | 17.3 | 21.4 | 8.2 | 1.3† | 15.0 | 38.5 |
| 20–29 | 6.9 | 71.5 | 50.6 | 45.8 | 17.2 | 16.8 | 12.4 | 2.9† | 9.1 | 33.2 |
| 30–39 | 8.6 | 76.9 | 54.0 | 49.7 | 15.6 | 23.1 | 10.7 | 7.2 | 13.9 | 39.0 |
| 40–49 | 7.2 | 75.3 | 50.3 | 46.8 | 14.8 | 22.1 | 11.7 | 5.6 | 11.9 | 38.4 |
| 50–59 | 5.1 | 79.1 | 59.3 | 50.5 | 8.7 | 21.4 | 19.7 | 9.2 | 19.8 | 27.2 |
| 60–69 | 3.9 | 76.1 | 56.6 | 53.6 | 11.5 | 21.4 | 21.5 | 5.6 | 16.7 | 29.3 |
| 70 and over | 5.1 | 83.0 | 66.6 | 63.2 | 16.4 | 30.8 | 17.5 | 4.9† | 22.4 | 19.8 |
| 20 and over | 36.8 | 76.6 | 55.4 | 50.8 | 14.5 | 22.4 | 14.5 | 5.9 | 14.9 | 32.5 |
| All individuals | 100.0 | 78.6 | 60.1 | 55.1 | 19.4 | 25.4 | 11.5 | 4.1 | 16.1 | 33.0 |

†Estimates based on small cell sizes may tend to be less statistically reliable than estimates based on larger cell sizes. Cell size refers to the unweighted number of individuals in a given sex-age group or demographic group.

Note: Excludes breast-fed children.

SOURCE: "Milk and milk products: Percentages of individuals consuming foods from various food groups, by sex and age, 1 day, 1996," in *Results From USDA's 1996 Continuing Survey of Food Intakes by Individuals and 1996 Diet and Health Knowledge Survey,* U.S. Agricultural Research Service, Beltsville, MD, 1997

health practitioners about cutting fat from diets, many people continue to eat red meat (beef, pork, veal, lamb, and mutton), although more and more of them are choosing leaner cuts. According to ERS data, in 2001, the average American consumed a total of 192.2 pounds of red meat, poultry, and fish, 68 pounds above the 1909 per capita consumption level. Red meat consumption per capita in 2001 accounted for 111.3 pounds (see Figure 2.2), but per-person consumption of red meat decreased 18 percent from its peak of 136.1 pounds per capita in 1971. Poultry consumption increased dramatically (491 percent), from 11.2 pounds in 1909 to 66.2 pounds in 2001. In fact, in the years 1975–1994, per capita poultry consumption increased 91 percent. Fish and shellfish per capita consumption increased 34 percent from 1909 to 2001, from 11.0 pounds to 14.7 pounds, although fish has yet to become a major part of the American diet.

Concerns about fat and cholesterol have led to the production of leaner meat, the practice of trimming outside fat before retail sale, and the introduction of processed meat products with lower fat contents. Health concerns relating to beef consumption have helped boost the sale of poultry.

The poultry industry responded to consumer demand by introducing new products, including boneless, skinless chicken and turkey; chicken and turkey franks, sausages, and deli meats; and ground chicken and turkey. During the 1990s, and into 2001, beef and poultry consumption were nearly equal in per capita food consumption, but beginning in 1997, per capita consumption of poultry consistently outranked per capita consumption of beef by Americans. (See Figure 2.3.)

The growing numbers of working women and single-parent families have influenced meat consumption. Hamburger, which can be prepared quickly, accounted for 40 percent of the beef consumed in 1995, compared with 26 percent in 1970. Roasts, which require longer preparation time, experienced a sharp decline in sales. In addition Americans now eat out more often, especially in fast-food restaurants that feature hamburgers, chicken, and pizza. As the total per capita consumption of chicken has climbed, the share provided by food-service establishments has almost doubled, from 25 percent in 1970 to 46 percent in 1996.

Nutrition: A Key to Good Health

TABLE 2.6

**Percent of individuals consuming various types of beverages over the course of one day, by sex and age, 1996**

| Sex and age (years) | Percentage of population | Total | Alcoholic Total | Wine | Beer and ale | Nonalcoholic Total | Coffee | Tea | Fruit drinks and -ades Total | Regular | Low calorie | Carbonated soft drinks Total | Regular | Low calorie |
|---|---|---|---|---|---|---|---|---|---|---|---|---|---|---|
| | Percent | | | | | | | Percent | | | | | | |
| Males and females: | | | | | | | | | | | | | | |
| Under 1 | 1.1 | 8.0† | 0.0† | 0.0† | 0.0† | 8.0† | 0.0† | .7† | 7.3† | 4.3† | 2.4† | 0.0† | 0.0† | 0.0† |
| 1–2 | 3.0 | 49.5 | 0.0† | 0.0† | 0.0† | 49.5 | .2† | 7.9 | 31.4 | 26.2 | 4.0 | 19.5 | 17.9 | 1.8† |
| 3–5 | 4.7 | 70.7 | 0.0† | 0.0† | 0.0† | 70.7 | .9† | 8.2 | 40.4 | 38.3 | 2.8 | 36.1 | 32.2 | 4.0 |
| 5 and under | 8.8 | 55.4 | 0.0† | 0.0† | 0.0† | 55.4 | .6† | 7.1 | 33.1 | 29.8 | 3.2 | 25.9 | 23.2 | 2.7 |
| Males: | | | | | | | | | | | | | | |
| 6–11 | 4.6 | 71.8 | .5† | 0.0† | 0.0† | 71.8 | 1.5† | 7.4 | 36.1 | 32.9 | 3.9† | 46.0 | 41.7 | 6.1 |
| 12–19 | 5.9 | 86.4 | 3.8† | 0.0† | 2.4† | 85.9 | 5.4 | 16.6 | 32.1 | 23.0 | 9.1 | 67.2 | 64.5 | 4.3 |
| 20–29 | 7.2 | 90.3 | 24.9 | 2.5† | 21.5 | 85.8 | 24.9 | 16.0 | 19.3 | 16.0 | 3.6 | 67.8 | 63.0 | 6.8 |
| 30–39 | 8.1 | 92.8 | 22.4 | 2.6† | 18.2 | 91.1 | 49.2 | 24.9 | 14.2 | 10.8 | 3.4 | 63.2 | 52.8 | 13.0 |
| 40–49 | 7.0 | 95.0 | 26.0 | 7.5 | 15.8 | 92.7 | 63.0 | 25.1 | 18.5 | 14.9 | 3.8† | 54.2 | 42.0 | 14.9 |
| 50–59 | 4.7 | 95.3 | 22.2 | 4.6 | 14.9 | 94.1 | 67.1 | 31.6 | 12.2 | 8.7 | 2.4† | 51.1 | 34.8 | 18.2 |
| 60–69 | 3.4 | 97.5† | 18.9 | 7.7 | 9.7 | 96.8† | 74.7 | 30.0 | 9.2 | 8.4 | .9† | 38.5 | 24.6 | 15.3 |
| 70 and over | 3.4 | 91.8 | 14.6 | 7.1 | 3.6† | 89.7 | 77.1 | 23.8 | 11.3 | 9.6 | 2.7† | 22.4 | 12.7 | 9.7 |
| 20 and over | 33.9 | 93.5 | 22.5 | 4.8 | 15.6 | 91.2 | 54.8 | 24.4 | 15.1 | 12.1 | 3.1 | 54.1 | 43.3 | 12.7 |
| Females: | | | | | | | | | | | | | | |
| 6–11 | 4.4 | 69.4 | .5† | 0.0† | 0.0† | 69.4 | 1.3† | 7.7 | 32.2 | 30.3 | 1.9† | 45.2 | 41.2 | 6.3 |
| 12–19 | 5.6 | 86.7 | 1.7† | .5† | 1.1† | 86.7 | 4.9 | 17.1 | 25.5 | 21.3 | 4.1† | 62.8 | 58.0 | 5.9 |
| 20–29 | 6.9 | 88.9 | 10.7 | 1.2† | 7.4 | 87.0 | 26.2 | 23.5 | 22.4 | 18.4 | 3.5† | 64.3 | 52.9 | 14.1 |
| 30–39 | 8.6 | 88.5 | 14.0 | 4.0 | 7.0 | 87.9 | 43.9 | 27.6 | 19.9 | 18.0 | 1.9† | 55.0 | 39.6 | 18.9 |
| 40–49 | 7.2 | 93.8 | 15.9 | 7.9 | 6.8 | 93.4 | 60.1 | 30.4 | 15.0 | 13.0 | 2.2† | 57.0 | 35.1 | 24.3 |
| 50–59 | 5.1 | 92.9 | 11.5 | 5.1 | 2.5† | 91.9 | 63.3 | 37.9 | 13.4 | 11.2 | 1.0† | 44.2 | 28.7 | 18.9 |
| 60–69 | 3.9 | 95.8† | 12.8 | 6.5 | 1.9† | 94.4 | 74.9 | 31.9 | 12.1 | 9.2 | 2.9† | 40.2 | 20.9 | 19.9 |
| 70 and over | 5.1 | 87.5 | 5.7† | 5.2† | .5† | 87.5 | 71.6 | 21.8 | 13.7 | 12.3 | 1.4† | 19.5 | 11.3 | 7.3 |
| 20 and over | 36.8 | 90.9 | 12.1 | 4.8 | 5.0 | 90.0 | 53.6 | 28.5 | 16.8 | 14.5 | 2.2 | 49.2 | 33.8 | 17.6 |
| All individuals | 100.0 | 86.3 | 12.4 | 3.4 | 7.3 | 85.2 | 39.0 | 22.0 | 20.6 | 17.5 | 3.1 | 50.3 | 39.9 | 12.2 |

†Estimates based on small cell sizes may tend to be less statistically reliable than estimates based on larger cell sizes. Cell size refers to the unweighted number of individuals in a given sex-age group or demographic group.

Note: Excludes breast-fed children.

SOURCE: "Beverages: Percentages of individuals consuming foods from various food groups, by sex and age, 1 day, 1996," in *Results From USDA's 1996 Continuing Survey of Food Intakes by Individuals and 1996 Diet and Health Knowledge Survey*, U.S. Agricultural Research Service, Beltsville, MD, 1997

## Flour and Cereal Products

In 2001 per capita consumption of flour and cereal products totaled 195.7 pounds, a 47 percent increase since 1972. Figure 2.4 shows graphically how wheat flour and cereal consumption has changed over the period 1967–2001. The USDA attributes the increase in flour and grain use to a greater appreciation for variety breads and other in-store bakery items and to the fast-food sales of hamburger buns, other sandwich rolls, pizza dough, and tortillas. The popularity of ethnic foods, especially Mexican foods, has been responsible in part for the increased per capita consumption of flour and grains.

Wheat is the major grain product consumed in the United States. The per capita use of wheat flour increased 21 percent between 1980 and 2001. As rice, corn products, and oat products have gained in popularity, however, wheat's share of total grain consumption has declined.

## Fruits and Vegetables

Total per capita consumption of fruits and vegetables reached 689 pounds in 2001, up 13 percent from 1982.

Much of this increase occurred since 1982, the year the landmark report *Diet, Nutrition, and Cancer* (National Academy of Sciences [NAS], Washington, D.C., 1982) was published. In that report, a panel of scientists assembled by the NAS stressed the beneficial effects of fruits, vegetables, and whole-grain products on overall health. The experts also reported that these foods might help reduce the risk of cancer. The panel suggested using citrus fruits, vegetables in the cabbage family, and vegetables and fruits rich in carotene (e.g., carrots, cantaloupe, pumpkin, sweet potatoes, and tomatoes).

Consumers chose noncitrus fruits over citrus fruits from 1970 to 2001. (See Figure 2.5.) Per capita citrus fruit consumption decreased 16 percent, from 28.8 pounds in 1970 to 24.3 pounds in 2001. Per capita consumption of noncitrus fruits, such as apples, bananas, and plums, increased 40 percent, from 72.3 pounds in 1970 to 101.5 pounds in 2001.

Even though nutritionists and other health professionals recommend daily servings of dark green leafy

TABLE 2.7

**Percent of individuals consuming various types of eggs, legumes, nuts and seeds, fats and oils, and sugars and sweets over the course of one day, by sex and age, 1996**

| Sex and age (years) | Percentage of population | Eggs | Legumes | Nuts and seeds | Fats and oils | | | Sugars and sweets | | |
|---|---|---|---|---|---|---|---|---|---|---|
| | | | | | Total | Table fats | Salad dressings | Total | Sugars | Candy |
| | Percent | | | | Percent | | | | | |
| Males and females: | | | | | | | | | | |
| Under 1 | 1.1 | 9.4† | 19.7 | 1.8† | 5.3† | 5.3† | 0.0† | 9.5† | 1.3† | 0.0† |
| 1–2 | 3.0 | 25.5 | 10.2 | 15.9 | 35.0 | 26.4 | 10.8 | 45.7 | 10.6 | 14.7 |
| 3–5 | 4.7 | 17.3 | 7.8 | 19.5 | 37.6 | 25.8 | 16.2 | 62.6 | 14.0 | 26.9 |
| 5 and under | 8.8 | 19.1 | 10.2 | 16.0 | 32.5 | 23.3 | 12.3 | 50.0 | 11.2 | 19.3 |
| Males: | | | | | | | | | | |
| 6–11 | 4.6 | 11.2 | 10.1 | 11.4 | 45.2 | 29.4 | 23.4 | 55.0 | 12.2 | 28.0 |
| 12–19 | 5.9 | 16.7 | 11.8 | 8.8 | 40.6 | 16.4 | 29.2 | 43.3 | 9.0 | 21.4 |
| 20–29 | 7.2 | 21.8 | 13.7 | 6.9 | 46.6 | 17.8 | 32.3 | 39.4 | 19.1 | 16.1 |
| 30–39 | 8.1 | 20.1 | 17.5 | 7.5 | 56.4 | 24.7 | 31.9 | 49.3 | 32.4 | 12.3 |
| 40–49 | 7.0 | 21.9 | 15.6 | 6.5 | 60.8 | 32.3 | 31.7 | 53.8 | 36.9 | 10.2 |
| 50–59 | 4.7 | 24.4 | 16.0 | 11.9 | 60.0 | 36.7 | 32.6 | 56.8 | 42.3 | 8.4 |
| 60–69 | 3.4 | 26.2 | 19.0 | 8.4 | 69.9 | 39.8 | 39.0 | 62.7 | 44.7 | 13.6 |
| 70 and over | 3.4 | 27.6 | 16.3 | 12.0 | 68.0 | 48.3 | 34.7 | 62.1 | 41.3 | 7.0 |
| 20 and over | 33.9 | 22.8 | 16.1 | 8.3 | 58.3 | 30.4 | 33.0 | 51.8 | 34.0 | 11.7 |
| Females: | | | | | | | | | | |
| 6–11 | 4.4 | 11.0 | 12.5 | 17.7 | 44.3 | 28.9 | 18.8 | 63.3 | 11.0 | 26.7 |
| 12–19 | 5.6 | 11.6 | 9.6 | 7.1 | 49.3 | 24.4 | 33.1 | 45.2 | 11.1 | 26.7 |
| 20–29 | 6.9 | 18.1 | 18.6 | 5.4 | 48.9 | 29.2 | 26.3 | 43.9 | 26.1 | 11.3 |
| 30–39 | 8.6 | 16.2 | 16.9 | 8.6 | 59.8 | 29.6 | 32.3 | 55.6 | 36.9 | 13.3 |
| 40–49 | 7.2 | 21.1 | 16.4 | 5.7 | 63.6 | 34.1 | 38.7 | 52.2 | 36.0 | 13.9 |
| 50–59 | 5.1 | 16.0 | 16.1 | 6.2 | 66.9 | 33.5 | 40.1 | 66.5 | 45.0 | 13.5 |
| 60–69 | 3.9 | 26.3 | 15.3 | 8.6 | 65.0 | 37.9 | 37.0 | 55.9 | 38.9 | 7.9 |
| 70 and over | 5.1 | 21.4 | 10.9 | 9.3 | 63.6 | 42.3 | 29.8 | 54.9 | 29.8 | 10.6 |
| 20 and over | 36.8 | 19.3 | 16.0 | 7.2 | 60.6 | 33.6 | 33.7 | 54.2 | 35.1 | 12.1 |
| All individuals | 100.0 | 19.1 | 14.5 | 9.1 | 54.1 | 29.7 | 30.1 | 52.3 | 27.6 | 15.4 |

†Estimates based on small cell sizes may tend to be less statistically reliable than estimates based on larger cell sizes. Cell size refers to the unweighted number of individuals in a given sex-age group or demographic group.

Note: Excludes breast-fed children.

SOURCE: "Eggs; legumes; nuts and seeds; fats and oils; sugars and sweets: Percentages of individuals consuming foods from various food groups, by sex and age, 1 day, 1996," in *Results From USDA's 1996 Continuing Survey of Food Intakes by Individuals and 1996 Diet and Health Knowledge Survey,* U.S. Agricultural Research Service, Beltsville, MD, 1997

vegetables to ensure a healthy diet, Americans prefer potatoes. While per capita consumption of vegetables increased 23 percent from 1970 to 2001, consumption of potatoes alone increased 13 percent over the same period. (See Figure 2.6.) However, per capita consumption of dark green and deep yellow vegetables (such as broccoli, carrots, and spinach) increased by 70 percent, from 20.7 pounds in 1970 to 35 pounds in 2001.

**Dairy Products**

In 2001 Americans drank an average of 20 percent less milk than they did in 1980. According to "Trends in U.S. Per Capita Consumption of Dairy Products, 1909 to 2001," published in the June 2003 issue of *Amber Waves* (USDA), in 1909 Americans consumed an average of 34 gallons of fluid milk per person—27 gallons of whole milk and 7 gallons of lower-fat milk, especially buttermilk. (See Figure 2.7.) Fluid milk consumption peaked at 45 gallons per person in 1945, but since has steadily declined, reaching a record low of just under 23 gallons per capita in 2001 (the latest year for which data are available). Consumption

of buttermilk and other lower-fat milks increased modestly—from 4 gallons per person in 1945 and 6 gallons per person in 1970 to 15 gallons per person in 2001. The USDA attributes these diet changes to concerns about cholesterol and fat, the declining numbers of teenage males, an increasing milk-sugar (lactose) intolerance due to the growing ethnic diversity in the country, and the growing preference for soft drinks.

The popularity of fluid cream products, however, increased dramatically. Consumption of fluid cream products—half-and-half, light and heavy cream, sour cream, eggnog, and dips—nearly doubled (89 percent) between 1980 and 2001.

According to USDA's "Trends in U.S. Per Capita Consumption of Dairy Products, 1909 to 2001," in 2001 Americans consumed 30 pounds of cheese per person, more than twice as much as in 1975. (See Figure 2.8.) Per capita consumption of cheese rose steadily from 1980 to 2001, increasing nearly three-quarters (71.4 percent), from 17.5 to 30 pounds. The continuing growth in cheese

TABLE 2.8

**Percent of young people consuming particular foods, by food group, sex, and age group, 1994–96, and 1998**

Based on a two-day average.[1]

| Category | Aged 9 years and under | Aged 19 years and under |
|---|---|---|
| **Grains** | **97.2** | **97.6** |
| Yeast breads and rolls | 61.6 | 62.4 |
| Cereals and pasta | 66.4 | 57.6 |
| Cakes, cookies, pastries, and pies | 48.9 | 46.1 |
| Crackers, popcorn, pretzels, and corn chips | 35.3 | 32.5 |
| **Vegetables** | **77.1** | **78.3** |
| Potatoes | 44.6 | 46.8 |
| Dark-green vegetables | 6.1 | 5.6 |
| Deep-yellow vegetables | 12.7 | 11.2 |
| Tomatoes | 30.7 | 34.6 |
| Lettuce, lettuce-based salads | 10.3 | 16.6 |
| Other vegetables | 25.2 | 29.4 |
| **Fruits** | **68.3** | **57.8** |
| Citrus fruits and juices | 25.2 | 24.8 |
| Apples | 20.9 | 15.2 |
| Bananas | 14.0 | 9.7 |
| Melons and berries | 7.1 | 6.2 |
| Noncitrus juices and nectars | 26.7 | 17.9 |
| **Dairy products** | **92.2** | **86.7** |
| Milk | 77.1 | 68.1 |
| Whole milk | 37.4 | 30.1 |
| Lowfat milk | 36.8 | 33.1 |
| Skim milk | 6.3 | 7.5 |
| Yogurt | 5.3 | 3.8 |
| Milk desserts | 20.1 | 18.6 |
| Cheese | 31.7 | 33.5 |
| **Meats** | **80.9** | **82.8** |
| Beef | 16.1 | 19.6 |
| Pork | 10.9 | 12.1 |
| Frankfurters, sausage, luncheon meats | 32.4 | 30.9 |
| Poultry | 24.3 | 22.7 |
| Fish | 5.6 | 5.5 |
| **Beverages** | **60.7** | **72.7** |
| Coffee | 0.6 | 2.4 |
| Tea | 7.8 | 11.9 |
| Fruit drinks and ades | 35.5 | 32.3 |
| Carbonated soft drinks | 32.4 | 47.8 |
| **Other categories mixed** | | |
| Eggs | 17.1 | 16.4 |
| Nuts and seeds | 16.9 | 13.2 |
| Fats and oils | 42.0 | 43.2 |
| Sugars and sweets | 52.8 | 50.8 |

[1] Figures are based on combined data from 1994-96 and 1998 for individuals 9 years of age and under and on 1994-96 data alone for those age 10 years and over.

SOURCE: Created by Information Plus with data from the *Continuing Survey of Food Intakes by Individuals* (CSFII 1994-96, 1998), U.S. Department of Agriculture, Agricultural Research Service, Beltsville, MD, October 2000

FIGURE 2.1

**Estimating food consumption: the supply-and-utilization commodity flow**

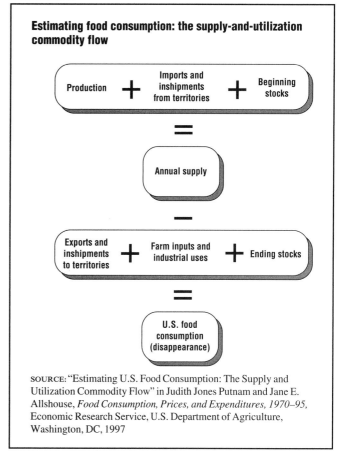

SOURCE: "Estimating U.S. Food Consumption: The Supply and Utilization Commodity Flow" in Judith Jones Putnam and Jane E. Allshouse, *Food Consumption, Prices, and Expenditures, 1970–95*, Economic Research Service, U.S. Department of Agriculture, Washington, DC, 1997

While per capita consumption of cheese continues to increase, specific types of cheese are showing dramatic increases in popularity. Consumption of cheddar cheese increased 43 percent from 1980 to 2001, from 6.9 to 9.9 pounds. Italian cheeses are by far the most popular choice—between 1980 and 2001 consumption of Italian cheeses increased 180 percent, from 4.4 to 12.3 pounds per capita. Mozzarella cheese consumption rose 221 percent between 1980 and 2001, from 3.02 pounds per capita to 9.7 pounds.

### Eggs

In 2001 each American, on average, consumed 251 eggs, a 14 percent decrease from 293 eggs per capita in 1909. (See Figure 2.9.) Since the 1980s eggs have been consumed not only as shell eggs but also as egg products (processed eggs that are sold to food manufacturers and food-service operators). Consumers use them as liquid eggs, which are sold in food stores. These liquid eggs are generally made from egg whites and are used as non-cholesterol substitutes for shell eggs. Consumers also use egg products as ingredients in processed foods and food-service menu items—for example, cake mixes, pasta, and baked goods. The decline in egg use seems to have leveled. Recently nutritionists have been recommending limited

consumption may be due to the proliferation of convenience food—two-thirds of cheese comes in commercially manufactured and prepared foods, such as pizzas, tacos, fast-food sandwiches, and packaged snack foods. Cheese is also offered in salad bars and in sauces for various vegetables, such as baked potatoes. New cheese products (in convenient, resealable containers), including cheese blends for the preparation of ethnic dishes, have also contributed to the increased per capita use.

FIGURE 2.2

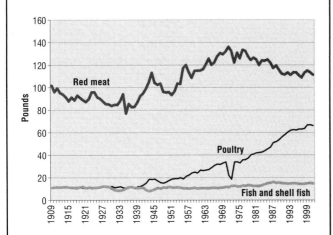

**Red meat, poultry, and fish consumption per capita, 1909–2001**

Note: The weight is for boneless or trimmed equivalent product. Prior to 1930, except for the war years, 1917–19, per capita figures are based on resident population only; from 1930 and thereafter, resident population plus Armed Forces located overseas.

SOURCE: Created by Information Plus from data in the food consumption data system, Economic Research Service (ERS), U.S. Department of Agriculture, Washington, DC [Online] http://www.ers.usda.gov/data/foodconsumption/ [accessed July 31, 2003]

FIGURE 2.3

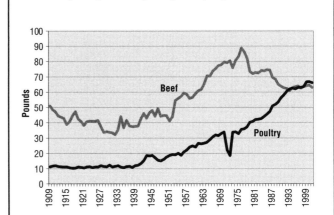

**Beef and poultry consumption per capita, 1909–2001**

Note: The weight is for boneless or trimmed equivalent product. Prior to 1930, except for the war years, 1917–19, per capita figures are based on resident population only; from 1930 and thereafter, resident population plus Armed Forces located overseas.

SOURCE: Created by Information Plus from data in the food consumption data system, Economic Research Service (ERS), U.S. Department of Agriculture, Washington, DC [Online] http://www.ers.usda.gov/data/foodconsumption/ [accessed July 31, 2003]

use of eggs rather than eliminating them from the diet completely.

**Fats and Oils**

Despite growing health concerns about the consumption of added fats and oils, Americans consumed 17 pounds more fats and oils per person in 2000 than in 1980, an increase of 28.3 percent. (See Figure 2.10.) Per capita consumption of shortening increased 63 percent from 1965 to 2001, and consumption of salad oils and cooking oils increased by 170 percent during the same period. This growth probably is due to the increased consumption of fried foods in restaurants and the increased use of salad dressings. According to the USDA the average woman 19–50 years old gets more fat from salad dressings than from any other food.

**Sweeteners**

Total per capita consumption of caloric sweeteners, mainly sucrose (table sugar made from cane and beets) and corn sweeteners (high-fructose corn syrup) increased 22 percent, from 120 pounds in 1980 to 147.1 pounds in 2001. Per capita consumption of cane and beet sugar decreased 34 percent between 1966 and 2001, but per capita consumption of corn sweeteners rose by 486 percent during the same period. (See Figure 2.11.) This amounted to over two-fifths of a pound of caloric sweeteners per person per day.

**COMPARISON OF PER CAPITA CONSUMPTION AND USDA RECOMMENDATIONS**

*A Dietary Assessment of the U.S. Food Supply: Comparing Per Capita Food Consumption with Food Guide Pyramid Serving Recommendations* (Linda Scott Kantor, Economic Research Service, USDA, Washington, D.C., 1998), the first study of its kind, compared average diets with the federal dietary recommendations. It used data from the food supply series *Food Consumption, Prices, and Expenditures, 1970–95* (Judith Jones Putnam and Jane E. Allshouse, Economic Research Service, USDA, Washington, D.C., 1997). The study was based on a sample diet of 2,200 calories, a daily energy intake considered by the USDA as appropriate for most children, teenage girls, active women, and sedentary men.

**Grain Group**

The study found that, in 1996, the grains group (bread, cereals, rice, and pasta) was the only food group that met the total servings recommended by the Food Guide Pyramid. (See Table 2.9.) On the other hand, although Americans were eating more grain products, these were mostly refined, rather than high-fiber, whole-grain products. In 2000, of the 146.3 pounds of wheat flour consumed per capita (see Table 2.10), less than 2 percent was whole-wheat flour. This finding was confirmed by the 1996 CSFII, which found that the mean daily intake of foods made from whole grains constituted just one serving of the Food Guide Pyramid recommendation.

FIGURE 2.4

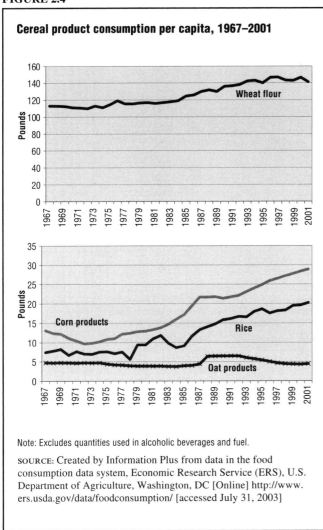

Cereal product consumption per capita, 1967–2001

Note: Excludes quantities used in alcoholic beverages and fuel.

SOURCE: Created by Information Plus from data in the food consumption data system, Economic Research Service (ERS), U.S. Department of Agriculture, Washington, DC [Online] http://www. ers.usda.gov/data/foodconsumption/ [accessed July 31, 2003]

FIGURE 2.5

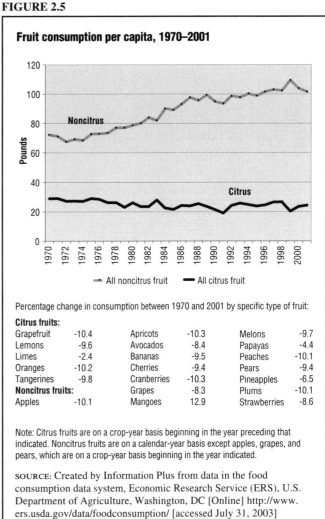

Fruit consumption per capita, 1970–2001

Percentage change in consumption between 1970 and 2001 by specific type of fruit:

| Citrus fruits: | | | | | |
|---|---|---|---|---|---|
| Grapefruit | -10.4 | Apricots | -10.3 | Melons | -9.7 |
| Lemons | -9.6 | Avocados | -8.4 | Papayas | -4.4 |
| Limes | -2.4 | Bananas | -9.5 | Peaches | -10.1 |
| Oranges | -10.2 | Cherries | -9.4 | Pears | -9.4 |
| Tangerines | -9.8 | Cranberries | -10.3 | Pineapples | -6.5 |
| **Noncitrus fruits:** | | Grapes | -8.3 | Plums | -10.1 |
| Apples | -10.1 | Mangoes | 12.9 | Strawberries | -8.6 |

Note: Citrus fruits are on a crop-year basis beginning in the year preceding that indicated. Noncitrus fruits are on a calendar-year basis except apples, grapes, and pears, which are on a crop-year basis beginning in the year indicated.

SOURCE: Created by Information Plus from data in the food consumption data system, Economic Research Service (ERS), U.S. Department of Agriculture, Washington, DC [Online] http://www. ers.usda.gov/data/foodconsumption/ [accessed July 31, 2003]

In its October 2000 report *Pyramid Servings Intakes by U.S. Children and Adults, 1994–96, 1998* the Community Nutrition Research Group of the Agricultural Research Service reported that 52 percent of individuals age 2 and older consumed at least the minimum daily number of servings of grain (6) recommended under the Food Guide Pyramid. (See Table 2.11.) Thirty-eight percent of individuals consumed the recommended daily number of servings based on caloric intake. Only one percent of this population did not consume at least one serving of food in the grain group. (See Figure 2.12.)

During the processing and refining of whole grains, the bran and germ (fiber) are removed, as well as such nutrients as vitamins and minerals. Even when the finished product has been "enriched" with some vitamins and minerals or with fiber, many of the initial nutrients may have been lost.

Whole-grain products always list whole wheat or another whole grain (oats, whole rye, brown and wild rice) as the first ingredient. Descriptions, such as "100 percent wheat," "multigrain," or "7-grain," may not necessarily mean the product is made from whole grains. Oatmeal bread, for example, may not necessarily be a whole-grain product unless oats are listed as the first ingredient.

### Vegetable Group

In 1996 the daily per capita consumption of 3.8 servings of vegetables almost equaled the Food Guide Pyramid recommendation of 4 servings. *The Food Guide Pyramid* bulletin (Center for Nutrition Policy and Promotion, USDA, 1996) further suggests dividing daily vegetable servings among deep yellow vegetables, dark green leafy vegetables, and starchy vegetables, including dry beans, peas, and lentils. Out of about 80 different vegetables considered by the ERS data, just 5 vegetables—head lettuce, 16.3 percent; frozen potatoes, 11.4 percent; fresh potatoes, 10 percent; potatoes for chips, 6.1 percent; and canned tomatoes, 5.9 percent—accounted for half of the total servings.

*Pyramid Servings Intakes by U.S. Children and Adults 1994–96, 1998* reported that 45 percent of individuals consumed at least the minimum daily number of servings (3) from the vegetable group. (See Table 2.12.) Thirty-

FIGURE 2.6

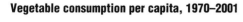

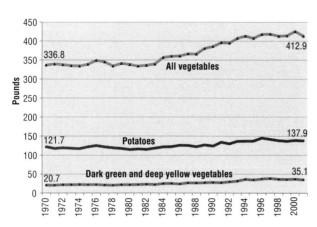

**Vegetable consumption per capita, 1970–2001**

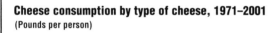

Note: Weights are based on farm weight.

SOURCE: Created by Information Plus from data in the food consumption data system, Economic Research Service (ERS), U.S. Department of Agriculture, Washington, DC [Online] http://www.ers.usda.gov/data/foodconsumption/ [accessed July 31, 2003]

FIGURE 2.7

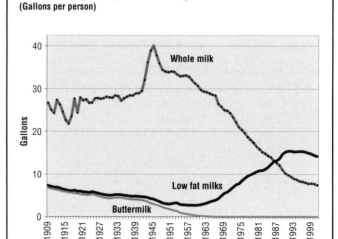

**Milk consumption by fat content, patterns 1909–2001**
(Gallons per person)

Note: Low fat milks include buttermilk (1.5 percent fat), plain and flavored reduced fat milk (2 percent fat), low-fat milk (1 percent fat), nonfat milk, and yogurt made from these milks (except frozen yogurt).

SOURCE: Adapted from Judy Putnam and Jane Allshouse, "Americans are switching to lower fat milks," in *Trends in U.S. Per Capita Consumption,* U.S. Department of Agriculture, Economic Research Service, Washington, DC, June 2003

FIGURE 2.8

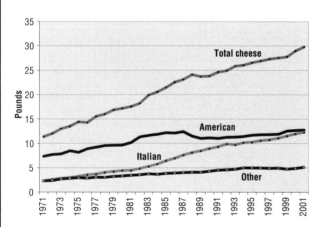

**Cheese consumption by type of cheese, 1971–2001**
(Pounds per person)

Note: American cheese includes Cheddar, Colby, Washed or Stirred Curd, Monterey, and Jack. Italian cheeses include Mozzarella, Ricotta, Provolone, Romano, Parmesan, and other Italian cheeses. Other natural cheese includes Swiss (including imports of Gruyere and Emmenthaler), Brick, Cream, Neufchatel, Blue, Gorgonzola, Edam, Gouda, and all others.

SOURCE: Adapted from Judy Putnam and Jane Allshouse, "Cheese consumption continues to rise," in *Trends in U.S. Per Capita Consumption,* U.S. Department of Agriculture, Economic Research Service, Washington, DC, June 2003

eight percent had consumed the daily number of servings that are recommended based on caloric intake. Twelve percent of us in the mid and late 1990s did not consume even one serving of food from the vegetable group. (See Figure 2.12.)

Daily per capita consumption provided only one-tenth of a daily serving of dark green leafy vegetables (mostly from broccoli and romaine lettuce) and less than one-quarter of a daily serving of deep yellow vegetables (more than 75 percent of which were from fresh, frozen, and canned carrots). Similarly, the 1996 CSFII data reported that survey participants satisfied just 6 percent of the Food Guide Pyramid recommendation for dark green leafy vegetables.

**Fruit Group**

The 1996 daily per capita consumption of fruits provided just 1.3 servings, not even half the Food Guide Pyramid recommendation of 3 servings. Moreover, consumers limited themselves to a few fruits, with half of the fruit servings coming from orange juice, 18 percent; bananas, 9.8 percent; fresh apples, 7.9 percent; watermelon, 6.5 percent; apple juice, 5.8 percent; and fresh grapes, 5.1 percent.

*Pyramid Servings Intakes by U.S. Children and Adults, 1994–96, 1998* reported that only 28 percent of individuals age 2 and older consumed at least the minimum daily number of servings of fruit recommended (2) per day. (See Table 2.13.) Twenty-three percent consumed the recommended number of servings based on caloric intake. Despite the recommendations under the Food Guide Pyramid, about half (49 percent) of individuals in this age group consumed less than one serving of fruit per day. (See Figure 2.12.)

**FIGURE 2.9**

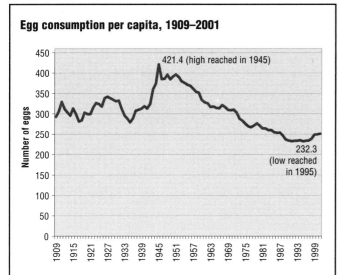

Egg consumption per capita, 1909–2001

Note: Prior to 1930, except for the war years, 1917–19, per capita figures are based on resident population only; from 1930 and thereafter, resident population plus Armed Forces located overseas.

SOURCE: Created by Information Plus from data in the food consumption data system, Economic Research Service (ERS), U.S. Department of Agriculture, Washington, DC [Online] http://www.ers.usda.gov/data/foodconsumption/ [accessed July 31, 2003]

**FIGURE 2.10**

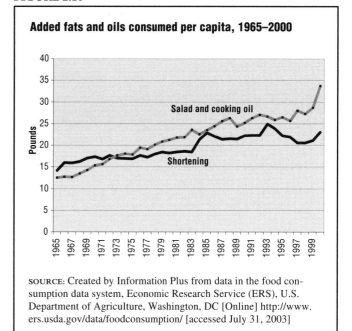

Added fats and oils consumed per capita, 1965–2000

SOURCE: Created by Information Plus from data in the food consumption data system, Economic Research Service (ERS), U.S. Department of Agriculture, Washington, DC [Online] http://www.ers.usda.gov/data/foodconsumption/ [accessed July 31, 2003]

**FIGURE 2.11**

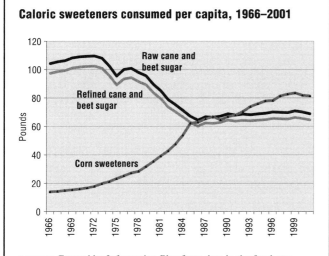

Caloric sweeteners consumed per capita, 1966–2001

SOURCE: Created by Information Plus from data in the food consumption data system, Economic Research Service (ERS), U.S. Department of Agriculture, Washington, DC [Online] http://www.ers.usda.gov/data/foodconsumption/ [accessed July 31, 2003]

## Milk, Yogurt, and Cheese Group (Dairy Group)

The dairy group is the only food group whose recommendations are weighted based on age and physiological status rather than the total energy intake. Three servings are recommended for teenagers, young adults up to 24 years old, and pregnant and lactating women. For children and other adults, the Food Guide Pyramid recommendation is two daily servings from the dairy group.

In 1996 the daily per capita consumption provided 1.7 servings of dairy products, somewhat short of the Pyramid recommendation of 2.2 servings daily. More than half of the dairy products consumed came from natural and processed cheese (38 percent) and whole milk (16 percent), which included dry and condensed milk. One-quarter of the servings were provided by skim milk (16 percent); low fat, or 1 percent milk (5 percent); and yogurt and buttermilk (2 percent, most of which were low fat). Reduced-fat, or 2 percent milk, made up 15 percent of the servings, and ice cream and other frozen dairy desserts accounted for 4 percent of the total servings.

*Pyramid Servings Intakes by U.S. Children and Adults, 1994–96, 1998* reported that only 27 percent of individuals consumed the recommended number of servings of dairy products based on age. (See Table 2.14.) Older children and teenagers (ages 9–18) and adults over 50 need 3 servings of dairy products per day. Others need 2 servings of dairy products per day. Despite the minimum recommendation (2 servings per day) 41 percent of individuals did not consume at least one serving of dairy products per day. (See Figure 2.12.)

Dairy foods are typically high in fat content. USDA experts, in light of the steep rise in cheese consumption since 1970 (see Figure 2.8), surmise that consumers are probably substituting one high-fat dairy food (cheese) for another (whole milk). They caution those who wish to increase their servings of dairy products to watch their total fat intake, since regular cheese generally has a higher proportion of total and saturated fat than whole milk.

**TABLE 2.9**

**Average food supply servings compared with Food Guide Pyramid serving recommendations, selected years, 1970–96**

| Food group | Servings | | | | Food Guide Pyramid serving recommendation[1] |
|---|---|---|---|---|---|
| | 1970–75 | 1980–85 | 1990–95 | 1996 | |
| Grains | 6.8 | 7.5 | 9.2 | 9.7 | 9 |
| Vegetables | 3.1 | 3.2 | 3.6 | 3.8 | 4 |
| Fruits | 1.1 | 1.2 | 1.3 | 1.3 | 3 |
| Milk, yogurt, and cheese[2] | 1.6 | 1.5 | 1.6 | 1.7 | 2.2 |
| Meat, poultry, fish, dry beans, eggs, and nuts (ounces) | 5.4 | 5.5 | 5.6 | 5.6 | 6.0 |
| Added fats and oils (grams of fat)[3] | 49 | 55 | 62 | 60 | 38 |
| Added sugars (teaspoons)[4] | 27 | 26 | 31 | 32 | 12 |

[1] Recommendation based on a 2,200-calorie diet. A 2,200-calorie diet is close to the 2,247 calories recommended as an average caloric intake for the population in 1995. Recommended servings for other years may differ.

[2] Three servings of milk, yogurt, and cheese are appropriate for teenagers and young adults to age 24 and for pregnant and breastfeeding women. Two servings are recommended for other adults.

[3] *The 1996 Dietary Guidelines* recommend that consumers choose a diet that provides no more than 30 percent of total calories from fat. The upper limit on the grams of fat in a consumer's diet will depend on calorie intake. For example, for a person consuming 2,200 calories per day, the upper limit on total daily fat intake is 660 calories. Seventy-three grams of fat contribute about 660 calories (73 grams x 9 calories per gram of fat = 660 calories). According to food supply data for 1994, added fats and oils account for 52 percent of the total fat provided by the food supply in that year. The recommendation shown here assumes that added fats and oils account for 52 percent of total fat intake for a daily upper limit of 38 grams of added fats and oils (73 * 0.52) = 38.

[4] To avoid getting too many calories from sugar, dietary guidance suggests that consumers on a 2,200-calorie diet try to limit added sugars to the daily quantity listed.

SOURCE: Linda Scott Kantor, *A Dietary Assessment of the U.S. Food Supply: Comparing Per Capita Food Consumption with Food Guide Serving Recommendations,* U.S. Department of Agriculture, Economic Research Service, Washington, DC, 1998

## Meat Group

In 1996 the daily per capita consumption (5.6 ounces, cooked) of foods in the meat group—red meat, poultry, fish, dry beans, eggs, and nuts—nearly equaled the Food Guide Pyramid's recommended 6 ounces. (See Table 2.9.) The red-meat share (52 percent) of the total meat servings was nearly twice that of poultry (29 percent). Fish and shellfish made up 7 percent, and eggs accounted for 9 percent of the meat-group servings. Peanut butter comprised another 2 percent of the recommended servings.

*Food Pyramid Intakes by U.S. Adults and Children 1994–96, 1998* reported that 41 percent of individuals consumed at least the minimum recommended quantity of meat servings per day. (See Table 2.15.) Thirty-six percent consumed the number of ounce equivalents recommended based on caloric intake, and 4 percent did not consume at least one serving per day. (See Figure 2.12.)

Although dry beans, peas, and lentils belong to the vegetable group, they are also included in the meat group because they are an excellent source of protein. They are low in fat, high in fiber, and cost less than meat, poultry, or fish.

## Added Fats and Oils

In 1996 the typical American consumed 60 grams of overall added fats and oils a day. Since the 1980s salad oil, cooking oil, and shortening have accounted for more than two-thirds of the total added fat and oil servings in the diet, and have accounted for almost the entire increase in added fat and oil use.

## Added Sugars

In 1996 the daily per capita consumption of added sugars was 32 teaspoons of caloric sweeteners. Caloric sweetener consumption rose 26 percent from 1970 to 1997, with 85 percent of that increase occurring since 1986. Part of that increase is due to the consumption of nondiet carbonated soft drinks, which increased 47 percent from 1986 to 1997. According to the *Food Guide Pyramid* bulletin, persons on a 1,600-calorie diet should limit their added sugar intake to 6 teaspoons per day, a mere fifth of the number of teaspoons of added sugar consumed per person in the United States in 1996. The suggested upper limit for a person whose diet equals 2,200-calorie a day was 12 teaspoons, and for a person who eats a 2,800-calorie diet each day the suggested upper limit was 18 teaspoons of added sugar.

TABLE 2.10

## Per capita consumption of major food commodities, selected years, 1980–2000

(In pounds, retail weight, except as indicated. Consumption represents the residual after exports, nonfood use and ending stocks are subtracted from the sum of beginning stocks, domestic production, and imports. Based on Census Bureau estimated population.)

| Commodity | Unit | 1980 | 1985 | 1990 | 1995 | 1998 | 1999 | 2000 |
|---|---|---|---|---|---|---|---|---|
| Red meat, total (boneless, trimmed weight)[1][2] | Pounds | 126.4 | 124.9 | 112.3 | 115.1 | 115.6 | 115.1 | 113.5 |
| Beef | Pounds | 72.1 | 74.6 | 63.9 | 64.4 | 64.9 | 64.4 | 64.4 |
| Veal | Pounds | 1.3 | 1.5 | 0.9 | 0.8 | 0.7 | 0.6 | 0.5 |
| Lamb and mutton | Pounds | 1.0 | 1.1 | 1.0 | 0.9 | 0.9 | 0.8 | 0.8 |
| Pork | Pounds | 52.1 | 47.7 | 46.4 | 49.0 | 49.2 | 49.4 | 47.7 |
| Poultry (boneless, trimmed weight)[2] | Pounds | 40.8 | 45.5 | 56.3 | 62.9 | 65.0 | 66.8 | 66.5 |
| Chicken | Pounds | 32.7 | 36.4 | 42.4 | 48.8 | 50.8 | 52.9 | 52.9 |
| Turkey | Pounds | 8.1 | 9.1 | 13.8 | 14.1 | 14.2 | 13.8 | 13.6 |
| Fish and shellfish (boneless, trimmed weight) | Pounds | 12.4 | 15.0 | 15.0 | 14.9 | 14.8 | 14.9 | 15.2 |
| Eggs | Number | 271 | 255 | 234 | 235 | 244 | 249 | 250 |
| Shell | Number | 236 | 217 | 186 | 175 | 176 | 177 | 177 |
| Processed | Number | 35 | 38 | 48 | 61 | 58 | 72 | 73 |
| Dairy products, total[3] | Pounds | 543.2 | 593.7 | 568.4 | 583.9 | 582.3 | 584.9 | 593.0 |
| Fluid milk products[4] | Gallons | 27.9 | 27.1 | 26.2 | 24.9 | 24.3 | 23.7 | 23.2 |
| Beverage milks | Gallons | 27.6 | 26.7 | 25.7 | 24.3 | 23.7 | 23.1 | 22.6 |
| Plain whole milk | Gallons | 16.5 | 13.9 | 10.2 | 8.4 | 8.0 | 7.9 | 7.8 |
| Plain reduced-fat milk (2%) | Gallons | 6.3 | 7.9 | 9.1 | 8.2 | 7.5 | 7.3 | 7.1 |
| Plain light and skim milks | Gallons | 3.1 | 3.2 | 4.9 | 6.2 | 6.6 | 6.3 | 6.1 |
| Flavored whole milk | Gallons | 0.6 | 0.4 | 0.3 | 0.3 | 0.3 | 0.4 | 0.4 |
| Flavored milks other than whole | Gallons | 0.6 | 0.7 | 0.8 | 0.8 | 1.0 | 1.0 | 1.0 |
| Buttermilk | Gallons | 0.5 | 0.5 | 0.4 | 0.3 | 0.3 | 0.3 | 0.3 |
| Yogurt (excl. frozen) | 1/2 pints | 4.6 | 7.3 | 7.4 | 9.4 | 9.3 | 9.0 | 9.9 |
| Fluid cream products[5] | 1/2 pints | 10.5 | 13.5 | 14.3 | 15.9 | 17.3 | 17.9 | 18.6 |
| Cream [6] | 1/2 pints | 6.3 | 8.2 | 8.7 | 9.5 | 10.9 | 11.4 | 11.8 |
| Sour cream and dips | 1/2 pints | 3.4 | 4.3 | 4.7 | 5.5 | 5.7 | 5.7 | 6.2 |
| Condensed and evaporated milks | Pounds | 7.0 | 7.5 | 7.9 | 6.9 | 6.4 | 6.5 | 5.8 |
| Whole milk | Pounds | 3.8 | 3.6 | 3.2 | 2.3 | 2.2 | 2.1 | 1.8 |
| Skim milk | Pounds | 3.3 | 3.8 | 4.8 | 4.5 | 4.1 | 4.4 | 3.8 |
| Cheese [7] | Pounds | 17.5 | 22.5 | 24.6 | 27.3 | 28.4 | 29.0 | 29.8 |
| American | Pounds | 9.6 | 12.2 | 11.1 | 11.8 | 12.2 | 12.6 | 12.7 |
| Cheddar | Pounds | 6.9 | 9.8 | 9.0 | 9.1 | 9.6 | 10.1 | (NA) |
| Italian | Pounds | 4.4 | 6.5 | 9.0 | 10.4 | 11.3 | 11.8 | (NA) |
| Mozzarella | Pounds | .0 | 4.6 | 6.9 | 8.1 | 8.7 | 9.2 | (NA) |
| Other[8] | Pounds | 3.4 | 3.9 | 4.5 | 5.0 | 4.8 | 5.0 | (NA) |
| Swiss | Pounds | 1.3 | 1.3 | 1.4 | 1.1 | 1.0 | 1.1 | (NA) |
| Cream and Neufchatel | Pounds | 1.0 | 1.2 | 1.7 | 2.1 | 2.3 | 2.4 | (NA) |
| Cottage cheese, total | Pounds | 4.5 | 4.1 | 3.4 | 2.7 | 2.7 | 2.6 | 2.6 |
| Lowfat | Pounds | 0.8 | 1.0 | 1.2 | 1.2 | 1.3 | 1.3 | 1.3 |
| Frozen dairy products | Pounds | 26.4 | 27.9 | 28.4 | 29.4 | 29.6 | 28.6 | 27.8 |
| Ice cream | Pounds | 17.5 | 18.1 | 15.8 | 15.7 | 16.6 | 16.7 | 16.5 |
| Lowfat ice cream | Pounds | 7.1 | 6.9 | 7.7 | 7.5 | 8.3 | 7.5 | 7.3 |
| Sherbet | Pounds | 1.2 | 1.3 | 1.2 | 1.3 | 1.4 | 1.3 | 1.2 |
| Frozen yogurt | Pounds | (NA) | (NA) | 2.8 | 3.5 | 1.9 | 1.9 | 1.8 |
| Fats and oils: | | | | | | | | |
| Total, fat content only | Pounds | 56.9 | 64.1 | 63.0 | 66.4 | 65.3 | 67.0 | 74.5 |
| Butter (product weight) | Pounds | 4.5 | 4.9 | 4.4 | 4.5 | 4.2 | 4.7 | 4.6 |
| Margarine (product weight) | Pounds | 11.3 | 10.8 | 10.9 | 9.2 | 8.3 | 7.9 | 8.2 |
| Lard (direct use) | Pounds | 2.3 | 1.6 | 1.6 | 1.7 | 2.0 | 2.0 | 1.9 |
| Edible beef tallow (direct use) | Pounds | 1.1 | 2.0 | 0.6 | 2.7 | 3.2 | 3.6 | 4.0 |
| Shortening | Pounds | 18.2 | 22.9 | 22.2 | 22.5 | 20.9 | 21.1 | 23.1 |
| Salad and cooking oils | Pounds | 21.3 | 23.6 | 25.3 | 26.9 | 27.9 | 28.8 | 33.7 |
| Other edible fats and oils | Pounds | 1.5 | 1.6 | 1.2 | 1.6 | 1.3 | 1.5 | 1.5 |
| Flour and cereal products[9] | Pounds | 144.7 | 156.5 | 181.5 | 190.7 | 196.8 | 196.9 | 199.9 |
| Wheat flour | Pounds | 116.9 | 124.6 | 136.0 | 141.9 | 147.8 | 144.0 | 146.3 |
| Rice, milled | Pounds | 9.4 | 9.1 | 15.8 | 18.9 | 18.9 | 19.5 | 19.7 |
| Corn products | Pounds | 12.9 | 17.2 | 21.9 | 21.8 | 22.3 | 27.8 | 28.4 |
| Oat products | Pounds | 3.9 | 4.0 | 6.5 | 6.5 | 6.6 | 4.4 | 4.3 |
| Breakfast cereals[10] | Pounds | 12.0 | 12.8 | 15.4 | 17.1 | (NA) | (NA) | (NA) |
| Ready-to-eat | Pounds | 9.7 | 10.5 | 12.6 | 14.6 | (NA) | (NA) | (NA) |
| Ready-to-cook | Pounds | 2.3 | 2.3 | 2.9 | 2.5 | (NA) | (NA) | (NA) |
| Caloric sweeteners, total[11] | Pounds | 123.0 | 128.8 | 137.0 | 149.8 | 155.1 | 152.6 | 152.4 |
| Sugar, refined cane and beet | Pounds | 83.6 | 62.7 | 64.4 | 65.5 | 67.0 | 65.0 | 65.6 |
| Corn sweeteners[12] | Pounds | 38.2 | 64.8 | 71.1 | 83.0 | 86.8 | 86.3 | 85.3 |
| High-fructose corn syrup | Pounds | 19.0 | 45.2 | 49.6 | 58.4 | 63.8 | 62.9 | 63.8 |
| Other: | | | | | | | | |
| Cocoa beans | Pounds | 3.4 | 4.6 | 5.4 | 4.6 | (NA) | 5.4 | 5.9 |
| Coffee (green beans) | Pounds | 10.3 | 10.5 | 10.3 | 8.0 | 9.5 | 9.3 | 10.3 |
| Peanuts (shelled) | Pounds | 4.8 | 6.3 | 6.0 | 5.7 | 5.9 | 5.8 | 5.7 |
| Tree nuts (shelled) | Pounds | 1.8 | 2.5 | 2.4 | 1.9 | 2.3 | 2.2 | 2.5 |

NA Not available. [1] Excludes edible offals. [2] Excludes shipments to Puerto Rico and the other U.S. possessions. [3] Milk-equivalent, milkfat basis. Includes butter. [4] Fluid figures are aggregates of commercial sales and milk produced and consumed on farms. [5] Includes eggnog, not shown separately. [6] Heavy cream, light cream, and half and half. [7] Excludes full-skim American, cottage, pot, and baker's cheese. [8] Includes other cheeses not shown separately. [9] Includes rye flour and barley products not shown separately. Excludes quantities used in alcoholic beverages. [10] Partially overlaps flour and cereal products category. [11] Dry weight. Includes edible syrups (maple, molasses, etc.) and honey not shown separately. [12] Includes glucose and dextrose not shown separately.

SOURCE: Adapted from "Table 195. Per Capita Consumption of Major Food Commodities: 1980 to 2000" in *Statistical Abstract of the United States, 2002*, U.S. Census Bureau, Washington, DC, December 2002

TABLE 2.11

## Grain consumption by number of Pyramid Servings per day, by sex and age, 1994–96, and 1998

Based on a two-day average for individuals two years of age and over.[1]

| Sex and age (years) | Percent of Population | Percent consuming | | |
|---|---|---|---|---|
| | | Less than 1 serving a day[3] | At least minimum number of servings recommended | Number of servings recommended based on caloric intake[2] |
| **Males** | | | | |
| 2-5 | 3.3 | 0 | 53 | 53 |
| 6-11 | 4.7 | 0 | 61 | 47 |
| 12-19 | 5.9 | 0 | 77 | 48 |
| 20-29 | 7.5 | 1 | 71 | 46 |
| 30-39 | 8.5 | -[4] | 70 | 41 |
| 40-49 | 7.1 | 1 | 68 | 40 |
| 50-59 | 4.8 | 1 | 59 | 36 |
| 60-69 | 3.5 | 0 | 58 | 41 |
| 70 and over | 3.4 | 1 | 49 | 38 |
| 20 and over | 34.8 | 0 | 65 | 41 |
| **Females** | | | | |
| 2-5 | 3.1 | 0 | 43 | 43 |
| 6-11 | 4.5 | 0 | 46 | 39 |
| 12-19 | 5.7 | 0 | 49 | 35 |
| 20-29 | 7.2 | 1 | 41 | 32 |
| 30-39 | 9.0 | 1 | 41 | 33 |
| 40-49 | 7.1 | 1 | 39 | 33 |
| 50-59 | 5.3 | 1 | 37 | 31 |
| 60-69 | 4.3 | 2 | 28 | 25 |
| 70 and over | 4.9 | 1 | 28 | 26 |
| 20 and over | 37.8 | 1 | 37 | 31 |
| **All individuals aged 2 years or older** | 100.0 | 1 | 52 | 38 |

Note: Grain consumption includes the consumption of yeast breads and rolls; quick breads such as muffins, biscuits, pancakes and tortillas; rice; pasta; breakfast cereals; grain-based snacks; and baked goods made from flour.

[1] Figures are based on combined data from 1994–96 and 1998 for individuals 9 years of age and under, and on 1994–96 data alone for those age 10 years and over. Data for individuals 10 to 19 years of age have been reweighted.

[2] Recommended servings were derived from sample patterns in "The Food Guide Pyramid" (USDA 1992) and from the children's Pyramid (USDA 1999).

[3] Based on data that is less statistically reliable than the other data presented.

[4] Value less than 0.05 but greater than 0.

SOURCE: Adapted from Annetta Cook and James E. Friday "Table 7B. Grain group: Percentages of individuals consuming specified numbers of Pyramid Servings per day, by sex and age, individuals 2 years of age and over, 2-day average, 1994-96, 1998," in *Pyramid Servings Intakes by U.S. Children and Adults 1994-96, 1998,* U.S. Department of Agriculture, Agricultural Research Service, Beltsville, MD, October 2000

FIGURE 2.12

## Percent of individuals who do not consume one serving of specific foods daily, by food group, 1994–96, and 1998

(Based on a two-day average for individuals two years of age and over)

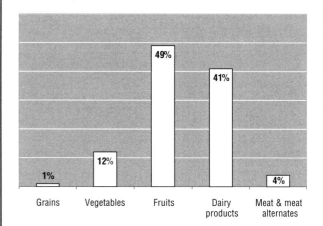

Note: Grains include yeast breads and rolls; quick breads such as muffins, biscuits, pancakes and tortillas; rice; pasta; breakfast cereals; grain-based snacks; and baked goods made from flour. Dairy products include milk, yogurt, and cheese. Dairy foods that are excluded are those which are primarily fats, namely butter, cream, sour cream, and cream cheese. Meats and meat alternate products include beef, pork, lamb, veal, game, poultry, fish, shellfish, frankfurters, sausage, bacon, luncheon meats, organ meats, eggs, soy-based products, nuts, and seeds. According to the Pyramid, dry beans and peas can count as a vegetable or as a meat alternative.

SOURCE: Created by Information Plus from data in a report by Annetta Cook and James E. Friday "Tables 7B, 8B, 9B, 10B, and 11B," in *Pyramid Servings Intakes by U.S. Children and Adults 1994-96, 1998,* U.S. Department of Agriculture, Agricultural Research Service, Beltsville, MD, October 2000

**TABLE 2.12**

## Vegetable consumption by number of Pyramid Servings per day, sex, and age, 1994–96, and 1998

Based on a two-day average for individuals two years of age and over.[1]

| Sex and age (years) | Percent of population | Percent consuming | | |
|---|---|---|---|---|
| | | Less than 1 serving a day | At least minimum number of servings recommended | Number of servings recommended based on caloric intake[2] |
| **Males** | | | | |
| 2-5 | 3.3 | 24 | 24 | 24 |
| 6-11 | 4.7 | 21 | 24 | 18 |
| 12-19 | 5.9 | 11 | 51 | 33 |
| 20-29 | 7.5 | 8 | 64 | 45 |
| 30-39 | 8.5 | 6 | 65 | 50 |
| 40-49 | 7.1 | 10 | 58 | 43 |
| 50-59 | 4.8 | 9 | 62 | 51 |
| 60-69 | 3.5 | 8 | 56 | 48 |
| 70 and over | 3.4 | 13 | 48 | 42 |
| 20 and over | 34.8 | 8 | 60 | 47 |
| **Females** | | | | |
| 2-5 | 3.1 | 23 | 21 | 21 |
| 6-11 | 4.5 | 23 | 22 | 19 |
| 12-19 | 5.7 | 15 | 34 | 26 |
| 20-29 | 7.2 | 13 | 39 | 35 |
| 30-39 | 9.0 | 10 | 42 | 37 |
| 40-49 | 7.1 | 10 | 46 | 42 |
| 50-59 | 5.3 | 11 | 46 | 44 |
| 60-69 | 4.3 | 10 | 43 | 41 |
| 70 and over | 4.9 | 11 | 37 | 36 |
| 20 and over | 37.8 | 11 | 42 | 39 |
| **All individuals aged 2 years or older** | 100.0 | 12 | 45 | 38 |

[1] Figures are based on combined data from 1994–96 and 1998 for individuals 9 years of age and under, and on 1994–96 data alone for those age 10 years and over. Data for individuals 10 to 19 years of age have been reweighted.

[2] Recommended servings were derived from sample patterns in "The Food Guide Pyramid" (USDA 1992) and from the children's Pyramid (USDA 1999).

SOURCE: Adapted from Annetta Cook and James E. Friday "Table 8B. Vegetable group: Percentages of individuals consuming specified numbers of Pyramid Servings per day, by sex and age, individuals 2 years of age and over, 2-day average, 1994-96, 1998," in *Pyramid Servings Intakes by U.S. Children and Adults 1994-96, 1998,* U.S. Department of Agriculture, Agricultural Research Service, Beltsville, MD, October 2000

**TABLE 2.13**

## Fruit consumption by number of Pyramid Servings per day, sex, and age, 1994–96, and 1998

Based on a two-day average for individuals two years of age and over.[1]

| Sex and age (years) | Percent of population | Percent consuming | | |
|---|---|---|---|---|
| | | Less than 1 serving a day | At least minimum number of servings recommended | Number of servings recommended based on caloric intake[2] |
| **Males** | | | | |
| 2-5 | 3.3 | 27 | 50 | 50 |
| 6-11 | 4.7 | 44 | 28 | 23 |
| 12-19 | 5.9 | 54 | 22 | 14 |
| 20-29 | 7.5 | 60 | 23 | 15 |
| 30-39 | 8.5 | 59 | 23 | 16 |
| 40-49 | 7.1 | 53 | 27 | 18 |
| 50-59 | 4.8 | 48 | 30 | 21 |
| 60-69 | 3.5 | 40 | 36 | 29 |
| 70 and over | 3.4 | 35 | 43 | 37 |
| 20 and over | 34.8 | 52 | 28 | 20 |
| **Females** | | | | |
| 2-5 | 3.1 | 29 | 46 | 46 |
| 6-11 | 4.5 | 44 | 27 | 24 |
| 12-19 | 5.7 | 53 | 24 | 18 |
| 20-29 | 7.2 | 57 | 20 | 18 |
| 30-39 | 9.0 | 55 | 23 | 20 |
| 40-49 | 7.1 | 53 | 23 | 21 |
| 50-59 | 5.3 | 45 | 31 | 29 |
| 60-69 | 4.3 | 38 | 35 | 33 |
| 70 and over | 4.9 | 33 | 36 | 36 |
| 20 and over | 37.8 | 49 | 27 | 25 |
| **All individuals aged 2 years or older** | 100.0 | 49 | 28 | 23 |

[1] Figures are based on combined data from 1994–96 and 1998 for individuals 9 years of age and under, and on 1994–96 data alone for those age 10 years and over. Data for individuals 10 to 19 years of age have been reweighted.

[2] Recommended servings were derived from sample patterns in "The Food Guide Pyramid" (USDA 1992) and from the children's Pyramid (USDA 1999).

SOURCE: Adapted from Annetta Cook and James E. Friday "Table 9B. Fruit group: Percentages of individuals consuming specified numbers of Pyramid Servings per day, by sex and age, individuals 2 years of age and over, 2-day average, 1994-96, 1998," in *Pyramid Servings Intakes by U.S. Children and Adults 1994-96, 1998,* U.S. Department of Agriculture, Agricultural Research Service, Beltsville, MD, October 2000

**TABLE 2.14**

## Dairy product consumption by number of Pyramid Servings per day, sex, and age, 1994–96, and 1998

Based on a two-day average for individuals two years of age and over.[1]

| Sex and age (years) | Percent of Population | Percent consuming | | |
|---|---|---|---|---|
| | | Less than 1 serving a day | At least minimum number of servings recommended | Number of servings recommended based on caloric intake[2] |
| **Males** | | | | |
| 2-5 | 3.3 | 17 | 45 | 45 |
| 6-11 | 4.7 | 12 | 53 | 40 |
| 12-19 | 5.9 | 21 | 51 | 30 |
| 20-29 | 7.5 | 37 | 30 | 30 |
| 30-39 | 8.5 | 39 | 31 | 31 |
| 40-49 | 7.1 | 42 | 29 | 29 |
| 50-59 | 4.8 | 50 | 20 | 10 |
| 60-69 | 3.5 | 45 | 23 | 7 |
| 70 and over | 3.4 | 43 | 24 | 6 |
| 20 and over | 34.8 | 42 | 27 | 22 |
| **Females** | | | | |
| 2-5 | 3.1 | 19 | 41 | 41 |
| 6-11 | 4.5 | 20 | 41 | 29 |
| 12-19 | 5.7 | 39 | 26 | 12 |
| 20-29 | 7.2 | 44 | 17 | 17 |
| 30-39 | 9.0 | 53 | 19 | 19 |
| 40-49 | 7.1 | 56 | 16 | 16 |
| 50-59 | 5.3 | 56 | 14 | 4 |
| 60-69 | 4.3 | 59 | 12 | 3 |
| 70 and over | 4.9 | 56 | 15 | 3 |
| 20 and over | 37.8 | 53 | 16 | 12 |
| **All individuals aged 2 years or older** | 100.0 | 41 | 27 | 21 |

Note: Dairy product consumption includes the consumption of milk, yogurt, and cheese. Dairy foods that are excluded are those which are primarily fats, namely butter, cream, sour cream, and cream cheese.

[1] Figures are based on combined data from 1994–96 and 1998 for individuals 9 years of age and under, and on 1994–96 data alone for those age 10 years and over. Data for individuals 10 to 19 years of age have been reweighted.

[2] The recommendation for an individual is based on age. Older children and teenagers (ages 9 through 18) and adults over the age of 50 need 3 servings daily. Others need 2 servings daily.

SOURCE: Adapted from Annetta Cook and James E. Friday "Table 10B. Dairy group: Percentages of individuals consuming specified numbers of Pyramid Servings per day, by sex and age, individuals 2 years of age and over, 2-day average, 1994-96, 1998," in *Pyramid Servings Intakes by U.S. Children and Adults 1994-96, 1998,* U.S. Department of Agriculture, Agricultural Research Service, Beltsville, MD, October 2000

---

**TABLE 2.15**

## Meat and meat alternative product consumption by number of Pyramid Servings per day, sex, and age, 1994–96, and 1998

Based on a two-day average for individuals two years of age and over.[1]

| Sex and age (years) | Percent of Population | Percent consuming | | |
|---|---|---|---|---|
| | | Less than 1 serving a day | At least minimum number of servings recommended | Number of servings recommended based on caloric intake[2] |
| **Males** | | | | |
| 2-5 | 3.3 | 9 | 22 | 22 |
| 6-11 | 4.7 | 5 | 24 | 21 |
| 12-19 | 5.9 | 2[3] | 55 | 44 |
| 20-29 | 7.5 | 2[3] | 65 | 54 |
| 30-39 | 8.5 | 1[3] | 69 | 60 |
| 40-49 | 7.1 | 1[3] | 68 | 59 |
| 50-59 | 4.8 | 1[3] | 64 | 57 |
| 60-69 | 3.5 | 1[3] | 58 | 52 |
| 70 and over | 3.4 | 2[3] | 40 | 36 |
| 20 and over | 34.8 | 1 | 63 | 55 |
| **Females** | | | | |
| 2-5 | 3.1 | 11 | 18 | 18 |
| 6-11 | 4.5 | 6 | 13 | 12 |
| 12-19 | 5.7 | 7 | 26 | 22 |
| 20-29 | 7.2 | 7 | 29 | 25 |
| 30-39 | 9.0 | 4 | 30 | 28 |
| 40-49 | 7.1 | 5 | 30 | 28 |
| 50-59 | 5.3 | 4 | 29 | 27 |
| 60-69 | 4.3 | 3 | 29 | 29 |
| 70 and over | 4.9 | 5 | 20 | 20 |
| 20 and over | 37.8 | 5 | 28 | 26 |
| **All individuals aged 2 years or older** | 100.0 | 4 | 41 | 36 |

Note: Meats and meat alternative products include beef, pork, lamb, veal, game, poultry, fish, shellfish, frankfurters, sausage, bacon, luncheon meats, organ meats, eggs, soy-based products, such as tofu and meat analogs, nuts, and seeds. According to the Pyramid, dry beans and peas can count as a vegetable or as a meat alternative.

[1] Figures are based on combined data from 1994–96 and 1998 for individuals 9 years of age and under, and on 1994–96 data alone for those age 10 years and over. Data for individuals 10 to 19 years of age have been reweighted.

[2] The recommendation for an individual is based on age. Older children and teenagers (ages 9 through 18) and adults over the age of 50 need 3 servings daily. Others need 2 servings daily.

[3] Based on data that is less statistically reliable than the other data presented due to size of the sample responding.

SOURCE: Adapted from Annetta Cook and James E. Friday "Table 11B. Meat group: Percentages of individuals consuming specified numbers of Pyramid Servings per day, by sex and age, individuals 2 years of age and over, 2-day average, 1994-96, 1998," in *Pyramid Servings Intakes by U.S. Children and Adults 1994-96, 1998,* U.S. Department of Agriculture, Agricultural Research Service, Beltsville, MD, October 2000

# CHAPTER 3
# THE ROLE OF FOODS

*Unless care is exercised in selecting food, a diet may result which is one-sided or badly balanced—that is, one in which either protein or fuel ingredients (carbohydrate and fat) are provided in excess. . . . The evils of overeating may not be felt at once, but sooner or later they are sure to appear—perhaps in an excessive amount of fatty tissue, perhaps in general debility, perhaps in actual disease.*

— W. O. Atwater, author of the first USDA dietary guide, the *Farmers' Bulletin,* 1902

For centuries people have understood that there is a connection between the food they eat and their health, but diets have generally been limited to locally available foods and, for the poor, foods they could grow or catch. It is only in modern times and in developed countries that a broad range of foods has been available, giving people the option of eating a diversified, healthy diet.

As recently as a generation ago, good nutrition primarily meant preventing vitamin and mineral deficiencies and the diseases that stemmed from them. Today consumers expect more; they hope that their diets will help them remain active, live longer, and avoid illness. As more research has been done, our understanding of nutrition has had to change. What may have been considered solid scientific knowledge 10 years ago is questioned today, and what we accept today may well be wrong tomorrow. Nonetheless nutritionists in the United States generally agree on what to eat and not eat to promote health and avoid disorders such as coronary heart disease, cancer, hypertension, and obesity.

## DIETARY GUIDELINES FOR AMERICANS

*Nutrition and Your Health: Dietary Guidelines for Americans,* popularly referred to as *Dietary Guidelines,* was initially released jointly by the U.S. Department of Agriculture (USDA) and the U.S. Department of Health and Human Services (HHS) in 1980. Under the National Nutrition Monitoring and Related Research Act of 1990

**TABLE 3.1**

**Dietary guidelines for Americans**

- Aim for a healthy weight.
- Be physically active each day.

- Let the Pyramid guide your food choices.
- Choose a variety of grains daily, especially whole grains.
- Choose a variety of fruits and vegetables daily.
- Keep food safe to eat.

- Choose a diet that is low in saturated fat and cholesterol and moderate in total fat.
- Choose beverages and foods to moderate your intake of sugars.
- Choose and prepare foods with less salt.
- If you drink alcoholic beverages, do so in moderation.

SOURCE: "Dietary Guidelines for Americans," in *Nutrition and Your Health: Dietary Guidelines for Americans,* U.S. Department of Agriculture, Washington, DC, May 2000

(PL 101-445), Congress mandated that the *Dietary Guidelines* be reviewed and revised, as needed, every five years. The act also required that every federal agency promote these guidelines.

The latest *Dietary Guidelines* was issued in 2000. Based on current scientific knowledge, the guidelines "are designed to help Americans choose diets that will meet nutrient requirements, promote health, support active lives, and reduce chronic disease risks." Table 3.1 presents the basic recommendations.

The Dietary Guidelines 2000 Advisory Committee was formed to revise the 1995 edition as mandated by Public Law 101-445. At its March 1999 meeting the committee spoke of possible changes to the guidelines—focusing on "adequacy" of foods instead of variety and introducing different versions of the Food Guide Pyramid, such as Asian and Mediterranean versions. Other possible changes included identifying the benefits of mono- and polyunsaturated fats and creating two guidelines for plant foods: one for grains and another for fruits and vegetables.

FIGURE 3.1

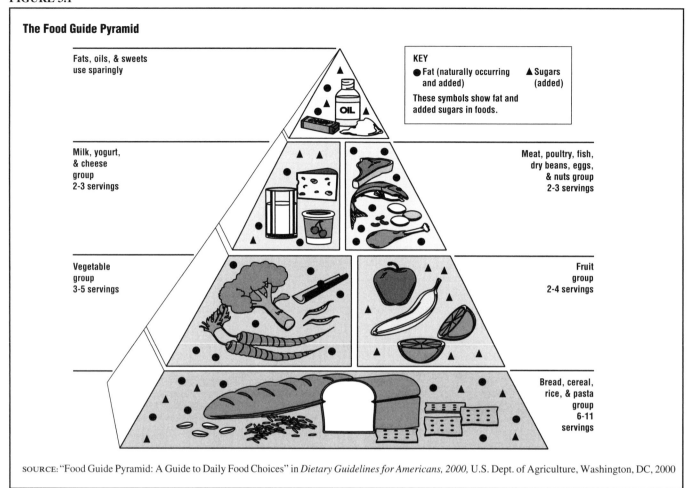

**The Food Guide Pyramid**

Fats, oils, & sweets use sparingly

**KEY**
● Fat (naturally occurring and added)  ▲ Sugars (added)
These symbols show fat and added sugars in foods.

Milk, yogurt, & cheese group
2-3 servings

Meat, poultry, fish, dry beans, eggs, & nuts group
2-3 servings

Vegetable group
3-5 servings

Fruit group
2-4 servings

Bread, cereal, rice, & pasta group
6-11 servings

SOURCE: "Food Guide Pyramid: A Guide to Daily Food Choices" in *Dietary Guidelines for Americans, 2000,* U.S. Dept. of Agriculture, Washington, DC, 2000

## THE FOOD GUIDE PYRAMID

Two other federal guidelines—the Food Guide Pyramid and the Nutrition Guide Label—serve as educational tools to help consumers put the *Dietary Guidelines* into practice. The Food Guide Pyramid graphic (see Figure 3.1) is published as part of a larger bulletin of dietary guidance, *The Food Guide Pyramid* bulletin, which explains the graphic's recommendations comprehensively.

The Food Guide Pyramid is not a rigid prescription, but a general guide to help consumers implement the *Dietary Guidelines* by suggesting both the types of food needed and the number of servings. The servings are only a general guide; there is no need for exact measurements. (See Table 3.2.) Nonetheless, if a person eats a significantly larger portion of food, he or she should count it as more than a serving. Table 3.3 shows how many servings of each food group are needed for several daily calorie intakes. If a person's calorie consumption falls between categories, the number of servings can be estimated.

Some confusion about servings exists in the public mind, as shown by a story in *Nutrition News* ("Servings: Size Matters," May 3, 1999). The story points out that the same "serving" may have a different weight as labeled by

the manufacturer, depending on the food group. A serving of bread is one ounce of bread but a serving of pasta may be two ounces. Fruit servings are measured by unit—one apple is a serving of fruit. And so on. The value of the *Dietary Guidelines* lies, among other things, in specifying what constitutes a serving with some precision.

The Food Guide Pyramid favors foods from the broader base of the pyramid—bread, cereal, rice, and pasta group (6–11 servings), the vegetable group (3–5 servings), and fruit group (2–4 servings). Once the caloric base is established from the lowest level of the pyramid, most people need to eat more fruit and vegetable servings in order to increase their intake of fiber, vitamins, and minerals.

Americans need only moderate amounts (2–3 servings each) from the milk group and the meat and beans group. Most foods in these groups come from animal sources.

The small tip of the pyramid represents those foods that should be eaten sparingly. The fats, oils, and sweets group supplies calories but little or no vitamins and minerals.

**SOME RETHINKING IS UNDERWAY.** Some nutrition experts are not convinced that the 2000 Food Guide Pyramid

TABLE 3.2

## What counts as a serving?

**Bread, cereal, rice, and pasta group (grains group)—whole grain and refined**
- 1 slice of bread
- About 1 cup of ready-to-eat cereal
- 1/2 cup of cooked cereal, rice, or pasta

**Vegetable group**
- 1 cup of raw leafy vegetables
- 1/2 cup of other vegetables—cooked or raw
- 3/4 cup of vegetable juice

**Fruit group**
- 1 medium apple, banana, orange, pear
- 1/2 cup of chopped, cooked, or canned fruit
- 3/4 cup of fruit juice

**Milk, yogurt, and cheese group (milk group)[1]**
- 1 cup of milk[2] or yogurt[2]
- 1 1/2 ounces of natural cheese[2] (such as Cheddar)
- 2 ounces of processed cheese[2] (such as American)

**Meat, poultry, fish, dry beans, eggs, and nuts group (meat and beans group)**
- 2–3 ounces of cooked lean meat, poultry, or fish
- 1/2 cup of cooked dry beans[3] or 1/2 cup of tofu counts as 1 ounce of lean meat
- 2 1/2-ounce soyburger or 1 egg counts as 1 ounce of lean meat
- 2 tablespoons of peanut butter or 1/3 cup of nuts counts as 1 ounce of lean meat

Note: Many of the serving sizes given above are smaller than those on the nutrition facts label. For example, 1 serving of cooked cereal, rice, or pasta is 1 cup for the label but only 1/2 cup for the Pyramid.

[1] This includes lactose-free and lactose-reduced milk products. One cup of soy-based beverage with added calcium is an option for those who prefer a non-dairy source of calcium.

[2] Choose fat-free or reduced-fat dairy products most often.

[3] Dry beans, peas, and lentils can be counted as servings in either the meat and beans group or the vegetable group. As a vegetable, 1/2 cup of cooked, dry beans counts as 1 serving. As a meat substitute, 1 cup of cooked, dry beans counts as 1 serving (2 ounces of meat).

SOURCE: "What Counts as a Serving?" in *Dietary Guidelines for Americans, 2000*, U.S. Department of Agriculture, Washington, DC, 2000

TABLE 3.3

## Daily sample diets, by calorie level

| | Lower about 1,600 | Moderate about 2,200 | Higher about 2,800 |
|---|---|---|---|
| Grain group servings | 6 | 8 | 11 |
| Vegetable group servings | 3 | 4 | 5 |
| Fruit group serving | 2 | 3 | 4 |
| Milk group servings | 2-3[1] | 2-3[1] | 2-3[1] |
| Meat group[2] (ounces) | 5 | 6 | 7 |
| Total fat (grams) | 53 | 73 | 93 |
| Total added sugars (teaspoons) | 6 | 12 | 18 |

[1] Women who are pregnant or breast-feeding, teenagers, and young adults to age 24 need 3 servings.

[2] Meat group amounts are in total ounces.

SOURCE: "Sample Diets for a Day at 3 Calorie Levels," in *Food Guide Pyramid Booklet 2000*, Center for Nutrition Policy and Promotion, U.S. Department of Agriculture, Washington, DC, 2000

is the final word on nutrition and good health. Nutrition scientists have felt for some time that the pyramid is outdated, according to an article in *USA Today* ("Scales Tip in Favor of New Pyramid," November 4, 2002). Scientists who have criticized the pyramid have offered several alternatives, including the Mediterranean Pyramid, the Healthy Eating Pyramid, and the Soul Food Pyramid, among others. According to the article, Walter Willett, chairman of the department of nutrition at the Harvard School of Public Health, believes that the pyramid does not incorporate the latest research on nutrition and weight control, and suggests that it may be a factor in obesity and other health problems. Willett developed the Healthy Eating Pyramid, in which he places daily exercise and weight control at the bottom of the pyramid and recommends eating more whole-grain foods and vegetables. He also points out that the government's pyramid does not distinguish between types of fat and, instead, puts all fats at the tip of the pyramid with the recommendation to limit intake. Willett asserts that monounsaturated and polyunsaturated fats are good for the heart.

The Center for Nutrition Policy and Promotion (CNPP) of the USDA is reviewing the recent nutrient recommendations from the National Academies' Institute of Medicine to determine if servings in the Food Guide Pyramid meets those requirements. The CNPP pointed out that many people use the graphic image of the pyramid but neglect to study the accompanying text, which explains that recommendations in the graphic are based on daily calorie consumption. The CNPP will make its decision on possible changes to the pyramid sometime in 2004, but has no plans to change the graphic design.

In August 2003 the federal government was expected to announce which scientists and other experts would be appointed to revise the nation's dietary guidelines ("Expect a Food Fight as U.S. Revises Dietary Guidelines," *Wall Street Journal,* August 8, 2003, B1). According to the article, members of the committee must include experts in the fields of pediatrics, obesity, cardiovascular disease, and public health. Food industry groups are submitting scientific reports and other data in support of claims the industry makes about its products. The Wine Institute, for example, is expected to resubmit scientific reports that discuss the beneficial cardiovascular effects of alcohol consumption. The committee is expected to meet in the fall of 2003.

## THE FOOD GUIDE PYRAMID FOR YOUNG CHILDREN

In March 1999 the USDA introduced the Food Guide Pyramid for Young Children, intended to serve children ages 2–6. (See Figure 3.2.) The new daily food guide is an offshoot of the original pyramid, with an emphasis on balanced meals, moderation, and variety in food choices, especially from the grain, fruit, and vegetable groups.

The child pyramid is based on the eating patterns of young children. Not surprisingly, 2- to 6-year-olds eat a different diet than older children and adults. More of their servings from the meat group come from ground beef and luncheon meat, and fewer from fish. They are more likely

**FIGURE 3.2**

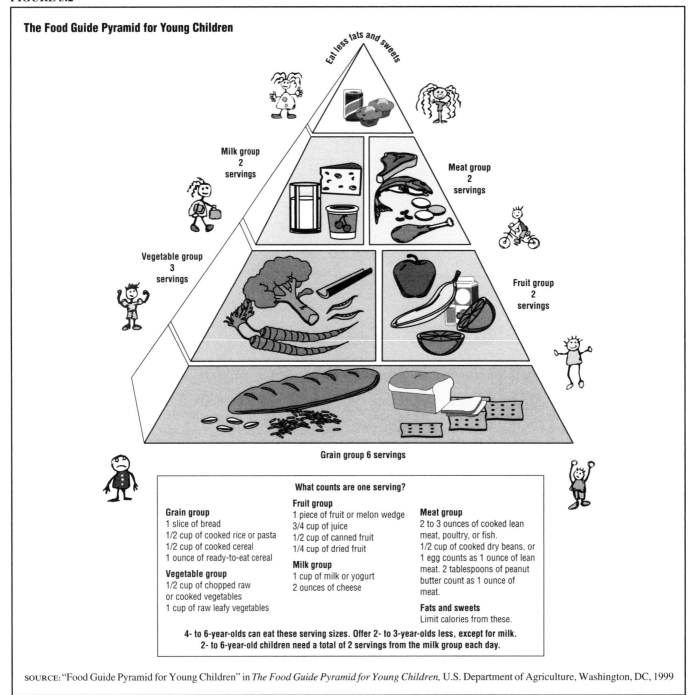

**The Food Guide Pyramid for Young Children**

Eat less fats and sweets

Milk group
2
servings

Meat group
2
servings

Vegetable group
3
servings

Fruit group
2
servings

Grain group 6 servings

**What counts are one serving?**

**Grain group**
1 slice of bread
1/2 cup of cooked rice or pasta
1/2 cup of cooked cereal
1 ounce of ready-to-eat cereal

**Vegetable group**
1/2 cup of chopped raw
or cooked vegetables
1 cup of raw leafy vegetables

**Fruit group**
1 piece of fruit or melon wedge
3/4 cup of juice
1/2 cup of canned fruit
1/4 cup of dried fruit

**Milk group**
1 cup of milk or yogurt
2 ounces of cheese

**Meat group**
2 to 3 ounces of cooked lean
meat, poultry, or fish.
1/2 cup of cooked dry beans, or
1 egg counts as 1 ounce of lean
meat. 2 tablespoons of peanut
butter count as 1 ounce of
meat.

**Fats and sweets**
Limit calories from these.

**4- to 6-year-olds can eat these serving sizes. Offer 2- to 3-year-olds less, except for milk.**
**2- to 6-year-old children need a total of 2 servings from the milk group each day.**

SOURCE: "Food Guide Pyramid for Young Children" in *The Food Guide Pyramid for Young Children,* U.S. Department of Agriculture, Washington, DC, 1999

to drink fruit juices than to eat whole fruits. They are less likely to eat lettuce and more likely to eat green beans. Young children are also more likely to consume ready-to-eat cereals.

The child pyramid has been simplified by shortening the name of food groups. Single numbers, instead of ranges, are used for servings. In addition the graphic illustrates food items in single servings, when possible. The table at the bottom of the pyramid shows what constitutes a single serving, picturing the types of food most often eaten by children. Moreover, to encourage children to be physically active, the pyramid features children at play.

Since some fats are needed for early growth and development, the bulletin accompanying the Food Guide Pyramid for Young Children does not stress fat restrictions. Rather, it advises gradually changing from whole milk to lower-fat dairy products, such as 2 percent or 1 percent or fat-free milk, by age five. It also suggests eating lower-fat and lean meats instead of higher-fat varieties. The *Dietary Guidelines for Americans* suggests that, by age five, fat in preschoolers' diets gradually be reduced from the children's earlier levels (34 percent of total calories) to the level recommended for most people (no more than 30 percent of total calories).

**TABLE 3.4**

## Trends and changes in girls' (6 to 11 years) percentages using items from selected food groups, 1977–98

| Food group | 1977–78 | 1989–91 | 1994–96, 1998 | Change[1] | Trend[2] |
|---|---|---|---|---|---|
| | | Percentage using | | | |
| **Grain products** | 99 | 100[3,4] | 99[4] | | |
| Yeast breads and rolls | 79 | 73 | 71 | -8 | |
| Ready-to-eat cereals | 51 | 48 | 46 | | |
| Cakes, cookies, pastries, pies | 51 | 45 | 55 | | |
| Crackers, popcorn, pretzels, corn chips | 18 | 22 | 37 | +19 | |
| Mixtures mainly grain | 29 | 40 | 46 | +17 | |
| **Vegetables** | 87 | 81 | 82 | | |
| White potatoes | 54 | 51 | 51 | | |
| Fried white potatoes | 30 | 37 | 39 | +9 | |
| Dark-green vegetables | 7 | 7 | 5 | | |
| Deep-yellow vegetables | 9 | 10 | 11 | | |
| Tomatoes | 21 | 27 | 33 | +12 | |
| Green beans | 14 | 8 | 8 | -6 | |
| Corn, green peas, lima beans | 24 | 17 | 15 | -9 | |
| **Fruits** | 62 | 67 | 62 | | |
| Citrus juices | 31 | 24 | 22 | -9 | |
| Apples | 18 | 21 | 16 | | |
| Melons and berries | 4 | 3 | 7 | | |
| Noncitrus juices and nectars | 6 | 16 | 15 | +9 | |
| **Milk and milk products** | 95 | 93 | 90 | -5 | |
| Fluid milk | 90 | 82 | 76 | -14 | * |
| Whole milk | 58 | 44 | 33 | -25 | ** |
| Lowfat milk | 17 | 39 | 38 | +21 | |
| Skim milk | 4 | 5 | 8 | +5 | |
| Milk desserts | 24 | 21 | 22 | | |
| Cheese | 17 | 28 | 32 | +14 | |
| **Meat, poultry, and fish** | 94 | 90 | 86 | -7 | |
| Beef | 35 | 22 | 20 | -15 | |
| Pork | 20 | 15 | 10 | -10 | * |
| Frankfurters, sausages, luncheon meats | 32 | 34 | 33 | | |
| Chicken | 16 | 18 | 20 | | |
| Fish and shellfish | 8 | 7 | 6 | | |
| Mixtures mainly meat, poultry, fish | 31 | 36 | 33 | | |
| **Eggs** | 22 | 21 | 13 | -8 | |
| **Legumes** | 13 | 15 | 11 | | |
| **Fats and oils** | 54 | 56 | 49 | | |
| **Sugars and sweets** | 56 | 55 | 60 | | |
| Candy | 11 | 16 | 29 | +18 | * |
| **Beverages** | 60 | 60 | 73 | +12 | |
| Tea | 16 | 11 | 11 | | |
| Fruit drinks and ades | 27 | 25 | 36 | +9 | |
| Carbonated soft drinks | 30 | 37 | 45 | +14 | * |

[1] Change = percentages in 1977–78 and 1994–96, 1998 are significantly different at p <0.001.
[2] Trend = percentage rose or fell progressively from 1977–78 through 1989–91 to 1994–96, 1998.
[3] Estimate is based on small sample size or coefficient of variation ≥ 30 percent.
[4] Value is between 99.5 and 100.
* = trend significant at p < 0.05.
** = trend significant at p < 0.01.

SOURCE: Cecilia Wilkinson Enns et al., "Table 3. Trends and changes in girls' (6 to 11 years) percentages using items from selected food groups," in "Trends in Food and Nutrient Intakes by Children in the United States," *Family Economics and Nutrition Review,* vol. 14, no. 2, 2002

---

**TABLE 3.5**

## Trends and changes in boys' (6 to 11 years) percentages using items from selected food groups, 1977–98

| Food group | 1977–78 | 1989–91 | 1994–96, 1998 | Change[1] | Trend[2] |
|---|---|---|---|---|---|
| | | Percentage using | | | |
| **Grain products** | 100[3,4] | 100[3,4] | 99[3] | | |
| Yeast breads and rolls | 81 | 68 | 69 | -12 | |
| Ready-to-eat cereals | 52 | 51 | 52 | | |
| Cakes, cookies, pastries, pies | 52 | 39 | 52 | | |
| Crackers, popcorn, pretzels, corn chips | 16 | 22 | 34 | +18 | |
| Mixtures mainly grain | 26 | 46 | 45 | +19 | |
| **Vegetables** | 85 | 80 | 79 | | |
| White potatoes | 56 | 46 | 49 | | |
| Fried white potatoes | 31 | 31 | 38 | | |
| Dark-green vegetables | 5 | 5 | 6 | | |
| Deep-yellow vegetables | 10 | 8 | 12 | | |
| Tomatoes | 18 | 28 | 39 | +21 | ** |
| Green beans | 13 | 10 | 7 | -6 | |
| Corn, green peas, lima beans | 24 | 16 | 14 | -10 | |
| **Fruits** | 59 | 63 | 57 | | |
| Citrus juices | 28 | 22 | 22 | | |
| Apples | 16 | 19 | 18 | | |
| Melons and berries | 4 | 5 | 7 | | |
| Noncitrus juices and nectars | 7 | 12 | 13 | +6 | |
| **Milk and milk products** | 94 | 90 | 92 | | |
| Fluid milk | 90 | 79 | 79 | -10 | |
| Whole milk | 58 | 40 | 31 | -27 | * |
| Lowfat milk | 17 | 41 | 43 | +26 | |
| Skim milk | 3 | 5 | 9 | +6 | |
| Milk desserts | 22 | 18 | 25 | | |
| Cheese | 15 | 25 | 32 | +17 | ** |
| **Meat, poultry, and fish** | 95 | 88 | 88 | -7 | |
| Beef | 33 | 18 | 22 | -11 | |
| Pork | 22 | 15 | 12 | -10 | |
| Frankfurters, sausages, luncheon meats | 33 | 30 | 36 | | |
| Chicken | 17 | 18 | 20 | | |
| Fish and shellfish | 7 | 9 | 5 | | |
| Mixtures mainly meat, poultry, fish | 31 | 35 | 36 | | |
| **Eggs** | 23 | 20 | 16 | -8 | |
| **Legumes** | 14 | 9 | 10 | | |
| **Fats and oils** | 55 | 46 | 47 | | |
| **Sugars and sweets** | 56 | 49 | 60 | | |
| Candy | 9 | 16 | 29 | +20 | ** |
| **Beverages** | 62 | 64 | 74 | +12 | |
| Tea | 15 | 11 | 9 | | |
| Fruit drinks and ades | 27 | 27 | 39 | +12 | |
| Carbonated soft drinks | 31 | 38 | 47 | +16 | |

[1] Change = percentages in 1977–78 and 1994–96, 1998 are significantly different at p <0.001.
[2] Trend = percentage rose or fell progressively from 1977–78 through 1989–91 to 1994–96, 1998.
[3] Estimate is based on small sample size or coefficient of variation ≥ 30 percent.
[4] Value is between 99.5 and 100.
* = trend significant at p < 0.05.
** = trend significant at p < 0.01.

SOURCE: Cecilia Wilkinson Enns et al., "Table 4. Trends and changes in boys' (6 to 11 years) percentages using items from selected food groups," in "Trends in Food and Nutrient Intakes by Children in the United States," *Family Economics and Nutrition Review,* vol. 14, no. 2, 2002

TABLE 3.6

**Consequence of inadequate and excessive intake of selected nutrients**

| Nutrient | Function in body | Consequence of inadequate intake | Consequence of excessive intake |
|---|---|---|---|
| Food energy | Metabolic processes; supports physical activity and growth, repairs bones and tissues, and maintains body temperature. | Underweight, semi-starvation, growth retardation in children. | Overweight and obesity (risk factors for heart disease, stroke, diabetes, hypertension, cancers). |
| Fiber | Promotes normal laxation. | Constipation; may increase risk of heart disease and some cancers. | Possible decrease in mineral absorption. |
| Calcium | Formation and maintenance of bone and teeth; muscle contraction; blood clotting; integrity of cell membranes. | May increase risk of osteoporosis. | Renal calculi; possible soft tissue calcification. |
| Iron | Carrier of oxygen in body; red blood cell formation. | Iron deficiency and iron deficiency anemia; functional impairments in intellectual development and learning, behavior, work performance, and resistance to infection. | Iron overload; may increase risk of stroke and some cancers in men. |
| Total fat, saturated fat, cholesterol | Concentrated sources of energy; carrier for fat-soluble vitamins; structural and functional components of cell membranes; precursors of compounds involved in many aspects of metabolism. | No public health problem; clinical deficiencies of essential fatty acids and fat-soluble nutrients have occurred. | Associated with elevated levels of blood cholesterol and of low-density lipoprotein (LDL) cholesterol, major risk factors for coronary heart disease. |
| Sodium | Regulation of body fluid volume and acid-base balance of blood; transmission of nerve impulses. | — | Edema; associated with high incidence of hypertension (risk factor for stroke and heart disease). |

SOURCE: Biing-Hwan Lin, Elizabeth Frazão, and Joanne Guthrie, "Table 1: Consequence of inadequate and excessive intake of selected nutrients," in *Away-From-Home Foods Increasingly Important to Quality of American Diet,* U.S. Department of Agriculture, Economic Research Service, Food and Drug Administration, Agricultural Information Bulletin #749, 2000

FIGURE 3.3

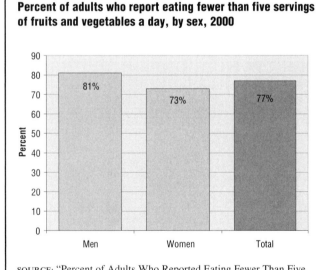

**Percent of adults who report eating fewer than five servings of fruits and vegetables a day, by sex, 2000**

SOURCE: "Percent of Adults Who Reported Eating Fewer Than Five Servings of Fruits and Vegetable a Day, by Sex, 2000," in *Physical Activity and Good Nutrition: Essential Elements to Prevent Chronic Diseases and Obesity 2003,* U.S. Centers for Disease Control and Prevention, National Center for Chronic Disease Prevention and Health Promotion, Atlanta, GA, 2003

An analysis of trends in food and nutrient intakes of American children between 1978 and 1998 demonstrated that nutrition education for children must be more strongly emphasized. In "Trends in Food and Nutrient Intakes by Children in the United States" (*Family Economics and Nutrition Review,* vol. 14, no. 2, 2002), researchers at the USDA Agricultural Service found that for any given pyramid group, less than one-half of children between the ages of 6 and 11 consumed the recommended number of servings. Moreover, children's consumption of added fats and added sugars was much higher than recommended.

Researchers noted increases between 1977 and 1998 in consumption of soft drinks, total grain products, grain mixtures, crackers, candy, fried potatoes, and other snack foods and beverages. They also noted decreases in consumption of whole milk, yeast breads, green beans, corn, green peas, lima beans, beef, pork, and eggs. Table 3.4 shows trends and changes in girls' consumption of foods from selected groups. Table 3.5 shows trends and changes in boys' consumption of foods from selected groups.

Children ages 6–11 drank about four times as much fluid milk as any other beverage in 1977–78, but by 1994–96, and in 1998, as shown by USDA's supplemental study, they drank only about 1.5 times as much milk as soft drinks. In addition, in 1994–96 and 1998, only 24 percent of girls and 23 percent of boys ages 6–11 consumed the number of servings of fruit recommended in the Food Guide Pyramid based on their caloric intake.

**DIET AND ILLNESS**

Poor diet has long been known to be a contributor to poor health. Table 3.6 outlines some consequences of over- and underconsumption of various nutrients. Poor diet also has been linked to several of the leading causes of death in the United States—diseases of the heart (coronary heart disease and stroke) and malignant neoplasms (cancer). Diet also plays a major role in the development of diabetes—the fifth (women) and sixth (men) leading cause of death, according to the Centers for Disease Control and Prevention in 2000—as well as hypertension and overweight. In 1994 coronary heart disease, cancer, stroke, and diabetes cost society an estimated $70.9 billion in diet-related medical costs, lost productivity due to disability, and premature deaths (although factors suggest that this is a low estimate). Studies have shown that improved dietary habits could reduce deaths from coronary heart disease and stroke by at least 20 percent, and cancer and diabetes mortality by at least 30 percent.

The Centers for Disease Control and Prevention (CDC) reported that chronic diseases such as cardiovascular disease (primarily heart disease and stroke), cancer, and diabetes are among the most prevalent, costly, and preventable of all heath problems ("Chronic Disease Overview," National Center for Chronic Disease Prevention and Health Promotion). The CDC cited unhealthy eating habits as one of the factors contributing to the incidence of chronic disease. For example, even though the Food Guide Pyramid recommends a minimum of five servings of fruits and vegetables per day, more than three-fourths (77 percent) of adults eat less than that. (See Figure 3.3.)

In "High Costs of Poor Eating Patterns in the United States" (*America's Eating Habits: Changes and Consequences,* USDA, Washington, D.C., 1999) Elizabeth Frazão notes that improving Americans' dietary habits would decrease morbidity and mortality associated with chronic health conditions. According to Frazão, in the United States, 14 percent of all deaths can be attributed to poor diets and/or sedentary lifestyles.

Black American men are particularly vulnerable to diet-related diseases, according to the National Cancer Institute (NCI) ("HHS and NCI Launch National Campaign to Address Diet-Related Diseases Affecting African-American Men," NCI press release, July 21, 2003). The NCI is trying to motivate black males to eat 9 servings of fruits and vegetables per day. The press release concludes that black men:

> Overall, have the highest cancer incidence and mortality rates, as well as the highest rates for certain cancers of any ethnic or racial group.
>
> Have the highest rates of prostate cancer and high blood pressure in the world.
>
> Are twice as likely as white men to develop diabetes.
>
> Develop diabetes and high blood pressure earlier in life than other men, and are more likely to suffer serious side-effects from these diseases.
>
> Have higher mortality rates from heart disease and obesity than other ethnic groups.

The NCI continues: "[A]lthough black men are the most seriously affected by diet-related chronic diseases, they have the lowest consumption of fruits and vegetables overall, eating an average of only 3.1 servings per day of the 9 recommended for men by federal nutrition policy. Only three percent of black men are aware that they should eat 9 servings of fruits and vegetables per day for better health." The NCI is working with a number of African American groups and other health organizations to get what it calls the "9 A Day" message out to black men.

## DIETARY REFERENCE INTAKES (DRIs)

In the past, Recommended Dietary Allowances (RDAs), prepared by the Food and Nutrition Board of the National Research Council under the National Academy of Sciences (NAS), served as the only standard of nutritional adequacy in the United States. Established in 1941 RDAs are revised about every five years to reflect current scientific knowledge.

Because of the growing amount of scientific knowledge concerning the roles of nutrients, the NAS's Institute of Medicine, in partnership with the Canadian government, has revised nutrient reference intakes. The new revised recommendations, called Dietary Reference Intakes (DRIs), include four reference values:

- Estimated Average Requirement (EAR)—the intake that meets the estimated nutrient need of half the individuals in a specific group. This figure is used as the basis for developing new RDAs for some nutrients.

- Recommended Dietary Allowance (RDA)—the intake of essential nutrients that meets the known nutrient needs of practically all healthy persons in a specific age (life stage) and gender group. Derived from the EAR the RDA can change allowances to permit variation within a particular group.

- Adequate Intake (AI)—the recommended intake of a nutrient where no RDA exists. AIs are established when sufficient scientific evidence is not available to estimate an average requirement. For example, AIs have been set for infants through one year of age, using as the standard the average observed nutrient intake of populations of healthy breast-feeding infants.

- Tolerable Upper Intake Level (TUIL)—the maximum intake unlikely to pose risks of adverse health effects in almost all healthy individuals in a specific group. Because of the popular use of dietary supplements and food fortification, the NAS, for the first time, sets these maximum-level guidelines to prevent overconsumption of a nutrient.

In August 1997 the Institute of Medicine released the first of the new DRIs for calcium, phosphorus, magnesium, vitamin D, fluoride, folates, B vitamins, and several other

TABLE 3.7

## Dietary reference intakes: Recommended levels for individual intake[a]

| Life-Stage Group | Calcium mg/day | Phosphorus mg/day | Magnesium mg/day | Vitamin D μg [b][c] | Flouride mg/day | Thiamine mg/day | Riboflavin mg/day | Niacin[d] mg/day | Vitamin B-6 mg/day | Folate[e] μg/day | Vitamin B-12 μg/day | Pantothenic Acid mg/day | Biotin μg/day | Choline[f] mg/day |
|---|---|---|---|---|---|---|---|---|---|---|---|---|---|---|
| **Infants** | | | | | | | | | | | | | | |
| 0–6 mo. | 210* | 100* | 30* | 5* | 0.01* | 0.2* | 0.3* | 2* | 0.1* | 65* | 0.4* | 1.7* | 5* | 125* |
| 7–12 mo. | 270* | 275* | 75* | 5* | 0.5* | 0.3* | 0.4* | 4* | 0.3* | 80* | 0.5* | 1.8* | 6* | 150* |
| **Children** | | | | | | | | | | | | | | |
| 1–3 y | 500* | 460 | 80 | 5* | 0.7* | 0.5 | 0.5 | 6 | 0.5 | 150 | 0.9 | 2* | 8* | 200* |
| 4–8 y | 800* | 500 | 130 | 5* | 1* | 0.6 | 0.6 | 8 | 0.6 | 200 | 1.2 | 3* | 12* | 250* |
| **Males** | | | | | | | | | | | | | | |
| 9–13 y | 1,300* | 1,250 | 240 | 5* | 2* | 0.9 | 0.9 | 12 | 1 | 300 | 1.8 | 4* | 20* | 375* |
| 14–18 y | 1,300* | 1,250 | 410 | 5* | 3* | 1.2 | 1.3 | 16 | 1.3 | 400 | 2.4 | 5* | 25* | 550* |
| 19–30 y | 1,000* | 700 | 400 | 5* | 4* | 1.2 | 1.3 | 16 | 1.3 | 400 | 2.4 | 5* | 30* | 550* |
| 31–50 y | 1,000* | 700 | 420 | 5* | 4* | 1.2 | 1.3 | 16 | 1.3 | 400 | 2.4 | 5* | 30* | 550* |
| 51–70 y | 1,200* | 700 | 420 | 10* | 4* | 1.2 | 1.3 | 16 | 1.7 | 400 | 2.4 [g] | 5* | 30* | 550* |
| >70 y | 1,200* | 700 | 420 | 15* | 4* | 1.2 | 1.3 | 16 | 1.7 | 400 | 2.4 [g] | 5* | 30* | 550* |
| **Females** | | | | | | | | | | | | | | |
| 9–13 y | 1,300* | 1,250 | 240 | 5* | 2* | 0.9 | 0.9 | 12 | 1 | 300 | 1.8 | 4* | 20* | 375* |
| 14–18 y | 1,300* | 1,250 | 360 | 5* | 3* | 1 | 1 | 14 | 1.2 | 400 [h] | 2.4 | 5* | 25* | 400* |
| 19–30 y | 1,000* | 700 | 310 | 5* | 3* | 1.1 | 1.1 | 14 | 1.3 | 400 [h] | 2.4 | 5* | 30* | 425* |
| 31–50 y | 1,000* | 700 | 320 | 5* | 3* | 1.1 | 1.1 | 14 | 1.3 | 400 [h] | 2.4 | 5* | 30* | 425* |
| 51–70 y | 1,200* | 700 | 320 | 10* | 3* | 1.1 | 1.1 | 14 | 1.5 | 400 | 2.4 [g] | 5* | 30* | 425* |
| >70 y | 1,200* | 700 | 320 | 15* | 3* | 1.1 | 1.1 | 14 | 1.5 | 400 | 2.4 [g] | 5* | 30* | 425* |
| **Pregnancy** | | | | | | | | | | | | | | |
| <18 y | 1,300* | 1,250 | 400 | 5* | 3* | 1.4 | 1.4 | 18 | 1.9 | 600 [i] | 2.6 | 6* | 30* | 450* |
| 19–30 y | 1,000* | 700 | 350 | 5* | 3* | 1.4 | 1.4 | 18 | 1.9 | 600 [i] | 2.6 | 6* | 30* | 450* |
| 31–50 y | 1,000* | 700 | 360 | 5* | 3* | 1.4 | 1.4 | 18 | 1.9 | 600 [i] | 2.6 | 6* | 30* | 450* |
| **Lactation** | | | | | | | | | | | | | | |
| <18 y | 1,300* | 1,250 | 360 | 5* | 3* | 1.5 | 1.6 | 17 | 2 | 500 | 2.8 | 7* | 35* | 550* |
| 19–30 y | 1,000* | 700 | 310 | 5* | 3* | 1.5 | 1.6 | 17 | 2 | 500 | 2.8 | 7* | 35* | 550* |
| 31–50 y | 1,000* | 700 | 320 | 5* | 3* | 1.5 | 1.6 | 17 | 2 | 500 | 2.8 | 7* | 35* | 550* |

(a) Recommended Dietary Allowances (RDAs) are presented in bold type and Adequate Intakes (AIs) in ordinary type followed by an asterisk (*). RDAs and AIs may both be used as goals for individual intake. RDAs are set to meet the needs of almost all (97% to 98%) individuals in a group. For healthy breast-fed infants, the AI is the mean intake. The AI for other life-stage and gender groups is believed to cover needs of all individuals in the group, but lack of data or uncertainty in the data prevent being able to specify with confidence the percentage of persons covered by this intake. Source: The Natural Academy of Sciences, Copyright 1998.

(b) As cholecalciferol. 1 μg cholecalciferol = 40 IU vitamin D.

(c) In the absence of adequate exposure to sunlight.

(d) As niacin equivalents (NE). 1 mg niacin = 60 mg tryptothan; 0 to 6 mo = preformed niacin (not NE).

(e) As dietary folate equivalent (DFE). 1 DFE = 1 μg food folate = 0.6 μg folic acid (from fortified food or supplement) consumed with food = 0.5 μg synthetic (supplemental) folic acid taken on an empty stomach.

(f) Although AIs have been set for choline, there are few data to assess whether a dietary supply of choline is needed at all stages of the life cycle, and it may be that the choline requirement can be met by endogenous synthesis at some of these stages.

(g) Because 10% to 30% of older people may malabsorb food-bound vitamin B-12, it is advisable for those older than 50 years to meet their RDA mainly by consuming foods fortified with vitamin B-12 or a supplement containing vitamin B-12.

(h) In view of evidence linking folate intake with neural tube defects in the fetus, it is recommended that all women capable of becoming pregnant consume 400 μg synthetic folic acid from fortified foods and/or supplements in addition to intake of food folate from a varied diet.

(i) It is assumed that women will continue consuming 400 μg folic acid until their pregnancy is confirmed and they enter prenatal care, which ordinarily occurs after the end of the periconceptional period- the critical time for formation of the neural tube.

SOURCE: "Dietary Reference Intakes (RDIs)," Food and Nutrition Board, National Academy of Sciences, Washington, DC, 1998

TABLE 3.8

**Recommended daily intake of selected dietary components**

| Gender and age | Dietary Recommendations | | | | | | | |
|---|---|---|---|---|---|---|---|---|
| | Calories [1] | Fat [2] | Saturated fat [2] | Cholesterol [3] | Sodium [4] | Fiber [5] | Calcium [1] | Iron [1] |
| | *Calories* | *Percent* | *Percent* | *Mg* | *Mg* | *Grams* | *Mg* | *Mg* |
| **Children** | | | | | | | | |
| 2–3 | 1,300 | ≤ 30 | < 10 | 300 | 2,400 | Age+5/day | 800 | 10 |
| 4–6 | 1,800 | ≤ 30 | < 10 | 300 | 2,400 | Age+5/day | 800 | 10 |
| 7–10 | 2,000 | ≤ 30 | < 10 | 300 | 2,400 | Age+5/day | 800 | 10 |
| **Males** | | | | | | | | |
| 11–14 | 2,500 | ≤ 30 | < 10 | 300 | 2,400 | Age+5/day | 1,200 | 12 |
| 15–18 | 3,000 | ≤ 30 | < 10 | 300 | 2,400 | Age+5/day | 1,200 | 12 |
| 19–20 | 2,900 | ≤ 30 | < 10 | 300 | 2,400 | Age+5/day | 1,200 | 10 |
| 21–24 | 2,900 | ≤ 30 | < 10 | 300 | 2,400 | 11.5/1,000 calories | 1,200 | 10 |
| 25–50 | 2,900 | ≤ 30 | < 10 | 300 | 2,400 | 11.5/1,000 calories | 800 | 10 |
| 51+ | 2,300 | ≤ 30 | < 10 | 300 | 2,400 | 11.5/1,000 calories | 800 | 10 |
| **Females** | | | | | | | | |
| 11–14 | 2,200 | ≤ 30 | < 10 | 300 | 2,400 | Age+5/day | 1,200 | 15 |
| 15–18 | 2,000 | ≤ 30 | < 10 | 300 | 2,400 | Age+5/day | 1,200 | 15 |
| 19–20 | 2,000 | ≤ 30 | < 10 | 300 | 2,400 | Age+5/day | 1,200 | 15 |
| 21–24 | 2,000 | ≤ 30 | < 10 | 300 | 2,400 | 11.5/1,000 calories | 1,200 | 15 |
| 25–50 | 2,000 | ≤ 30 | < 10 | 300 | 2,400 | 11.5/1,000 calories | 800 | 15 |
| 51+ | 1,900 | ≤ 30 | < 10 | 300 | 2,400 | 11.5/1,000 calories | 800 | 10 |

[1] National Research Council's *Recommended Dietary Allowances.*
[2] U.S. Department of Health and Human Services and U.S. Department of Agriculture's *1995 Nutrition and Your Health: Dietary Guidelines for Americans.*
[3] U.S. Food and Drug Administration's (FDA) Daily Values (Kurtzweil).
[4] National Research Council's *Diet and Health* (National Academy Press, 1989).
[5] American Health Foundation for "age plus 5" per day (Williams) and FDA's Daily Value for 11.5 grams per 1,000 calories (Kurtzweil).

SOURCE: Biing-Hwan Lin, Elizabeth Frazão, and Joanne Guthrie, "Table 4: Recommended daily intake of selected dietary components," in *Away-From-Home Foods Increasingly Important to Quality of American Diet,* U.S. Department of Agriculture, Economic Research Service, Food and Drug Administration, Agricultural Information Bulletin #749, 2000

vitamins. In subsequent years, it issued DRIs for other nutrients and elements, and for macronutrients such as protein, fat, and carbohydrate. Table 3.7 illustrates DRIs for select nutrients, and Table 3.8 presents Recommended Daily Intakes (used by the Food and Drug Administration) for some dietary components.

## VITAMINS

Vitamins are organic (carbon-containing) substances derived from animals or plants that are necessary in small amounts for growth and maintenance of life. Together with minerals, they are called micronutrients, because, compared with macronutrients (carbohydrate, protein, fat, and water), they are needed in relatively small amounts.

The effects of vitamins have been understood on some level for thousands of years. In about 1500 A.D. some people realized that eating certain foods could affect the development of certain diseases. From this, theories developed as to which foods cured deficiency diseases such as scurvy, rickets, and night blindness. Eventually vitamins were isolated and their biochemical functions and required amounts determined. Traditionally scientists have recognized 13 vitamins as needed by the human body. In April 1998 the National Academy of Sciences added the vitamin choline to the new DRIs.

Vitamins are either fat-soluble or water-soluble. Fat-soluble vitamins (A, D, E, and K), as their name suggests, dissolve in fat. They can be stored in the body for long periods and not excreted, leading to toxicity if a person takes large doses of supplements. Because they do not dissolve in water, fat-soluble vitamins are generally retained in foods during preparation. Vitamin C and the eight B-complex vitamins—thiamin, riboflavin, niacin, pyridoxine, cobalamin, pantothenic acid, biotin, and folate (folic acid)—are water-soluble. They are more likely to be destroyed during food preparation. Since the body excretes excess quantities of these vitamins, dangerous buildups in the body are unlikely.

Today researchers have moved beyond the link between vitamins and deficiency diseases to a greater recognition of the role of vitamins in disease prevention. American scientists no longer emphasize getting enough vitamins to prevent deficiency diseases, such as scurvy or rickets. Instead, studies focus on the role of vitamins in preventing cancer, heart disease, cataracts, and other chronic diseases.

## VITAMINS AS ANTIOXIDANTS

In order to sustain life the body uses oxygen to convert food into energy, in a process called metabolism. As the body cells consume oxygen they produce unstable oxygen molecules, known as free radicals. These unstable

**TABLE 3.9**

**Fruits and vegetables recommended by the National Cancer Institute**

In selecting your daily intake of fruits and vegetables, the National Cancer Institute recommends choosing:
• At least one serving of a vitamin A-rich fruit or vegetable a day.
• At least one serving of a vitamin C-rich fruit or vegetable a day.
• At least one serving of a high-fiber fruit or vegetable a day.
• Several serving of cruciferous vegetables a week. Studies suggest that these vegetables may offer additional protection against certain cancers, although further research is needed.

| High in vitamin A* | High in vitamin C* | High in fiber or good source of fiber* | Cruciferous vegetables |
|---|---|---|---|
| apricots | apricots | apple | bok choy |
| cantaloupe | broccoli | banana | broccoli |
| carrots | brussels sprouts | blackberries | brussels sprouts |
| kale, collards | cabbage | blueberries | cabbage |
| leaf lettuce | cantaloupe | brussel sprouts | cauliflower |
| mango | cauliflower | carrots | |
| mustard greens | chili peppers | cherries | |
| pumpkin | collards | cooked beans and peas | |
| romaine lettuce | grapefruit | (kidney, navy, lima, | |
| spinach | honeydew melon | and pinto beans, lentils | |
| sweet potato | kiwi fruit | black-eyed peas) | |
| winter squash | mango | dates | |
| (acorn, hubbard) | mustard greens | figs | |
| | orange | grapefruit | |
| | orange juice | kiwi fruit | |
| | pineapple | orange | |
| | plum | pear | |
| | potato with skin | prunes | |
| | spinach | raspberries | |
| | strawberries | spinach | |
| | bell peppers | strawberries | |
| | tangerine | sweet potato | |
| | tomatoes | | |
| | watermelon | | |

*Based on FDA's food labeling regulations.

SOURCE: Paula Kurtzweil, "Fruits and Vegetables: Eating Your Way to Five a Day," in *FDA Consumer,* U.S. Food and Drug Administration, Washington, DC, March 1997, revised August 1998

molecules, which have one or more unpaired electrons, are drawn toward molecules in cells in order to combine with their electrons. In this ongoing process enough molecules may be damaged to cause cell death. Scientists believe that free radicals may cause the development of cancer through this destructive behavior and may even be responsible for the development of heart disease.

Environmental factors, including ultraviolet light, radiation, cigarette smoke, alcohol, and certain pollutants, such as ozone, also produce free radicals in the body. The body makes its own antioxidants that combine with free radicals, neutralizing their harmful actions. Scientists, however, believe that there are more free radicals than the body can handle. A group of nutrients found in food— mainly vitamins C and E and carotenoids—have been found to act as antioxidants, helping the body's defense against free radicals.

## Vitamin C

A special report, "Can Antioxidants Save Your Life?" (*University of California at Berkeley Wellness Letter,* vol. 14, issue 10, July 1998), describes how vitamins C and E and carotenoids function as antioxidants. Vitamin C (also known as ascorbic acid) not only fights free radicals, but also interferes with the formation of nitrosamines (cancer-causing compounds) from nitrites found in such foods as hot dogs, ham, and sausages. Low vitamin C in the diet has been linked to an increased risk of stomach, esophagus, lung, breast, cervical, colon, and bladder cancer.

Vitamin C's antioxidant action can also help prevent cataracts. Scientists have found that eye fluids contain large amounts of vitamin C and other antioxidants, which may protect the eye from free radicals produced by sunlight. Moreover, vitamin C plays an important role in preventing heart disease and birth defects.

**VITAMIN C'S OTHER FUNCTIONS.** Vitamin C performs other important functions, as well. Consumed in adequate amounts, it helps prevent scurvy, the disease most associated with vitamin C deficiency. (Scurvy is rare in the United States and other developed countries, where fresh fruits and vegetables, the highest sources of vitamin C, are consumed in sufficient amounts.) Vitamin C also helps in the formation of collagen (connective tissue) and bones, the absorption of iron and excretion of lead, and the production of certain antibodies.

Vitamin C stimulates the production of epinephrine (formerly called adrenalin) and norepinephrine (noradrenalin), hormones released in times of danger to strengthen and prepare a person for "fight or flight." Vitamin C also helps convert folic acid to its active form and "regenerates" vitamin E oxidized during cell metabolism. Scientists describe "regeneration" as the process by which an antioxidant revives another antioxidant that has been oxidized (combined with a free radical). Nutritionists advise consumers to get vitamin C from fruits and vegetables. (See Table 3.9.)

## Vitamin E

Scientists at the University of California at Berkeley discovered vitamin E in 1922. During the 1990s, a growing body of research worldwide suggested that vitamin E may prevent heart disease; reduce the risk of cancer, including prostate cancer; delay aging; and prevent or postpone the development of cataracts. Vitamin E may also help reduce the symptoms of Parkinson's disease, a degenerative disorder of the brain's nerve centers.

University of California at Berkeley researchers believe that vitamin E may reduce the risk of heart disease because it prevents the oxidation of low-density lipoprotein (LDL), often referred to as "bad" cholesterol. When LDL cholesterol is attacked, or oxidized, by free radicals, it is predisposed to accelerate the buildup of plaque, a condition called atherosclerosis, which may result in a heart

TABLE 3.10

## Which fruits and vegetables provide the most nutrients?

The lists below show which fruits and vegetables are
the best sources of vitamin A (carotenoids), vitamin
C, folate, and potassium. Eat at least 2 servings of
fruits and at least 3 servings of vegetables each day:

**Sources of vitamin A (carotenoids)**
- Orange vegetables like carrots, sweet potatoes, pumpkin
- Dark-green leafy vegetables such as spinach, collards, turnip greens
- Orange fruits like mango, cantaloupe, apricots
- Tomatoes

**Sources of vitamin C**
- Citrus fruits and juices, kiwi fruit, strawberries, cantaloupe
- Broccoli, peppers, tomatoes, cabbage, potatoes
- Leafy greens such as romaine lettuce, turnip greens, spinach

**Sources of folate**
- Cooked dry beans and peas, peanuts
- Oranges, orange juice
- Dark-green leafy vegetables like spinach and mustard greens, romaine lettuce
- Green peas

**Sources of potassium**
- Baked white or sweet potato, cooked greens (like spinach), winter (orange) squash
- Bananas, plantains, dried fruits such as apricots and prunes, orange juice
- Cooked dry beans (such as baked beans) and lentils

Note: Read nutrition facts labels for product-specific information, especially for processed fruits and vegetables.

SOURCE: "Which Fruits and Vegetables Provide the Most Nutrients?" in
*Dietary Guidelines for Americans, 2000,* U.S. Department of Agriculture,
Washington, DC, 2000

attack or a stroke. Vitamin E traps free radicals quickly because it is carried in the bloodstream by LDL.

In a 2001 report, "Should You Take Vitamin C and E Supplements?" (*University of California at Berkeley Wellness Letter,* June 2001), editors revised their recommendations for intake of vitamin C and E supplements. Citing a finding by the Food and Nutrition Board of the National Academy of Sciences that taking antioxidant supplements served no purpose, the editorial board provided amended vitamin intake recommendations. For intake of vitamin E the board recommended decreasing the daily dosage to 200–400 IU (international units) per day from up to 800 IU per day. While still recommending daily intake of 250–500 milligrams of vitamin C, the board suggested that this amount be obtained from food.

## Carotenoids

Carotenoids are the pigments that give plants their red, orange, and yellow colors. Once valued only as provitamins, or precursors of vitamin A (they can be converted by the liver to vitamin A, as needed), these compounds have been found to possess nutritional values of their own. Scientists have discovered more than 600 carotenoids; the body can convert about 50 into active vitamin A. Beta-carotene is the best known of the group, but other important carotenoids include alpha-carotene, gamma-carotene, beta-cryptoxanthin, lycopene, lutein, and zeaxanthin. Table 3.10 shows fruits and vegetables that are good sources of different carotenoids.

There is growing evidence that carotenoids may play an important role against such diseases as cancer and heart disease. Lycopene, found in tomatoes and tomato products, such as pizza sauce and ketchup, has been linked to the prevention of prostate cancer. Like vitamin E, it prevents the oxidation of LDL cholesterol. Alpha-carotene, found abundantly in carrots, is associated with reduced risk of lung cancer. Cryptoxanthin, found in many orange-colored fruits, may decrease the risk of cervical cancer.

**CONTROVERSIES OVER BETA-CAROTENE.** Beta-carotene, the most popular of carotenoids, is said to boost the immune system, partly because of its antioxidant activity. It has also been linked to decreased risk of lung and oral cancers. However, two large clinical trials sponsored by the National Cancer Institute (NCI) questioned the potential health benefits of beta-carotene.

The first study involved a collaboration between the NCI and the National Public Health Institute of Finland (the results of the study were released in 1994). The purpose of the *Alpha-Tocopherol, Beta-Carotene Cancer Prevention Trial* (ATBC Trial) was to determine if certain supplements would prevent lung cancer and other cancers in a group of over 29,000 male smokers in Finland. After 5–8 years, 18 percent more lung cancers were diagnosed, and 8 percent more overall deaths occurred in the study participants taking beta-carotene than in those taking a placebo.

Once the study was completed, all participants stopped taking beta-carotene. The NCI, however, continued to follow the group for an additional eight years by monitoring Finnish health registries and closely following some individuals. The NCI released results of this second trial in July 2003 (available online at http://www.cancer.gov/ newscenter/pressreleases/ATBCfollowup). The follow-up study showed that individuals who had taken beta-carotene continued to have a 7 percent higher overall death rate than did those on the placebo for a period of 6 years after the first trial ended. The higher mortality rate, however, was from cardiovascular diseases rather than lung cancer. After 6 years, the death rate of those taking beta-carotene came to match that of those who had taken a placebo. Results of both trials, however, supported the recommendation that smokers should avoid beta-carotene supplements.

The second study, the *Beta Carotene and Retinol Efficacy Trial* (CARET), was conducted to find out if a combination of beta-carotene and vitamin A would prevent lung and other cancers in men and women who were smokers or former smokers, as well as in men exposed to asbestos. In 1996, after an average of four years of taking the supplements, the more than 18,000 participants were told to stop taking them. About 28 percent more lung cancers were diagnosed, and 17 percent more deaths occurred in CARET participants taking beta-carotene and vitamin A than in

## TABLE 3.11

**Food sources of folate**

| Food | Micrograms dietary folate equivalents | % DV* |
|---|---|---|
| Ready to eat cereal, fortified with 100% of the DV, 3/4 cup | 400 | 100 |
| Beef liver, cooked, braised, 3 oz | 185 | 45 |
| Cowpeas (blackeyes), immature, cooked, boiled, 1/2 cup | 105 | 25 |
| Breakfast cereals, fortified with 25% of the DV, 3/4 cup | 100 | 25 |
| Spinach, frozen, cooked, boiled,1/2 cup | 100 | 25 |
| Great Northern beans, boiled, 1/2 cup | 90 | 20 |
| Asparagus, boiled, 4 spears | 85 | 20 |
| Wheat germ, toasted, 1/4 cup | 80 | 20 |
| Orange juice, chilled, includes concentrate, 3/4 cup | 70 | 20 |
| Turnip greens, frozen, cooked, boiled, 1/2 cup | 65 | 15 |
| Vegetarian baked beans, canned, 1 cup | 60 | 15 |
| Spinach, raw, 1 cup | 60 | 15 |
| Green peas, boiled, 1/2 cup | 50 | 15 |
| Broccoli, chopped, frozen, cooked, 1/2 cup | 50 | 15 |
| Egg noodles, cooked, enriched, 1/2 cup | 15 | 50 |
| Rice, white, long-grain, parboiled, cooked, enriched, 1/2 cup | 45 | 10 |
| Avocado, raw, all varieties, sliced 1/2 c sliced | 45 | 10 |
| Peanuts, all types, dry roasted, 1 oz | 40 | 10 |
| Lettuce, romaine, shredded, 1/2 cup | 40 | 10 |
| Tomato juice, canned, 6 oz | 35 | 10 |
| Orange, all commercial varieties, fresh, 1 small | 30 | 8 |
| Bread, white, enriched, 1 slice | 25 | 6 |
| Egg, whole, raw, fresh, 1 large | 25 | 6 |
| Cantaloupe, raw, 1/4 medium | 25 | 6 |
| Papaya, raw, 1/2 c cubes | 25 | 6 |
| Banana, raw, 1 medium | 20 | 6 |
| Broccoli, raw, 1 spear (about 5 inches long) | 20 | 6 |
| Lettuce, iceberg, shredded,1/2 cup | 15 | 4 |
| Bread, whole wheat, 1 slice | 15 | 4 |

*DV = Daily Value. DVs are reference numbers based on the Recommended Dietary Allowance (RDA). They were developed to help consumers determine if a food contains a lot or a little of a specific nutrient. The DV for folic acid is 400 micrograms (mcg). The percent DV (%DV) listed on the nutrition facts panel of food labels tells adults what percentage of the DV is provided by one serving. Percent DVs are based on a 2,000 calorie diet. Your Daily Values may be higher or lower depending on your calorie needs. Foods that provide lower percentages of the DV also contribute to a healthful diet.

SOURCE: "Table of Selected Food Sources of Folate" in *Facts About Dietary Supplements,* Clinical Nutrition Services, Office of Dietary Supplements, National Institutes of Health, Washington, DC, 2000

those taking placebos. Both studies found no significant evidence of any benefit in taking beta-carotene.

The *Physicians' Health Study* (National Institutes of Health, Bethesda, MD, 1999), a 12-year study of 22,000 U.S. male physicians, found no significant evidence of either beneficial or harmful effects of beta-carotene on cancer or heart disease.

The NCI reported one consistent finding from both the ATBC Trial and CARET: participants with the highest levels of *blood-borne* beta-carotene, obtained from consumption of foods containing beta-carotene, developed fewer

lung cancers. The NCI, however, does not recommend that Americans take dietary supplements of beta-carotene. Rather, the institute recommends that those who wish to reduce their risk of cancer adopt a low-fat diet containing plenty of fruits, vegetables, and grains. It continues to stress its "Five-A-Day" program of eating five servings of fruits and vegetables daily. (See Table 3.9.)

## FOLATE (FOLIC ACID)

Folate, or folacin, is a B vitamin added to many vitamin and mineral supplements in the form of folic acid. In its April 1998 report on Dietary Reference Intakes (DRIs) the Institute of Medicine recommended that all adult men and women (14 and over) include 400 micrograms of folate in their diets daily. (See Table 3.7.) The institute claimed that, although folate can be found in many food items, such as enriched bread, pasta, flour, breakfast cereal, crackers, and rice, many Americans still do not take enough folic acid. Consequently, starting in January 1998, the Food and Drug Administration required manufacturers of grain products to fortify their foods with folic acid.

Every year in the United States about 4,000 pregnancies are affected by neural tube defects. About 2,500 of these pregnancies involve infants born with the two most common neural tube defects—anencephaly (absence of a major part of the brain, skull, and scalp) or spina bifida (incomplete closure of the spinal column). These conditions result from the disruption of the fetus's central nervous system in the first month of pregnancy, when many women may not realize that they are pregnant.

To reduce the risk of neural tube defects, the Institute of Medicine recommends that women capable of becoming pregnant should consume 400 micrograms of folic acid daily from fortified foods and/or supplements in addition to folate from a varied diet. For pregnant women the institute recommends 600 micrograms. (See Table 3.7.) However, the February 1999 *University of California at Berkeley Wellness Letter* (vol. 15, issue 5) reported that a number of studies show that folic acid in vitamin supplements, and folic acid used to fortify foods, are better absorbed by the body than the folate naturally occurring in food. Table 3.11 shows some good sources of folate.

### Knowledge and Use of Folic Acid

The Centers for Disease Control and Prevention, in "Knowledge and Use of Folic Acid by Women of Childbearing Age—United States, 1995 and 1998" (*Morbidity and Mortality Weekly Report,* vol. 48, no. 16, April 30, 1999), reported that a 1998 nationwide survey by the March of Dimes Birth Defects Foundation found that over two-thirds (68 percent) of women ages 18–45 (prime childbearing years) had heard of or read about folic acid, up from 52 percent in 1995. (See Table 3.12.)

**TABLE 3.12**

**Knowledge and use of folic acid among women of childbearing age, 1995 and 1998\***

| Characteristic | 1995 | 1998 |
|---|---|---|
| **Knowledge** | | |
| Heard of folic acid | 52% | 68% |
| Knew folic acid can help prevent birth defects | 5% | 13% |
| Knew folic acid should be taken before pregnancy | 2% | 7% |
| **Behavior** | | |
| Take folic acid daily (nonpregnant women) | 25% | 29% |
| Take folic acid daily (all women) | 28% | 32% |
| **Source of knowledge** | | |
| Magazine/newspaper | 35% | 31% |
| Radio/television | 10% | 23% |
| Health-care provider | 13% | 19% |

\*The margin of error for estimates based on the total sample size was ± 3%

SOURCE: "Knowledge, behavior, and source of knowledge regarding folic acid among childbearing-aged women–United States, 1995 and 1998" in "Knowledge and Use of Folic Acid by Women of Childbearing Age—United States, 1995 and 1998," *Morbidity and Mortality Weekly Report,* vol. 48, no. 16, April 30, 1999

In 1998, 13 percent of all respondents knew folic acid can help prevent birth defects, up from 5 percent in 1995, while 7 percent knew folic acid should be taken before pregnancy, up from 2 percent in 1995. In 1998, among women not pregnant at the time of the survey, 29 percent were taking a vitamin supplement containing folic acid, compared with 25 percent in 1995. Nearly one-third (32 percent) of all women reported taking a vitamin supplement containing folic acid, compared with 28 percent in 1995.

The proportion of women who obtained folic acid information from magazine or newspaper articles decreased from 35 percent in 1995 to 31 percent in 1998. On the other hand the proportion who learned about folic acid from radio or television increased from 10 to 23 percent, while the proportion who learned from health care providers rose from 13 to 19 percent during the same time period.

According to a CDC press release from October 27, 2000, blood folate levels for American women of childbearing age (ages 15–44) nearly tripled between 1988 and 1999. (See Table 3.13.) In the period between the Third National Health and Nutrition Examination Survey (NHANES III), conducted from 1988 to 1994, and NHANES 1999, mean serum folate concentrations for all women of childbearing age increased from 6.3 to 16.2 nanograms per milliliter (ng/ml). Mean serum folate levels of childbearing-age women who ranked in the 75th percentile increased from 7.8 to 19.5 ng/ml over the same period. For nonpregnant women, results were equally dramatic—from 6.0 ng/ml to 15.9 ng/ml. Red blood cell (RBC) folate, which the CDC considers to be a better measure of long-term folate status, increased from 181 to 315 ng/ml.

## RATING DIETARY SUPPLEMENTS

A recent review of several studies of vitamin supplements concluded that there is insufficient scientific evidence to support claims that the supplements help to prevent diseases such as cardiovascular disease and cancer ("Task Force Finds Little Evidence to Support Use of Vitamin Supplements to Prevent Cancer or Heart Disease," Agency for Healthcare Research and Quality, Rockville, MD, June 30, 2003).

The U.S. Preventive Task Force, sponsored by the Agency for Healthcare Research and Quality, is an independent panel of private-sector experts in prevention and primary health care. It assigns letter grades (A, B, C, D, and I) to studies, based on the strength of scientific evidence.

According to the press release, the task force reviewed randomized trials and observational studies to determine whether taking vitamins, A, C, or E, or multivitamins with folic acid, or antioxidant combinations, reduce the risk of heart disease, stroke, or various types of cancers. The best studies, according to the task force, "suggested no clear benefit of taking vitamins, but the number and length of the studies were insufficient to rule out possible benefits of long-term vitamin use."

The task force concentrated on the role of vitamins and other supplements in preventing cancer and did not review the role of vitamins/supplements used by people with nutritional deficiencies, by pregnant women, the aging, and individuals with chronic illnesses.

Studies in which cancer or cardiovascular disease was the focus of attention received an "I" rating from the task force, indicating that insufficient evidence existed either for or against recommending the use of vitamins/supplements.

Taking vitamins according to the Recommended Daily Allowance (RDA) caused no harm, according to the task force, but adverse effects could arise even from moderate doses. For example, moderate doses of vitamin A may affect bone density; high doses may affect the liver or can sometimes harm a fetus. The task force echoed the NCI's findings by recommending that smokers avoid taking beta-carotene. Overall, the task force gave beta-carotene a "D" rating, a negative recommendation.

## DIETARY FIBER

For centuries, human beings have recognized that dietary fiber is beneficial to the normal functioning of the digestive system. Formerly called roughage or bulk, fiber has always been considered invaluable in preventing constipation. Dr. Victor Herbert, in "Dietary Fiber" (*Total Nutrition: The Only Guide You'll Ever Need,* St. Martin's Press, New York, 1995), defines dietary fiber as

TABLE 3.13

**Mean and selected percentiles of serum and red blood cell (RBC) folate concentrations (in ng/mL) for women aged 15–44, 1988–94 and 1999**

| Folate | Sample size | Mean No. | Mean (95% CI) | 10th No. | 10th (95% CI) | 25th No. | 25th (95% CI) | 50th No. | 50th (95% CI) | 75th No. | 75th (95% CI) | 90th No. | 90th (95% CI) |
|---|---|---|---|---|---|---|---|---|---|---|---|---|---|
| **Serum** | | | | | | | | | | | | | |
| 1988–1994 | 5,261 | 6.3 | (6.1– 6.5) | 2.3 | (2.2–2.3) | 3.1 | (3.1–3.3) | 4.8 | (4.6–5.0) | 7.8 | (7.4–8.1) | 11.7 | (11.0–12.5) |
| 1999 | 658 | 16.2 | (14.2–18.2) | 6.7 | (6.3–7.5) | 9.6 | (8.1–11.3) | 14.5 | (11.9–17.0) | 19.5 | (17.8–24.6) | 28.6 | (24.6–34.4) |
| **RBC** | | | | | | | | | | | | | |
| 1988–1994 | 5,254 | 181 | (177–185) | 92 | (90– 94) | 120 | (116–122) | 160 | (156–164) | 223 | (216–231) | 296 | (286–309) |
| 1999 | 663 | 315 | (289–641) | 174 | (161–185) | 216 | (201–232) | 293 | (240–338) | 381 | (341–419) | 474 | (434–540) |

CI = Confidence interval.

SOURCE: "Table 1. Mean and selected percentiles of serum and red blood cell (RBC) folate concentrations (in ng/mL) for U.S. women aged 15–44 years—National Health and Nutrition Examination Surveys, United States, 1988–1994 and 1999," in "Folate Status in Women of Childbearing Age—United States, 1999," *Morbidity and Mortality Weekly Report,* vol. 49, no. 42, October 27, 2000

**FIGURE 3.4**

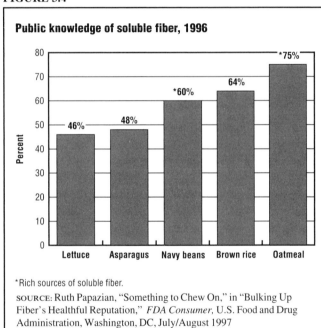

*Rich sources of soluble fiber.

SOURCE: Ruth Papazian, "Something to Chew On," in "Bulking Up Fiber's Healthful Reputation," *FDA Consumer,* U.S. Food and Drug Administration, Washington, DC, July/August 1997

"the sum of the unabsorbable crude fiber (mainly cellulose and lignin) remaining in the colon after digestion, plus the available (fermentable) fiber."

Dietary fibers are either soluble or insoluble:

• Soluble fibers—fibers that combine with water, forming gels. They include pectin, guar, mucilages, and most hemicelluloses. Foods containing soluble fibers include oat bran, barley, dried beans, other legumes, and some vegetables and fruits.

• Insoluble fibers—as their name suggests, fibers that do not dissolve in water. Therefore, they pass through the digestive tract, reduced in size by chewing but unchanged. These include cellulose, some

hemicelluloses, and lignin (which is found in the woody part of vegetables and fruit seeds). Whole-grain products, wheat bran, and the skins of fruits and vegetables contain insoluble fibers.

**A Lot to Learn**

Ruth Papazian, in "Bulking Up Fiber's Healthful Reputation" (*FDA Consumer,* July/August 1997), reported that, in 1996, when Americans were asked which foods—lettuce, asparagus, navy beans, brown rice, oatmeal—are the best sources of cholesterol-lowering soluble fibers, 60 percent chose navy beans and 75 percent chose oatmeal (correct answers). However, nearly half mistakenly identified lettuce (46 percent) and asparagus (48 percent), and almost two-thirds (64 percent) incorrectly chose brown rice, as sources of soluble fibers that help reduce blood cholesterol. (See Figure 3.4.)

**No Specific Dietary Allowance**

No Recommended Dietary Allowances (RDAs) currently exist for dietary fiber. The American Heart Association urges consumers to increase their intake to 25–30 grams of dietary fiber daily, although the typical American consumes only about 11 grams a day. The U.S. Food and Drug Administration (FDA), recognizing the growing numbers of studies showing the health benefits of fiber, now requires the inclusion of fiber on the Nutrition Facts food labels that list other important nutrients. The Daily Values on food labels recommend a dietary fiber intake of 25 grams for individuals consuming 2,000 calories daily and 30 grams for those consuming 2,500 calories. In addition the FDA has approved four health claims for dietary fiber on food labels. According to Ruth Papazian, recent studies show that dietary fiber may play a role in reducing the risk of certain cancers, diabetes, digestive disorders, and heart disease.

The Food and Nutrition Board of the Institute of Medicine issued its *Dietary Reference Intakes: Applications in Dietary Planning* (National Academies Press, Washington, DC) in 2003. According to this reference, men 50 and younger should consume 38 grams of fiber daily, and women in the same age group, 25 grams. Men over 50 should have a total daily intake of 30 grams, and women, 21 grams.

## Dietary Fiber and Health

CONSTIPATION AND DIVERTICULOSIS. The role of fiber in preventing constipation has long been recognized. Insoluble fiber, capable of absorbing as much as 15 times its weight in water, adds to the water-holding capacity of large intestine contents, increasing the bulk of stools. The passage of stool through the digestive track is expedited, thus preventing and relieving constipation.

Dietary fiber may also help reduce the risk of diverticulosis, a condition where diverticula, or small, abnormal pockets, form in the wall of the colon (the main part of the large intestine). These sac-like protrusions along the inner lining of the large intestine are usually caused by straining during bowel movement, or simply by aging. Kathleen Meister, in *Dietary Fiber* (American Council on Science and Health, New York, December 1996), reports that "one-third of all North Americans over the age of 45 and two-thirds of all persons over the age of 85 have diverticula in their colons."

While most cases of diverticulosis cause no symptoms, the diverticula may get inflamed, causing a condition called diverticulitis, characterized by fever and pain. Hospitalization and surgery may be needed, especially if perforations occur. Dietary fiber is not part of the treatment of diverticulitis.

CANCER. Scientists who have studied the relationship between a high-fiber diet and lower incidence of colon cancer believe that insoluble fiber not only adds bulk to stool, but also dilutes cancer-causing substances (carcinogens) in the stool. In addition, since stool bulk helps decrease its travel time through the digestive tract, it thereby reduces the colon's exposure to carcinogens.

Some studies suggest there may be a correlation between high-fiber intake and a reduced risk of breast cancer. Ruth Papazian reports, "In the early stages, some breast tumors are stimulated by excess amounts of estrogen circulating in the bloodstream." Some scientists think that dietary fiber may combine with estrogen in the intestine, reducing excess estrogen levels in the bloodstream and thus preventing further growth of breast tumors.

The role of dietary fiber in preventing cancer is still not well established. As in the case of beta-carotene, contrary data have begun to surface. In 2003 the Harvard School of Public Health reported that recent, large, and well-designed studies have not established a link between dietary fiber intake and reduced incidence of colon cancer ("Fiber: Start Roughing It!"; available online at http://www.hsph.harvard.edu/nutritionsource/fiber.html). One of the school's own studies followed more than 80,000 female nurses for 16 years and found that "dietary fiber was not strongly associated with a reduced risk for either colon cancer or colon polyps (a precursor to colon cancer)." The absence of a positive preventative link, however, according to the report, should not cause people to abandon a high-fiber diet.

HEART DISEASE. There is some evidence that a high intake of dietary fiber, especially soluble fiber, can reduce low-density lipoprotein (LDL) blood cholesterol. LDL, also called "bad" cholesterol, is responsible for forming the plaque that contributes to coronary heart disease (CHD). As soluble fiber passes through the digestive tract, it links with LDL and helps remove it from the body.

Heart disease is the leading killer of women. Alicja Wolk et al., in "Long-Term Intake of Dietary Fiber and Decreased Risk of Coronary Heart Disease Among Women" (*Journal of the American Medical Association,* vol. 281, no. 21, June 2, 1999), examined 68,782 women ages 37–64 who were enrolled in the 10-year longitudinal *Nurses' Health Study.*

The researchers found that, of the three sources of dietary fiber—cereals, fruits, and vegetables—only cereal fiber was strongly linked to decreased risk of CHD in women. Consumption of cold cereal five or more times per week, compared with nonconsumption, was linked to a 19 percent lower risk of CHD. Consumption of oatmeal (soluble fiber) was associated with a 29 percent lower risk of CHD. Eating fruit and vegetable fibers was not significantly related to the risk of CHD. Similar results have been found in studies among men.

A 2003 study discussed in the *Journal of the American Medical Association* (JAMA) demonstrated that the cardiovascular health benefits of dietary fiber intake apply to older Americans, too. The article, "Cereal, Fruit, and Vegetable Fiber Intake and the Risk of Cardiovascular Disease in Elderly Individuals" (*Journal of the American Medical Association,* vol. 289, 2003), described a study of 3,588 men and women age 65 and older. These individuals were free of cardiovascular disease at the outset of the study, from 1989 to 1990. Investigators determined the dietary fiber consumed by this group using a questionnaire describing 99 food items. Researchers followed the group for 8.6 years. During that time, 811 cardiovascular events were recorded for the group. After results were adjusted for other factors, including exercise and smoking, the study found that cardiovascular disease was lowest among those with high dietary fiber consumption. Those who

TABLE 3.14

**Sources of dietary fiber**

| | Rich sources of dietary fiber (4 or more grams of fiber per serving) | | | | Vegetables | Bean sprouts, raw | 1/2 cup |
|---|---|---|---|---|---|---|---|
| | | | | | | Beets, diced, canned | 1/2 cup |
| Breads and cereals | Cereals with 4 or more grams fiber per serving (check product Nutrition Facts Label) | 1/3 – 1/2 cup (varies) | | | | Broccoli, chopped, frozen, boiled | 1/2 cup |
| | | | | | | Brussels sprouts | 1/2 cup |
| Legumes (cooked) | Beans, brown | 1/2 cup | | | | Cabbage, cooked | 1/2 cup |
| | Beans, kidney | 1/2 cup | | | | Carrots | 1/2 cup |
| | Beans, large lima | 1/2 cup | | | | Cauliflower | 1/2 cup |
| | Beans, navy | 1/2 cup | | | | Corn | 1/2 cup |
| | Beans, pinto | 1/2 cup | | | | Eggplant | 1/2 cup |
| | Beans, white | 1/2 cup | | | | Kale, boiled | 1/2 cup |
| | Lentils | 1/2 cup | | | | Okra, frozen, boiled | 1/2 cup |
| | Peas, black-eyed | 1/2 cup | | | | Potatoes, baked or mashed | 1/2 cup |
| Vegetables | Artichoke, cooked | 1 each | | | | Spinach | 1/2 cup |
| Fruits | Blackberries | 1/2 cup | | | | Squash, winter or summer | 1/2 cup |
| | Prunes, dried | 4 each | | | | Sweet potatoes | 1/2 cup |
| | Raspberries | 1/2 cup | | | | Tomatoes, canned | 1/2 cup |
| | | | | | | Turnip greens | 1/2 cup |
| | | | | | | Yams | 1/2 cup |
| | | | | | | Zucchini, cooked | 1/2 cup |
| | Moderately rich sources of dietary fiber (1 to 3 grams of fiber per serving) | | | | Miscellaneous | Almonds | 2 tablespoons |
| | | | | | | Flour, whole wheat | 2 tablespoons |
| | | | | | | Peanuts | 2 tablespoons |
| Breads | Bagel, 3.5" diameter | 1 each | | | | Popcorn, popped | 1 cup |
| | Bread: whole wheat, cracked wheat, pumpernickel, or rye | 1 slice | | | | | |
| | Corn bread | 2" square | | | | Low sources of dietary fiber (less than 1 gram of fiber per serving) | | |
| | Crackers, whole wheat | 4 each | | | | | |
| | Muffin: bran, blueberry, cornmeal, or English | 1 each | | | Breads and cereals | Bread: white, raisin, or pita | 1 slice or 1 each |
| Cereals | Cereals with 1-3 grams of fiber per serving (check product Nutrition Facts Label) | 1/2 cup (varies) | | | | Cereals with less than 1 gram of fiber per serving (check product Nutrition Facts Label) | 1/2 cup (varies) |
| | Bran, rice, or wheat | 2 tablespoons | | | | Crackers, saltine | 4 each |
| | Wheat germ | 2 tablespoons | | | | Crackers, graham | 2 each |
| Fruits | Apple, 2 3/4" diameter | 1 each | | | | Rice, white | 1/2 cup |
| | Applesauce | 1/2 cup | | | | Roll, white dinner | 1 each |
| | Apricots, canned | 1/2 cup | | | Fruits | Cantaloupe | 1/6 each |
| | Banana | 1 each | | | | Grapes, Thompson seedless | 1/2 cup |
| | Cherries, canned or fresh | 1/2 cup | | | | Juices, grape, orange, etc. | 1/2 cup |
| | Cranberries, fresh | 1/2 cup | | | | Mandarin oranges | 1/2 cup |
| | Dates, whole | 3 each | | | | Watermelon | 1 cup |
| | Figs, fresh, medium | 2 each | | | Vegetables | Asparagus, cooked | 3 spears |
| | Fruit cocktail, canned | 1/2 cup | | | | Beans, green | 1/2 cup |
| | Grapefruit | 1 half | | | | Chestnuts, water | 1/2 cup |
| | Kiwi fruit | 1 each | | | | Lettuce, iceberg, chopped | 1 cup |
| | Orange, 2 5/8" diameter | 1 each | | | | Mushrooms, canned | 1/2 cup |
| | Peaches, canned | 1/2 cup | | | | Mustard greens, fresh | 1/2 cup |
| | Peaches, fresh | 1 each | | | | Onions, chopped, raw | 1/4 cup |
| | Pears, canned | 1/2 cup | | | | Pepper, sweet green | 1/2 cup |
| | Pears, fresh | 1/2 each | | | Miscellaneous | Flour, white | 2 tablespoons |
| | Plum, medium, 2 1/8" diameter | 1 each | | | | | |
| | Raisins | 1/4 cup | | | | | |
| | Strawberries, fresh | 1/2 cup | | | | | |
| | Tangerine | 1 each | | | | | |

SOURCE: "Rich Sources of Dietary Fiber," "Moderately Rich Sources of Dietary Fiber," and "Low Sources of Dietary Fiber" in Janice R. Hermann, *Dietary Fiber*, Oklahoma Cooperative Extension Service, Division of Agricultural Sciences and Natural Resources, Oklahoma State University, Stillwater, OK, May 1999

consumed the most cereal fiber had a 21 percent lower risk of cardiovascular disease.

**DIABETES.** In the late 1980s and early 1990s, when it was thought that dietary fiber (particularly soluble fiber) might help regulate blood sugar, health professionals prescribed a daily dietary fiber intake of up to 40 grams for diabetics. Further research has shown that an unusually large amount of fiber is needed to control blood sugar and that not all soluble fibers achieve the same antidiabetic result. In 1994 the American Dietetic Association recommended

that diabetics should consume the same amount of dietary fibers as nondiabetics.

Research, however, continues to unveil new findings. A 2000 article in the *New England Journal of Medicine* discussed a study that supports the beneficial health effects of fiber intake on diabetes (Manisha Chandalia et al., "Beneficial Effects of High Dietary Fiber Intake in Patients with Type 2 Diabetes Mellitus," May 11, 2000). Researchers assigned 13 patients with type 2 diabetes to follow two diets. Subjects ate each diet for six weeks. One

TABLE 3.15

**Composition of fats**

| Kind of fat | % Saturated | % Poly | % Mono |
|---|---|---|---|
| Canola oil | 6 | 32 | 62 |
| Safflower oil | 10 | 77 | 13 |
| Sunflower oil | 11 | 69 | 20 |
| Corn oil | 13 | 62 | 25 |
| Olive oil | 14 | 9 | 77 |
| Soybean oil | 15 | 61 | 24 |
| Margarine (tub) | 17 | 34 | 24 |
| Peanut oil | 18 | 33 | 49 |
| Cottonseed oil | 27 | 54 | 19 |
| Chicken fat | 31 | 22 | 47 |
| Lard | 41 | 12 | 47 |
| Beef fat | 52 | 4 | 44 |
| Palm kernel oil | 81 | 2 | 11 |
| Coconut oil | 92 | 2 | 6 |

SOURCE: *Composition of Foods,* U.S. Department of Agriculture, Washington, DC

consisted of moderate amounts of fiber (8 grams of soluble fiber, 16 grams of insoluble fiber, as recommended by the American Diabetes Association). The second diet (high-fiber) consisted of 25 grams of soluble fiber and 25 grams of insoluble fiber. The diets were otherwise the same. Subjects on the high-fiber diet had lower blood sugar and urinary sugar than those following the American Diabetes Association diet. The researchers concluded that high dietary fiber, especially soluble fiber, helps type 2 diabetics control their sugar levels.

Measuring the amount of fiber in food can be difficult, because scientists do not agree on which method is best. The amount of fiber can vary by as much as 30 percent, depending on the method of analysis. Oklahoma State University's Division of Agricultural Sciences provides a listing of rich and moderate sources of fiber. (See Table 3.14.)

### Caution in Using Dietary Fiber

Although Americans are encouraged to increase their intake of dietary fiber, they should not necessarily use dietary supplements to boost their intake. In fact, nutritionists generally discourage the use of dietary supplements. Experts also recommend that fiber should come from a variety of foods, be increased gradually, and be eaten throughout the day instead of during one sitting. Some people experience gas pains, bloating, and even diarrhea after eating a large amount of fiber. Excessive fiber consumption may also prevent the absorption of some minerals, such as calcium, zinc, and iron.

### Fiber in Children's Diets

Kathleen Meister, in *Dietary Fiber,* warns against adding too much fiber to children's diets. High-fiber foods tend to be bulky and low in caloric value, and children need many calories for normal growth and development. In addition, fiber may fill them up quickly, leaving little room for other foods. As with adults, children cannot afford to lose the minerals that may be combined with unabsorbed fiber excreted from the body. The American Academy of Pediatrics recommends 0.5 grams of dietary fiber for each kilogram of a child's body weight, while the American Health Foundation recommends that a child age 3 and older have a dietary fiber intake equivalent to his or her age, plus 5 grams, daily.

## DIETARY FATS AND CHOLESTEROL

All dietary fats are mixtures of saturated and unsaturated fatty acids. Fatty acids are the building blocks of dietary fats. Fatty acids are classified as saturated or unsaturated, based on their chemical composition—that is, the number of hydrogen atoms they contain.

Saturated fatty acids contain the most hydrogen atoms; in other words, they are "saturated" with hydrogen. Saturated fats, found in meat, egg yolks, and whole-milk dairy products, are generally solid at room temperature. Three vegetable fats—coconut oil, palm oil, and palm kernel oil—are very high in saturated fats. (See Table 3.15.)

Unsaturated fats, which are missing hydrogen atoms, are generally liquid at room temperature and are called oils. Plants and fish are the main sources of unsaturated fats. Unsaturated fats are classified as monounsaturated or polyunsaturated. Monounsaturated fats, such as olive, canola, and peanut oils, are missing a pair of hydrogen atoms, while polyunsaturated fats are missing two or more pairs of hydrogen atoms. Corn, soybean, safflower, and sesame seed oils are polyunsaturated fats. (See Table 3.15.)

### Fats, Cholesterol, and Heart Disease

Health professionals recommend limiting fat intake to 30 percent or less of total daily calories, and saturated fat intake to less than 10 percent of calories. The *Third National Health and Nutrition Examination Survey* (NHANES III) found that Americans currently consume about 34 percent of their total calories as fat, with 12 percent of their calories provided by saturated fats.

According to the CDC, data from the *National Health and Examination Survey 1999–2000* show that Americans consumed 33 percent of their daily intakes of calories as fat. Data were based on one 24-hour dietary interview ("Dietary Intake of Ten Key Nutrients for Public Health, United States: 1999–2000," Centers for Disease Control and Prevention, Augusta, GA, April 17, 2003).

Fat consumption in the United States has been rising steadily. In the 1970–74 period, daily per capita consumption of added fat—fat over and above that which occurs naturally in foods such as meats, milk, nuts, and avocados—was 47.9 grams (1.7 ounces). Intake increased almost without interruption in every 5-year period

**TABLE 3.16**

**Consumption of added fats, 2000**

| Item | 1970-74 | 1975-79 | 1980-84 | 1985-89 | 1990-94 | 1995-99 | 2000 | Change, 1970-74 to 2000 | 2000 food supply added fats per capita per day[1] |
|---|---|---|---|---|---|---|---|---|---|
| | _Pounds, product weight [2] (per capita annual averages)_ | | | | | | | _Percent_ | _Grams_ |
| **Fats and oils** | 55.7 | 57.4 | 61.7 | 66.1 | 69.1 | 67.5 | 77.1 | 38 | 63.0 |
| Salad and cooking oils | 16.7 | 19.5 | 22.2 | 24.8 | 26.2 | 27.2 | 33.7 | 102 | 29.8 |
| Shortening | 17.2 | 17.6 | 19.0 | 21.9 | 23.1 | 21.2 | 23.1 | 34 | 19.2 |
| Margarine | 11.0 | 11.4 | 10.8 | 10.6 | 10.6 | 8.5 | 8.2 | -25 | 4.8 |
| Butter | 5.0 | 4.4 | 4.6 | 4.6 | 4.5 | 4.4 | 4.6 | -8 | 3.6 |
| Lard (direct use)[3] | 3.6 | 2.5 | 2.1 | 1.5 | 1.4 | 1.8 | 1.9 | -47 | 1.2 |
| Edible beef tallow (direct use)[3] | na | .4 | 1.4 | 1.2 | 1.8 | 2.9 | 4.0 | na | 2.5 |
| Other edible fats and oils[4] | 2.2 | 1.9 | 1.6 | 1.4 | 1.4 | 1.4 | 1.5 | -32 | 1.8 |
| **Very high-fat diary foods that are included in total added fat:** | | | | | | | | | |
| Cream cheese | .6 | .8 | 1.1 | 1.4 | 2.0 | 2.2 | 2.4 | 300 | .7 |
| | _Half pints, product weight [2] (per capita annual averages)_ | | | | | | | | |
| Heavy cream | 1.0 | 1.1 | 1.5 | 2.2 | 2.5 | 3.4 | 3.7 | 270 | .6 |
| Light cream | .7 | .6 | .5 | .8 | .6 | .9 | 1.1 | 57 | .1 |
| Sour cream | 2.4 | 3.1 | 3.7 | 4.5 | 5.0 | 5.5 | 6.2 | 158 | .5 |
| Half and half | 5.0 | 4.5 | 4.8 | 5.8 | 5.8 | 6.1 | 6.9 | 38 | .3 |
| Eggnog | .7 | .8 | .8 | .9 | .8 | .7 | .6 | -14 | -- |
| | _Grams per capita per day, fat content basis[1]_ | | | | | | | | |
| **Total added fat (excludes naturally occuring fat in such foods as meats,** | 47.9 | 49.3 | 52.5 | 56.4 | 58.6 | 57.2 | 65.3 | 36 | 65.3 |
| | _Tablespoon per capita per day, fat content basis[1]_ | | | | | | | | |
| **beverage milks, nuts, and avocados)[1]** | 3.5 | 3.6 | 3.9 | 4.1 | 4.3 | 4.2 | 4.8 | 37 | na |

Note: na = not applicable or not available. -- = less than 0.05 grams. Totals may not add due to rounding.

[1] Adjusted for cooking losses, plate waste, and other losses. Includes only the cream portions of half and half and eggnog; the milk portions are included in the dairy group. Fat content of butter and margarine calculated at 80 percent. One tablespoon of fat equals approximately 13.6 grams of fat.

[2] Aggregate data, unadjusted for cooking losses, plate waste, and other losses.

[3] Excludes use in margarine and shortening.

[4] Specialty fats used mainly in confections and nondairy creamers.

SOURCE: Judy Putnam, Jane Allshouse, and Linda Scott Kantor, "Table 2–Americans Consume an Average of 65 Grams, or 600 Calories' Worth, of Added Fats Per Person Per Day in 2000," in "U.S. Per Capita Food Supply Trends: More Calories, Refined Carbohydrates, and Fats," in _FoodReview,_ U.S. Department of Agriculture, Economic Research Service, Washington, DC, Winter 2002

thereafter, reaching 65.3 grams (2.3 ounces) in 2000. (See Table 3.16.) During the roughly three decades between 1970 and 2000, added fat consumption rose 36 percent. In that entire period, fat consumption dropped only once, from 1990–94 to 1995–99, when it went from 58.6 to 57.2 grams.

Excess saturated fats in the diet have been found to elevate serum or blood cholesterol levels. High blood cholesterol has been recognized as a risk factor for coronary heart disease. Cholesterol is transported through the bloodstream by lipoproteins, a mixture of fats (lipids) and proteins. Excess blood cholesterol accumulates in the inner lining of the arterial walls, combining with fats and other substances to form plaque. (See Figure 3.5.) This condition is known as atherosclerosis. The arteries become narrowed because of these deposits, thereby reducing the flow of blood in these arteries. A thrombus (clot) may form when blood flow is sluggish. If a clot forms where the plaque is located, the blood flow to the heart may be blocked, causing a heart attack. If blood flow to the brain is blocked, a stroke results.

Two lipoproteins are believed to play major roles in the amount of blood cholesterol. Low-density lipoprotein (LDL) contains most of the cholesterol found in the blood and is said to be responsible for the "bad" cholesterol that forms plaque. High-density lipoprotein (HDL), or "good" cholesterol, is believed to carry cholesterol from the arteries to the liver, where it is excreted from the body. According to the American Heart Association's _Heart and Stroke A-Z Guide_ (2000), "Some experts believe HDL removes excess cholesterol from atherosclerotic plaques and thus slows their growth."

According to NHANES III, the average level of serum cholesterol in the U.S. population was 203

FIGURE 3.5

## Example of cholesterol plaque buildup in a blood vessel

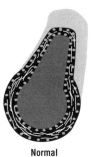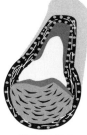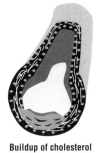

Normal     Buildup of cholesterol     Blockage from plaque formation

SOURCE: John Henkel, "The Plague of Plaque" in "Keeping Cholesterol Under Control," *FDA Consumer,* Jan-Feb, 1999

FIGURE 3.6

## Adults diagnosed at sometime with high blood cholesterol, 2001

(Median for all respondents aged 18 or older in a nationwide survey)

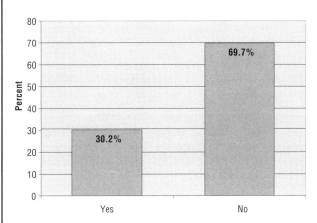

SOURCE: Adapted from "Diagnosed With High Cholesterol Nationwide – 2001," in *Behavioral Risk Factor Surveillance System, Prevalance Data,* an online data presentation tool from the Centers for Disease Control and Prevention, National Center for Chronic Disease Prevention & Health Promotion, Hyattsville, MD [Online] http://apps.nccd.cdc.gov/page.asp?cat=CA&yr=2001&state=US#CA [accessed August 11, 2003]

TABLE 3.17

## Cholesterol levels

| Type of cholesterol | Classification |
|---|---|
| **Total blood cholesterol** | |
| Less than 200 mg/dL | Desirable |
| 200-239 mg/dL | Borderline high |
| 240 mg/dL and over | High |
| **LDL cholesterol** | |
| Less than 130 mg/dL | Desirable |
| 130-159 mg/dL | Borderline high |
| 160 mg/dL or higher | High |
| **HDL cholesterol** | |
| 40-50 mg/dL(men) | Desirable |
| 50-60 mg/dL (women) | Desirable |
| Less that 35 mg/dL | Low |

LDL = Low-density lipoprotein.
HDL = High-density lipoprotein.

SOURCE: National Heart, Lung, and Blood Institute, National Institutes of Health, Washington, DC

In 2001 the CDC found that 30.2 percent of the U.S. adult population had, at some point, been diagnosed with high cholesterol. (See Figure 3.6.)

### Heart Benefits from Monounsaturated Fats

A number of studies have found that monounsaturated fats decrease bad cholesterol (LDL) levels and increase good cholesterol (HDL) levels. This does not mean, however, that people should indulge in large amounts of olive or canola oil, but that they would do better to choose monounsaturates over other fats, especially saturated fats.

A study in Lyon, France, has again called attention to the diets of Mediterranean countries, noted for their high intake of fruits, vegetables, and breads, their low consumption of meat, and their use of olive oil. The "Lyon Diet Heart Study (University of California at Berkeley Wellness Letter," vol. 15, issue 8, May 1999) found that, among people from the Greek island of Crete who had had a heart attack in the six months prior to the study, a change in fat in their diet cut the risk of a second heart attack and the overall death rate by as much as 70 percent over the course of four years. Margarine made from canola (rapeseed) oil was used in place of other fats. Blood tests revealed a high concentration of a polyunsaturated fatty acid called alpha-linoleic acid, which is present in canola oil.

High concentrations of alpha-linoleic acid are found in few foods—canola, soybean, and flaxseed oils, as well as walnuts and the leafy, green vegetable purslane. Researchers believe that alpha-linoleic acid, a "short-chain" omega-3 fatty acid related to the "longer-chain" omega-3 fatty acid found in fish, may be capable of reducing blood clotting and heart-rhythm defects and of exerting an anti-inflammatory effect in blood vessels. The researchers, however, did not discount the beneficial

milligrams/deciliter (mg/dl). Between 1988 and 1994, 18.9 percent of the population had high serum cholesterol. Somewhat more females (20 percent) than males (17.5 percent) had high serum cholesterol, with 2 in 5 females age 55 and older having high serum cholesterol. The National Cholesterol Education Program of the National Heart, Lung, and Blood Institute classifies the risk for coronary heart disease based on total serum cholesterol. Since the type of cholesterol also plays a major role in the risk of heart disease, the institute also provides a guideline. (See Table 3.17.)

**TABLE 3.18**

**Comparing saturated-fat content**

| Food category | Portion | Saturated fat content in (grams) |
|---|---|---|
| Cheese | | |
| Regular Cheddar cheese | 1 oz. | 6.0 |
| Low-fat Cheddar cheese* | 1 oz. | 1.2 |
| Ground beef | | |
| Regular ground beef | 3 oz. cooked | 7.2 |
| Extra lean ground beef* | 3 oz. cooked | 5.3 |
| Milk | | |
| Whole milk | 1 cup | 5.1 |
| Low-fat (1%) milk* | 1 cup | 1.6 |
| Breads | | |
| Croissant | 1 medium | 6.6 |
| Bagel* | 1 medium | 0.1 |
| Frozen desserts | | |
| Regular ice cream | 1/2 cup | 4.5 |
| Frozen yogurt* | 1/2 cup | 2.5 |
| Table spreads | | |
| Butter | 1 tsp. | 2.4 |
| Soft margarine* | 1 tsp. | 0.7 |

Note: The food categories listed are among the major food sources of saturated fat for U.S. adults and children.

* Choice that is lower in saturated fat.

SOURCE: "A Comparison of Saturated Fat in Some Foods" in *Dietary Guidelines for Americans, 2000,* U.S. Department of Agriculture, Washington, DC, 2000

effects the overall Mediterranean diet had on the patients' heart conditions.

Studies of the health benefits of the Mediterranean diet have been conducted in other countries, as well, not least in Italy. A study published in the April 2003 issue of the *European Journal of Clinical Nutrition* (summarized in *Nutrition News Focus* as "Today's Topic: Mediterranean Diet for Life," May 14, 2003) reported on follow-ups of people in 172 centers in Italy who had had a heart attack. They were told to eat the basic Mediterranean diet (fish, fruit, raw and cooked vegetables, and olive oil). Six and a half years later, researchers found that those who had followed the recommendations had a reduced mortality rate. Mortality and adherence to the diet had a direct, linear relationship.

**Hydrogenation and Trans Fats**

Food manufacturers use hydrogenation—the addition of hydrogen molecules to monounsaturated or polyunsaturated fatty acids—to prevent rancidity and to improve food textures. Fats normally break down when exposed to air and heat, becoming rancid. Hydrogenation stabilizes them, promoting freshness and helping to extend the shelf lives of hydrogenated foods. Hydrogenation also raises the melting point of oils, a characteristic useful in deep fat frying. It makes baked goods tender and flaky. Vegetable oils are often partially hydrogenated to create margarines and shortenings.

Food manufacturers use only as much hydrogenation as they need to achieve desired food tastes and textures,

but foods that are partially hydrogenated still contain more unsaturated than saturated fats.

Trans fatty acids (trans fats) form when unsaturated fats become hydrogenated. Some studies have found that trans fats raise the blood levels of LDL cholesterol, which increases the risk of heart disease. Until more studies confirm this, however, experts suggest that consumers use softer tub margarines instead of stick margarines and butter, and reduce their intake of fried foods.

Table 3.18 compares the saturated fat content of certain foods. See Table 3.8 for Recommended Daily Intakes for fat, saturated fat, and cholesterol.

## CALCIUM

### Calcium and Osteoporosis

Osteoporosis is a condition in which bones become porous and brittle. Those with the disease develop a thinning and weakening of the bones, which become much more prone to breakage. Osteoporosis is called the "silent disease" because the weakening of bones produces no visible symptoms. Physicians, however, can diagnose it before fractures occur, by using the bone density test.

The body's 206 bones are in a continuous process of building, breaking down, and rebuilding. In the first few decades of life, rebuilding outpaces breakdown of bones, resulting in greater bone density and strength. The body forms most of its bone mass before puberty, so that, during adolescence, about 75–85 percent of the skeleton is formed. Since the main mineral in bones is calcium, a growing body needs about 1,300 milligrams of calcium daily.

Peak bone mass (maximum bone density and strength) is achieved somewhere between the ages of 20 and 30. After 30, bones begin to break down faster than they can be replaced. Nonetheless, the body continues to draw on the calcium in bones for functions such as muscle contraction. Bones that have not attained optimal mass tend to become thinner and more brittle with each calcium withdrawal.

Not all the causes of osteoporosis are fully known. It is recognized, however, that women lose bone mass at an accelerated rate after menopause. The ovaries produce lower levels of estrogen, which is responsible for protecting against bone loss. Some women begin to lose bone mass as early as age 35. Men also suffer bone loss, but at a later age.

According to the National Osteoporosis Foundation, (available online at http://www.nof.org/osteoporosis/stats.htm) about 10 million people in the United States have osteoporosis, and another 34 million have low bone mass, putting them at increased risk for the disease. Osteoporosis is a threat to four out of five women.

FIGURE 3.7

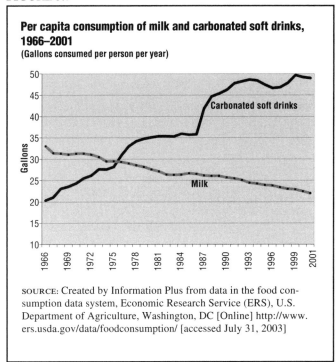

**Per capita consumption of milk and carbonated soft drinks, 1966–2001**

(Gallons consumed per person per year)

SOURCE: Created by Information Plus from data in the food consumption data system, Economic Research Service (ERS), U.S. Department of Agriculture, Washington, DC [Online] http://www.ers.usda.gov/data/foodconsumption/ [accessed July 31, 2003]

Osteoporosis is responsible for 1.5 million fractures a year—mostly of the spine, hip, and wrist. The most common fracture occurs in the spine. When several spinal bones, or vertebrae, are fractured, the spinal column collapses, eventually resulting in a stooped posture known as kyphosis, or dowager's hump. Although hip fractures occur most often in women, one-quarter of all hip fractures occur in men. Health care cost for these fractures was about $17 billion in 2001 and is expected to rise as the population ages.

**Preventing Osteoporosis**

INCREASED CALCIUM INTAKE. Osteoporosis can be prevented. In 1997 the Institute of Medicine released the new Dietary Reference Intakes (DRIs) for calcium, established at levels compatible with the body's capacity to retain the most calcium. The recommendation for adolescents is 1,200 milligrams (mg). Apparently, calcium may enhance bone building in growing children, and, starting at puberty, the body has a greater capacity to absorb and retain calcium.

Experts are especially concerned about growing girls, who generally have lower calcium intakes than boys. A USDA survey found that, while boys and young men ages 12–19 have average calcium intakes of 1,176 mg daily, girls and young women in the same age group consume just 777 mg of calcium per day. USDA studies have found that girls drink the least amount of fluid milk, tend to skip breakfast, depriving themselves of the calcium in cereals and milk, and consume the highest share of calories from fast foods, which have the lowest calcium contents compared with foods prepared at home, in schools, or restaurants.

The National Institute of Child Health and Development (NICHD) summarized the report's findings in a press release on December 10, 2001 ("'Calcium Crisis' Affects American Youth"; available online at http://www.nichd.nih.gov/new/releases/calcium_crisis.cfm). Boys between 12 and 19 consume 36 percent of their daily requirement, but girls of the same age consume only 14 percent, placing them at serious risk of osteoporosis and other bone diseases. The NICHD sees this situation as a calcium crisis:

"Osteoporosis is a pediatric disease with geriatric consequences," said Duane Alexander, M.D. [director of NICHD].... "Preventing this and other bone diseases begins in childhood. With low calcium intake levels during these important bone growth periods, today's children and teens are certain to face a serious public health problem in the future."

Rickets, a bone disease that is the consequence of low vitamin D levels, has also been on the rise, according to the NICHD. Dr. Alexander says that rickets became nearly nonexistent after vitamin D was added to milk in the 1950s, but it is now appearing at greater rates around the country. In an effort to get children to pay attention to their calcium needs, the NICHD has expanded its "Milk Matters" campaign and Web site to speak directly to children and their parents about the importance of calcium in children's diets.

The popularity of carbonated soft drinks may contribute to the decline in per capita consumption of beverage milk. A USDA analysis of data on per capita beverage consumption in the United States between 1947 and 2001 showed that carbonated soft drink consumption increased by 356 percent, while beverage milk per capita consumption decreased by 44 percent during the same period. Figure 3.7 shows the dramatic increase in consumption of carbonated soft drinks and the decline in milk consumption for the years 1966–2001.

Studies have also shown that the average American adult consumes just 500–700 mg of calcium daily, well below the new DRI of 1,000 mg. Postmenopausal women and older men also need to increase their calcium intakes. The DRI for those over 50 is 1,200 mg daily. As a person ages, his or her body becomes less efficient at absorbing calcium and other nutrients. Older adults also are more likely to have chronic medical problems and to use medications that may impair calcium absorption. Moreover, inadequate vitamin D intake also calls for additional calcium intake. Major sources of calcium are cheese, milk, yogurt, tofu (made with calcium sulfate), broccoli, spinach, perch, and salmon.

FIGURE 3.8

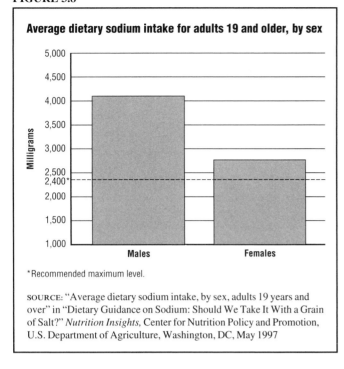

**Average dietary sodium intake for adults 19 and older, by sex**

*Recommended maximum level.

SOURCE: "Average dietary sodium intake, by sex, adults 19 years and over" in "Dietary Guidance on Sodium: Should We Take It With a Grain of Salt?" *Nutrition Insights,* Center for Nutrition Policy and Promotion, U.S. Department of Agriculture, Washington, DC, May 1997

TABLE 3.19

**Salt content, by food group**

| Food groups | Sodium, mg |
|---|---|
| **Bread, cereal, rice, and pasta** | |
| Cooked cereal, rice, pasta, unsalted, 1/2 cup | Trace |
| Ready-to-eat cereal,1 oz. | 100-360 |
| Bread, 1 slice | 110-175 |
| Popcorn, salted, 1 oz. | 100-420 |
| Pretzels, salted 1 oz | 130-880 |
| **Vegetable** | |
| Vegetables, fresh, or frozen, cooked without salt, 1/2 cup | Less that 70 |
| Vegetables, canned or frozen with sauce, 1/2 cup | 140-460 |
| Tomato juice, canned, 3/4 cup | 660 |
| Vegetable soup, canned, 1 cup | 820 |
| **Fruit** | |
| Fruit, fresh, frozen, canned, 1/2 cup | Trace |
| **Milk, yogurt, and cheese** | |
| Milk, 1 cup | 120 |
| Yogurt, 8 oz. | 160 |
| Natural cheeses, 1-1/2 oz. | 110-450 |
| Process cheeses, 2 oz. | 800 |
| **Meat, poultry, fish, dry beans, eggs, and nuts** | |
| Fresh meat, poultry, fish, 3 oz. | Less than 90 |
| Tuna, canned, water pack, 3 oz. | 300 |
| Bologna, 2 oz. | 580 |
| Ham, lean, roasted, 3 oz. | 1,020 |
| Peanuts, roasted in oil, salted, 1 oz. | 120 |
| **Other** | |
| Salad dressing, 1 tsp. | 75-220 |
| Ketchup, mustard, steak sauce, 1 tbsp. | 130-230 |
| Soy sauce, 1 tbsp. | 1,030 |
| Salt, 1 tsp. | 2,325 |
| Dill pickle, 1 medium | 930 |

SOURCE: "Where's the Salt?" in *Food Guide Pyramid Booklet 2000,* Center for Nutrition Policy and Promotion, U.S. Department of Agriculture, Washington, DC, 2000

**VITAMIN D.** Vitamin D helps prevent osteoporosis by assisting the body's absorption of calcium from the intestinal tract. More importantly, vitamin D helps maintain normal levels of calcium in the blood. By regulating the blood calcium levels, vitamin D helps make calcium available to bones for a process called mineralization. If the body has inadequate vitamin D, the bones are demineralized—they lose minerals to the blood in order to keep the calcium levels normal. Calcium is necessary for other body functions, including the contraction and relaxation of muscles (most notably the heart), nerve transmission, and blood clotting. If calcium is inadequate in the diet, it is withdrawn from the bones to maintain the levels of calcium in the blood and to regulate heartbeat.

In recent years experts have recognized that many elderly people get too little vitamin D. Skin conversion of vitamin D slows with age. About 10–15 minutes of exposure to sunlight three times a week is generally enough for the body to synthesize its own vitamin D, but older people need about 30 minutes of sun exposure. Those who are housebound or who live in nursing homes are not likely to get enough sun. In addition, while milk is the primary source of vitamin D, older people tend to become less tolerant of the lactose in milk, causing many to eliminate milk from their diets.

Those who take supplements must continue to do so. The Agricultural Research Service highlighted the importance of calcium and vitamin D intake among the elderly in a January 24, 2001, article ("Bone Gains Fade When Elders Cease Supplements"; available online at

http://www.ars.usda.gov/is/pr/2001/010124.htm). In the study 389 seniors participated in a three-year phase during which they took supplements; 295 were followed for two years thereafter. Researchers found that volunteers who stopped taking 500 mg of calcium and 700 IU of vitamin D daily lost the benefits that they had gained earlier in the spine and hip.

The USDA reported that fewer than one in ten U.S. elders meets the current recommendations for calcium intake (1,200 mg daily from food and supplements) and vitamin D intake (400–600 IU per day.)

New federal recommendations for vitamin D intake were issued in 1997. Guidelines for adults up to age 50 remained at 200 IU, but the Institute of Medicine set higher levels for those 51–70 years old (400 IU) and those over 70 (600 IU).

**EXERCISE.** Bones, like muscles, are living tissues; they become stronger with exercise. Regular, weight-bearing exercise builds bone strength and prevents bone loss. Exercise also helps prevent falls. People who exercise have a better sense of balance and better reflexes. They also build up more muscle padding to absorb the shock of a fall.

## SODIUM

Sodium can be found most commonly in table salt. It plays an important role in regulating body fluids and blood pressure. Currently there is no daily dietary requirement for sodium. Health authorities, including the American Heart Association and the National Academy of Sciences, recommend that sodium intake should be limited to no more than 2,400 mg—about a teaspoon of salt—a day. The Department of Agriculture has found that Americans consume much more than the recommended limit, even when salt added at the table or during food preparation is excluded. (See Figure 3.8.) Table 3.19 shows the concentrations of sodium in various foods.

More than 2,400 mg of sodium in the diet is often associated with elevated blood pressure. Increased blood pressure can lead to hypertension, heart disease, stroke, and renal (kidney) disease. In the United States, nearly one in four people has hypertension. Clinical studies have shown that decreasing sodium intake lowers blood pressure in persons with or without hypertension. According to a study from the Northwestern University Medical School in Chicago, lowering lifetime salt intake by about one teaspoon a day would mean a 16-percent drop in coronary heart disease deaths and 23 percent fewer stroke deaths at age 55. Table 3.6 presents some of the consequences of excess sodium intake.

In 2001 a study supported by the National Heart, Lung, and Blood Institute (NHLBI) confirmed the blood-pressure-lowering effects of reduced sodium intake ("NHLBI Study Finds DASH Diet and Reduced Sodium Lowers Blood Pressure for All," NIH News Release, December 17, 2001). DASH stands for Dietary Approaches to Stop Hypertension. The 412 participants in the study were 22 or older and had elevated blood pressure. The group was chosen to represent subgroups within the population.

Participants were separated into groups who ate the DASH diet or typical American diet. Salt intake was varied in a random order so that some took 3,300 mg a day (the U.S. average), others 2,400 mg (the highest level recommended by the National Blood Pressure Education Program), and yet others only 1,500 mg/day.

The best results in controlling blood pressure were achieved by those who followed the DASH diet and took the least amount of salt.

According to NHLBI:

The DASH diet is rich in fruits, vegetables, and lowfat dairy foods and reduced in total and saturated fat. It also is reduced in red meat, sweets, and sugar-containing drinks.

It is rich in potassium, calcium, magnesium, fiber, and protein. Prior studies found that the DASH diet lowers blood pressure and also lowers blood LDL-cholesterol (the "bad" cholesterol) and the amino acid homocysteine, which appears to increase the risk of heart disease. Prior studies also showed reducing dietary sodium lowers blood pressure, both with and without the DASH diet.

According to NHLBI director Dr. Claude Lenfant, earlier research on the link between sodium and blood pressure gave conflicting results in various population groups. But he says that the DASH results demonstrate that cutting back on dietary sodium will benefit Americans in general, not just those who have high blood pressure.

## VEGETARIAN AND VEGAN DIETS

For a number of different reasons, including health concerns, cultural and/or religious beliefs, and concern for animals, many Americans choose to follow vegetarian or vegan diets. According to a publication by the North Dakota State University Agricultural Service (*Vegetarian Diets,* HE-463, August 1994), a vegan diet consists exclusively of plant foods: vegetables, fruits, legumes, grains, nuts, and seeds. No foods of animal origin, including meat, fish, fowl, eggs, and dairy products, are consumed. Some vegetarian diets, however, include dairy products (lacto-vegetarian); some also permit eggs (lacto-ovo-vegetarian). There are other even more permissive semi-vegetarian diets, as well, that permit chicken or fish. According to *Vegetarian Diets,* vegetarian diets in the United States are high in fiber and low in total fat, saturated fat, cholesterol, and calories. Moreover, studies have suggested a positive relationship between vegetarian eating practices and risk reduction for such illnesses as coronary heart disease, high blood pressure, diabetes, and certain types of cancers.

Neal Barnard, president of the Physicians Committee for Responsible Medicine (PCRM), claims that studies have found that vegetarians get much better nutrition than nonvegetarians ("Vegetarian Diet on Solid Ground, Experts Say," *USA Today,* November 28, 2001). The vegetarian diet also provides for greater amounts of fiber, iron, vitamins, and cancer-fighting compounds than do nonvegetarian diets. Barnard asserts that vegetarians have a 40 percent less risk of cancer and a much lower risk of illnesses such as heart disease, diabetes, and hypertension.

The National Institute of Diabetes & Digestive & Kidney Diseases (NIDDK) reported that vegetarian diets can provide the recommended daily amount of all the important nutrients if foods are chosen carefully ("Weight-Loss and Nutrition Myths: How Much Do You Really Know?"; available online at http://www.niddk.nih.gov/health/nutrit/pubs/myths/index.htm). The institute points out that animal products provide most of the iron, calcium, vitamin D, vitamin B12, and zinc in the human diet. Getting these nutrients from a vegetarian diet requires special care, but it can be done. Ample supplies of protein can be obtained from such food as lentils, tofu, nuts, seed, tempeh, miso, and peas. Tempeh and miso are produced from soybeans.

According to a 2002 poll conducted by *Time* magazine, 10 million people in the U.S. considered themselves to be practicing vegetarians ("Should We All Be Vegetarians? Would We Be Healthier? Would the Planet? The Risks and Benefits of a Meat-Free Life," July 15, 2002). The actual number of serious vegetarians appears to be much smaller, however. The *Time* survey showed that 37 percent of those who identified themselves as vegetarian reported eating red meat in the 24-hour period before the survey; 60 percent reported that they had eaten meat, poultry, or seafood. A lower estimate is provided by the Vegetarian Resource Group (VRG). A national Zogby poll sponsored by the VRG in 2000 found that 2.5 percent of those polled (968 adults 18 and over) reported never eating meat/poultry, fish/seafood, dairy products, eggs, and honey ("How Many Vegetarians Are There?," August 30, 2000). The VGR extrapolated this percentage to the 2000 population, counting only the noninstitutionalized population, and arrived at an estimate of 4.8 million vegetarians and vegans.

# CHAPTER 4
# FOOD SPENDING

According to the Economic Research Service of the U.S. Department of Agriculture (USDA), in 2002 Americans spent $790.7 billion on food—a sum that equates to 10.1 percent of their total disposable personal income that year. (See Table 4.1.) (Disposable personal income is the sum of personal consumption expenditures—spending on goods and services—plus savings and other miscellaneous expenditures.) As huge as that figure seems, Americans do not have to spend as much of their money on food as they once did. In the early years of the twentieth century, Americans spent nearly a quarter of their income on food. In 1930 they spent 24.3 percent of their disposable personal income feeding themselves. By 2001 that percentage had dropped to 10.2 percent, a decline of 145 percent, leaving far more money available to be saved or spent on other things. (See Table 4.1.)

Spending on food at home in 2002 accounted for 6.2 percent of disposable personal income; spending on food away from home, 4.0 percent. (See Table 4.1.) Our taste for eating out has increased over the years. As a percentage of all food expenditures, eating out has grown over the years, from just 13 percent in 1930 to 32 percent in 1980, 37 percent in 1990, and 39 percent in 2002. (See Figure 4.1.) Worth noting is that, because the costs of restaurant meals include services (such as cooking and preparing the food, bringing it to your table, and washing dishes), as well as the cost of the food, money spent for food away from home does not purchase as much actual food as money spent on food eaten at home.

Overall spending on food increased at a slower rate during the 1990s than did overall household income. Expenditures for food increased 21 percent from 1993 to 2001, while before-tax income rose by 36 percent during the same period. (See Table 4.2.)

## DO AMERICANS SPEND MORE FOR FOOD THAN OTHERS?

In 1999 (the latest year for which comparable international data are available) Americans spent only 7.5 percent of their total personal consumption expenditures on food and alcoholic beverages consumed at home. (For international comparison, total personal consumption expenditures are used, instead of disposable personal income, because personal savings are seldom reported in the United Nations System of National Accounts, which furnished these data.) This compares with the 14 percent and 18 percent that Canada and the United Kingdom, respectively, spent on food and drink. (See Table 4.3.) The average Icelander, with the greatest per-person consumption expenditures outside of the United States ($17,813), spent 23 percent of total personal expenditures on food and alcoholic beverages.

In 1999, in less-developed countries, food spending accounted for a much larger proportion of personal income. In the Philippines, for example, a person had to work more than half of his or her time in order to pay for food, since food expenditures represented 51.3 percent of all personal consumption expenditures. (See Table 4.3.)

In relation to total personal consumption budgets, Americans spend the least on food. The United States, with its varied climate and huge expanses of arable land, is not as dependent on imported food as most countries. Also, the farm-to-consumer distribution system is highly successful at moving large quantities of perishable food long distances with minimum spoilage. Finally, many American farmers have the most current information and use state-of-the-art farming tools in their work.

## FOOD SPENDING IN AMERICAN HOUSEHOLDS

*Consumer Expenditures in 2001* (Bureau of Labor Statistics, Washington, D.C., 2003) found that, while

TABLE 4.1

**Food expenditures by families and individuals as a share of disposable personal income, selected years, 1930–2002**

| Years | Disposable personal income Billion dollars | Expenditures for food | | | | | |
|-------|---|---|---|---|---|---|---|
| | | At home[1] | | Away from home[2] | | Total[3] | |
| | | Billion dollars | Percent | Billion dollars | Percent | Billion dollars | Percent |
| 1930 | 74.6 | 15.8 | 21.2 | 2.3 | 3.1 | 18.1 | 24.3 |
| 1940 | 76.7 | 13.5 | 17.6 | 2.4 | 3.1 | 15.9 | 20.7 |
| 1950 | 210.6 | 35.7 | 16.9 | 7.6 | 3.6 | 43.3 | 20.5 |
| 1960 | 366.2 | 51.5 | 14.1 | 12.6 | 3.4 | 64.0 | 17.5 |
| 1970 | 736.5 | 75.5 | 10.3 | 26.4 | 3.6 | 102.0 | 13.8 |
| 1971 | 801.7 | 79.5 | 9.9 | 28.1 | 3.5 | 107.6 | 13.4 |
| 1972 | 868.6 | 86.0 | 9.9 | 31.3 | 3.6 | 117.3 | 13.5 |
| 1973 | 979.0 | 94.9 | 9.7 | 34.9 | 3.6 | 129.8 | 13.3 |
| 1974 | 1,072.3 | 107.3 | 10.0 | 38.5 | 3.6 | 145.8 | 13.6 |
| 1975 | 1,181.4 | 117.4 | 9.9 | 45.9 | 3.9 | 163.3 | 13.8 |
| 1976 | 1,299.9 | 125.1 | 9.6 | 52.6 | 4.0 | 177.7 | 13.7 |
| 1977 | 1,436.0 | 133.8 | 9.3 | 58.5 | 4.1 | 192.3 | 13.4 |
| 1978 | 1,614.8 | 147.3 | 9.1 | 67.5 | 4.2 | 214.8 | 13.3 |
| 1979 | 1,808.2 | 164.0 | 9.1 | 76.9 | 4.3 | 240.9 | 13.3 |
| 1980 | 2,019.8 | 180.8 | 8.9 | 85.2 | 4.2 | 266.0 | 13.2 |
| 1981 | 2,247.9 | 195.5 | 8.7 | 95.8 | 4.3 | 291.3 | 13.0 |
| 1982 | 2,406.8 | 201.0 | 8.4 | 104.5 | 4.3 | 305.5 | 12.7 |
| 1983 | 2,586.0 | 211.4 | 8.2 | 113.7 | 4.4 | 325.1 | 12.6 |
| 1984 | 2,887.6 | 224.0 | 7.8 | 121.9 | 4.2 | 345.8 | 12.0 |
| 1985 | 3,086.5 | 234.0 | 7.6 | 128.6 | 4.2 | 362.6 | 11.7 |
| 1986 | 3,262.5 | 242.7 | 7.4 | 137.9 | 4.2 | 380.6 | 11.7 |
| 1987 | 3,459.5 | 252.7 | 7.3 | 146.4 | 4.2 | 399.0 | 11.5 |
| 1988 | 3,752.4 | 268.3 | 7.2 | 157.5 | 4.2 | 425.9 | 11.3 |
| 1989 | 4,016.3 | 287.5 | 7.2 | 165.5 | 4.1 | 453.1 | 11.3 |
| 1990 | 4,293.6 | 302.5 | 7.0 | 177.7 | 4.1 | 480.3 | 11.2 |
| 1991 | 4,474.8 | 316.7 | 7.1 | 186.7 | 4.2 | 503.4 | 11.3 |
| 1992 | 4,754.6 | 316.5 | 6.7 | 190.8 | 4.0 | 507.3 | 10.7 |
| 1993 | 4,935.3 | 325.7 | 6.6 | 205.0 | 4.2 | 530.7 | 10.8 |
| 1994 | 5,165.4 | 339.7 | 6.6 | 215.8 | 4.2 | 555.5 | 10.8 |
| 1995 | 5,422.6 | 348.5 | 6.4 | 225.4 | 4.2 | 574.0 | 10.6 |
| 1996 | 5,677.7 | 364.1 | 6.4 | 232.9 | 4.1 | 597.0 | 10.5 |
| 1997 | 5,968.2 | 373.9 | 6.3 | 243.6 | 4.1 | 617.6 | 10.3 |
| 1998 | 6,355.6 | 388.2 | 6.1 | 257.1 | 4.0 | 645.3 | 10.2 |
| 1999 | 6,627.4 | 413.6 | 6.2 | 269.3 | 4.1 | 682.9 | 10.3 |
| 2000 | 7,120.2 | 435.9 | 6.1 | 287.7 | 4.0 | 723.6 | 10.2 |
| 2001 | 7,393.2 | 459.8 | 6.2 | 296.4 | 4.0 | 756.1 | 10.2 |
| 2002 | 7,815.5 | 481.4 | 6.2 | 309.3 | 4.0 | 790.7 | 10.1 |

[1] Food purchases from grocery stores and other retail outlets, including purchases made with food stamps, vouchers from the Women, Infants, and Children (WIC) program, and food produced and consumed on farms because the value of these foods is included in personal income. Excludes government donated foods.

[2] Purchases of meals and snacks by families and individuals, and food furnished to employees since it is included in personal income. Excludes food paid for by government and business, such as donated foods to schools, meals in prisons and other institutions, and expense-account meals.

[3] Total may not add due to rounding.

SOURCE: Adapted from "Table 7. Food expenditures by families and individuals as a share of disposable personal income," in *Consumption: Household Food Expenditures*, U.S. Department of Agriculture, Economic Research Service, Washington, DC, no date

FIGURE 4.1

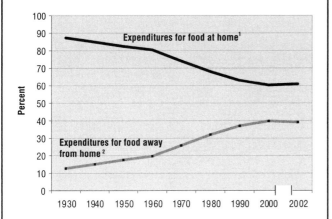

**Food expenditures at home and away from home as a percent of total food expenditures, selected years, 1930–2002**

¹ Food purchases from grocery stores and other retail outlets, including purchases made with food stamps, vouchers from the Women, Infants, and Children (WIC) program, and food produced and consumed on farms because the value of these foods is included in personal income. Excludes government donated foods.

² Purchases of meals and snacks by families and individuals, and food furnished to employees since it is included in personal income. Excludes food paid for by government and business, such as donated foods to schools, meals in prisons and other institutions, and expense-account meals.

SOURCE: Created by Information Plus from data in "Table 7. Food expenditures by families and individuals as a share of disposable personal income," in *Consumption: Household Food Expenditures,* U.S. Department of Agriculture, Economic Research Service, Washington, DC, no date

average annual expenditures rose 6.82 percent between 1999 and 2001, food expenditures rose somewhat less, at 5.76 percent. (See Table 4.4.)

Economists often describe food consumption as a relatively inelastic commodity. In other words, there is a limit to how much is spent on food. However, as income rises, the proportion spent on food declines and more money is spent on personal services and discretionary spending. Expenditures for food require a large share of income when income is relatively low.

The Economic Research Service (ERS) tracks the share of income that Americans spend on food. Over the years 1930–2002, expenditures on food eaten at home have decreased as a share of disposable income, while expenditures on food eaten away from home have increased. (See Figure 4.2.)

Not surprisingly, *Consumer Expenditures in 2001* reported that lower-income households spent the least money on food ($3,051), but spent the highest percentage of their disposable income (39.8 percent) on food. (See Figure 4.3. and Figure 4.4.) In contrast, the most affluent households—those with annual before-tax incomes of $70,000 or higher—spent the most money ($9,066) on food, but spent the lowest share (8.0 percent) of their total income on food.

## DO THE POOR PAY MORE FOR FOOD?

In designing food-assistance programs, the federal government generally considers providing sufficient food dollars to enable low-income households to buy nutritious foods. For example, the monthly food stamp benefits consider the cost of the USDA's Thrifty Food Plan (TFP), "a market basket of suggested amounts of foods that make up a nutritious diet and can be purchased at a relatively low cost." These food prices are what the government knows poor households actually spend. Moreover, food stamp benefits are adjusted each year to allow for changes in the costs of these food items. In 2002, for example, the average monthly benefit per person totaled $79.55, a 6.3 percent increase over 2001, and the largest annual increase in benefits in 11 years (*The Food Assistance Landscape,* ERS, Washington, D.C., March 2003).

In *Do the Poor Pay More for Food?: Item Selection and Price Differences Affect Low-Income Household Food Costs* (ERS, Washington, D.C., November 1997) Phillip R. Kaufman, James M. MacDonald, Steve M. Lutz, and David M. Smallwood analyzed a number of studies to compare what low-income households and other households paid for the same food items. The researchers evaluated store surveys of food prices, household food expenditures surveys, and information from the *Census of Retail Trade,* the *Census of Population,* and USDA food stamp redemption.

According to Kaufman and his group, some studies concluded that low-income households paid more for food items because they bought their foods in their neighborhoods—usually central cities or rural areas. Unlike suburban supermarkets, which generally offer lower prices, grocery stores in central cities and rural neighborhoods typically charge higher prices in order to cover higher business costs.

### Buying in Central City and Rural Areas

The findings above suggest that low-income shoppers are less likely to visit supermarkets, where prices are usually lower. However, the researchers found that the use of various food outlets by low-income persons was similar to that of the rest of the population, and in fact, the percentage of food spending in supermarkets by low-income households was similar to that of the general population. (See Figure 4.5.) For example, the USDA reported that 76.7 percent of food stamps were redeemed in supermarkets and other large retailers (warehouse clubs and mass merchandisers), while *Census of Retailing* data showed that supermarkets and other large retailers accounted for 77.7 percent of national food sales.

Researchers found, however, that food spending in supermarkets varied by location within urban areas. In urban locations overall, supermarkets accounted for 74.6

TABLE 4.2

## Household spending on food and alcoholic beverages, 1993–2001

(Annual spending per household in dollars)

| Items | 1993 | 1994 | 1995 | 1996 | 1997 | 1998 | 1999 | 2000 | 2001 |
|---|---|---|---|---|---|---|---|---|---|
| **Income:** | | | | | | | | | |
| Income before taxes | $34,868 | $36,181 | $36,918 | $38,014 | $39,926 | $41,622 | $43,951 | $44,649 | $47,507 |
| Income after taxes | 31,890 | 33,098 | 33,864 | 34,864 | 36,684 | 38,358 | 40,652 | 41,532 | 44,587 |
| **Average annual expenditures:** | $30,692 | $31,731 | $32,264 | $33,797 | $34,819 | $35,535 | $36,995 | $38,045 | $39,518 |
| **Food** | 4,399 | 4,411 | 4,505 | 4,698 | 4,801 | 4,810 | 5,031 | 5,158 | 5,321 |
| Food at home | 2,735 | 2,712 | 2,803 | 2,876 | 2,880 | 2,780 | 2,915 | 3,021 | 3,086 |
| Cereals and bakery products | 434 | 429 | 441 | 447 | 453 | 425 | 448 | 453 | 452 |
| Cereals and cereal products | 160 | 162 | 165 | 166 | 161 | 146 | 160 | 156 | 156 |
| Bakery products | 274 | 267 | 276 | 281 | 292 | 278 | 288 | 297 | 296 |
| Meats, poultry, fish, and eggs | 734 | 732 | 752 | 737 | 743 | 723 | 749 | 795 | 828 |
| Beef | 234 | 227 | 228 | 215 | 224 | 218 | 220 | 238 | 248 |
| Pork | 154 | 156 | 156 | 157 | 157 | 146 | 157 | 167 | 177 |
| Other meats | 98 | 94 | 104 | 99 | 96 | 92 | 97 | 101 | 102 |
| Poultry | 131 | 137 | 138 | 144 | 145 | 137 | 136 | 145 | 152 |
| Fish and seafood | 87 | 89 | 97 | 88 | 89 | 98 | 106 | 110 | 114 |
| Eggs | 30 | 30 | 30 | 34 | 33 | 32 | 32 | 34 | 35 |
| Dairy products | 295 | 289 | 297 | 312 | 314 | 301 | 322 | 325 | 332 |
| Fresh milk and cream | 128 | 127 | 123 | 132 | 128 | 120 | 122 | 131 | 136 |
| Other dairy products | 167 | 162 | 174 | 180 | 186 | 181 | 200 | 193 | 196 |
| Fruits and vegetables | 444 | 437 | 457 | 490 | 476 | 472 | 500 | 521 | 522 |
| Fresh fruits | 137 | 133 | 144 | 153 | 150 | 149 | 152 | 163 | 160 |
| Fresh vegetables | 132 | 135 | 137 | 147 | 143 | 145 | 149 | 159 | 162 |
| Processed fruits | 96 | 93 | 96 | 110 | 102 | 101 | 113 | 115 | 116 |
| Processed vegetables | 79 | 76 | 80 | 80 | 80 | 76 | 86 | 84 | 84 |
| Other food at home | 827 | 825 | 856 | 889 | 895 | 858 | 896 | 927 | 952 |
| Sugar and other sweets | 113 | 105 | 112 | 114 | 114 | 109 | 112 | 117 | 116 |
| Fats and oils | 78 | 79 | 82 | 83 | 81 | 77 | 84 | 83 | 87 |
| Miscellaneous foods | 365 | 362 | 377 | 391 | 403 | 388 | 420 | 437 | 455 |
| Nonalcoholic beverages | 225 | 233 | 240 | 252 | 245 | 231 | 242 | 250 | 256 |
| Food prepared for out of town trips | 46 | 46 | 45 | 49 | 52 | 53 | 39 | 40 | 38 |
| Food away from home | 1,664 | 1,698 | 1,702 | 1,823 | 1,921 | 2,030 | 2,116 | 2,137 | 2,235 |
| **Alcoholic beverages** | 268 | 278 | 277 | 309 | 309 | 309 | 318 | 372 | 349 |

SOURCE: Adapted from "Average annual expenditures and characteristics of all consumer units, Consumer Expenditure Survey, 1993-2001," in *Consumer Expenditure Survey,* U.S. Department of Labor, Bureau of Labor Statistics, Washington, DC [Online] http://www.bls.gov/cex/2001/standard/multiyr.pdf [accessed August 13, 2003]

percent of food stamp redemptions. However, within urban low-income neighborhoods, supermarkets accounted for only 64.3 percent of food stamp redemptions, and in low-income rural areas, supermarket food stamp redemptions accounted for just half (52.8 percent) of all redemptions. (See Table 4.5.) The authors surmised that many low-income persons had no means to get to the supermarkets and might have had to pay more at smaller food stores. Table 4.6 illustrates weekly food costs for various food plans. For a family of four (including two children aged 1–2 and 3–5) on the Thrifty Plan, weekly costs rose from $70.10 per week in 1990 to $91.10 per week in 2001, an increase of 30 percent. (See Table 4.6.)

According to data from the Food and Nutrition Service's *FY 2002 Annual Report,* supermarkets still account for the largest share of food stamp redemptions. (See Figure 4.6.) Supermarkets accounted for 84.8 percent of all food stamp redemptions in fiscal year 2002. Small- and medium-sized grocery stores accounted for 7.5 percent, and specialty food stores for 2.7 percent. Twenty-three percent of food stamp redemptions (valued at $4,025,046,802) occurred in the southeastern United States. Figure 4.7 and Figure 4.8 show the breakdown of food stamp redemptions and their value, by region.

### Spending Less

Despite the fact that low-income households may face higher food prices, their spending patterns help them offset these higher costs. Low-income households generally spend less than other households do for every food group, except fruit juices, vegetables, and eggs. Not surprisingly,

TABLE 4.3

## Personal consumption expenditures on food and alcoholic beverages at home in selected countries, 1999

| Country/Territory | Share of total personal consumption expenditures | | Personal consumption expenditures | |
|---|---|---|---|---|
| | Food[1] | Alcoholic beverages | Total[2] | Food |
| | Percent | | Dollars per person | |
| United States[3] | | | | |
| ERS estimate | 6.7 | 0.8 | 22,391 | 1,489 |
| PCE estimate | 8.6 | 1.8 | 22,391 | 1,923 |
| United Kingdom | 9.7 | 7.9 | 15,386 | 1,492 |
| Canada | 10.0 | 3.9 | 11,620 | 1,164 |
| Netherlands | 11.5 | 3.2 | 12,361 | 1,419 |
| Germany | 11.5 | 3.8 | 14,317 | 1,650 |
| Ireland | 12.1 | 6.3 | 11,696 | 1,418 |
| Sweden | 12.6 | 4.1 | 13,267 | 1,666 |
| Austria | 12.9 | 2.9 | 13,398 | 1,725 |
| Denmark | 12.9 | 4.8 | 16,159 | 2,086 |
| Belgium | 12.9 | 3.8 | 11,956 | 1,548 |
| Finland | 13.0 | 5.7 | 12,095 | 1,575 |
| Hong Kong S.A.R. | 13.4 | 0.8 | 12,463 | 1,669 |
| France | 14.6 | 3.5 | 13,140 | 1,921 |
| New Zealand[4] | 15.1 | NA | 9,180 | 1,387 |
| Puerto Rico | 15.2 | 3.6 | 8,970 | 1,360 |
| Italy | 15.2 | 2.5 | 11,276 | 1,718 |
| Korea, South | 16.5 | 2.4 | 4,731 | 782 |
| Greece | 17.9 | 4.8 | 8,353 | 1,491 |
| Iceland | 18.1 | 4.6 | 17,813 | 3,219 |
| Poland | 21.7 | 7.7 | 2,554 | 554 |
| Botswana | 29.8 | 13.4 | 916 | 273 |
| South Africa[4] | 30.8 | NA | 1,909 | 588 |
| Venezuela[5] | 33.4 | NA | 2,997 | 1,002 |
| Iran[4] | 35.1 | NA | 1,959 | 687 |
| Philippines | 51.3 | 2.1 | 696 | 357 |

NA = Not available.

[1] Includes nonalcoholic beverages.

[2] Consumer expenditures for goods and services.

[3] Two sets of figures are shown for the United States. The first set is based on the Economic Research Service (ERS) estimates of the U.S. food and beverage expenditures by families and individuals. The second set is based on the U.S. Department of Commerce estimates of personal consumption expenditures (PCE) for food and beverages, and is used by the United Nations (UN). The ERS estimate is lower than the PCE estimate partly because it excludes pet food, ice, and prepared feed, which are included in the PCE estimate. The ERS estimates also deduct more from grocery store sales for nonfoods, such as drugs and household supplies, in arriving at the estimate for food purchases for at-home consumption.

[4] Food includes nonalcoholic and alcoholic beverages and tobacco.

[5] Food includes nonalcoholic and alcoholic beverages.

SOURCE: Adapted from "Table 97. Share of personal consumption expenditures spent on food and alcoholic beverages consumed at home, by selected countries, 1999," in *Consumption: Household Food Expenditures,* U.S. Department of Agriculture, Economic Research Service, Washington, DC, no date

TABLE 4.4

## Average annual household expenditures by type, 1999 and 2001

| Item | 1999 | 2001 | Percent Change |
|---|---|---|---|
| **Number of households (000)** | 108,465 | 110,339 | |
| Income before taxes | $43,951 | $47,507 | |
| Averages: | | | |
| Age of reference person | 47.9 | 48.1 | |
| Number of persons in consumer unit | 2.5 | 2.5 | |
| Number of earners | 1.3 | 1.4 | |
| Number of vehicles | 1.9 | 1.9 | |
| Percent homeowners | 65 | 66 | |
| **Average annual expenditures** | $36,995 | $39,518 | 6.82 |
| Food | 5,031 | 5,321 | 5.76 |
| Food at home | 2,915 | 3,086 | 5.87 |
| Cereal and bakery products | 448 | 452 | 0.89 |
| Meats, poultry, fish, and eggs | 749 | 828 | 10.55 |
| Dairy products | 322 | 332 | 3.11 |
| Fruits and vegetables | 500 | 522 | 4.40 |
| Other foods | 896 | 952 | 6.25 |
| Food away from home | 2,116 | 2,235 | 5.62 |
| Alcoholic beverages | 318 | 349 | 9.75 |
| Housing | 12,057 | 13,011 | 7.91 |
| Shelter | 7,016 | 7,602 | 8.35 |
| Utilities, fuels, and public services | 2,377 | 2,767 | 16.41 |
| Household operations | 666 | 676 | 1.50 |
| Housekeeping supplies | 498 | 509 | 2.21 |
| Housefurnishings and equipment | 1,499 | 1,458 | -2.74 |
| Apparel and services | 1,743 | 1,743 | 0.00 |
| Transportation | 7,011 | 7,633 | 8.87 |
| Vehicle purchases | 3,305 | 3,579 | 8.29 |
| Gasoline and motor oil | 1,055 | 1,279 | 21.23 |
| Other vehicle expenses | 2,254 | 2,375 | 5.37 |
| Public Transportation | 397 | 400 | 0.76 |
| Health care | 1,959 | 2,182 | 11.38 |
| Entertainment | 1,891 | 1,953 | 3.28 |
| Personal care products and services | 408 | 485 | 18.87 |
| Reading | 159 | 141 | -11.32 |
| Education | 636 | 648 | 1.89 |
| Tobacco products and supplies | 300 | 308 | 2.67 |
| Miscellaneous | 867 | 750 | -13.49 |
| Cash contributions | 1,181 | 1,258 | 6.52 |
| Personal insurance and pensions | 3,436 | 3,737 | 8.76 |
| Life and other personal insurance | 394 | 410 | 4.06 |
| Pensions and Social Security | 3,042 | 3,326 | 9.34 |

SOURCE: Adapted from "Table A. Average annual expenditures on all consumer units and percent changes, Consumer Expenditures Survey, 1999–2001," in *Consumer Expenditures in 2001,* Report 966, U.S. Department of Labor, Bureau of Labor Statistics, Washington, DC, April 2003

## WHAT DID THE FOOD DOLLAR BUY IN 1999?

The money spent for food can be divided into the farm value (payment to farmers for the raw farm product) and the marketing bill. The marketing bill is the difference between the farm value of food produced on farms and the final cost to consumers at grocery stores and eating places. The marketing bill includes labor, packaging, transportation, depreciation, advertising, fuels and electricity, rent, taxes, and other expenses.

Consumers spent $618 billion on domestic farm foods in 1999. The estimated bill for marketing these foods was $498 billion, or 80 percent of total spending. The remaining $121 billion (20 percent) represents the farm value.

they often choose more economical foods and lower-quality items. The researchers also found that low-income households tend to get more nutrients for their money, compared with other households. Low-income households are more likely to buy unprocessed foods, such as beans and rice, and they are more likely to limit their purchases of convenience and prepared foods, which cost more money.

FIGURE 4.2

**Food expenditures at home and away from home as a percent of personal disposable income, selected years, 1930–2002**

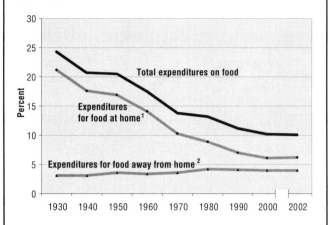

[1] Food purchases from grocery stores and other retail outlets, including purchases with food stamps, vouchers from the Women, Infants, and Children (WIC) program, and food produced and consumed on farms because the value of these foods is included in personal income. Excludes government donated foods.

[2] Purchases of meals and snacks by families and individuals, and food furnished to employees since it is included in personal income. Excludes food paid for by government and business, such as donated foods to schools, meals in prisons and other institutions, and expense-account meals.

SOURCE: Adapted from "Table 7. Food expenditures by families and individuals as a share of disposable personal income," in *Consumption: Household Food Expenditures,* U.S. Department of Agriculture, Economic Research Service, Washington, DC, no date

FIGURE 4.4

**Annual expenditures on food, by income level, 2001**

(In dollars)

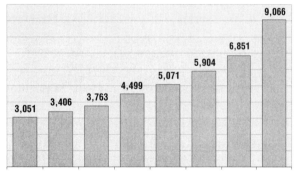

SOURCE: Compiled by Information Plus from data in "Table 2. Income before taxes: Average annual expenditures and characteristics, Consumer Expenditures Survey, 2001," in *Consumer Expenditures in 2001,* Report 966, U.S. Department of Labor, Bureau of Labor Statistics, Washington, DC, April 2003

FIGURE 4.3

**Annual expenditures on food as a percent of total income, by income level, 2001**

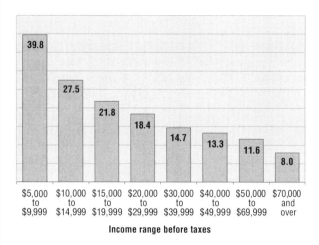

SOURCE: Compiled by Information Plus from data in "Table 2. Income before taxes: Average annual expenditures and characteristics, Consumer Expenditures Survey, 2001," in *Consumer Expenditures in 2001,* Report 966, U.S. Department of Labor, Bureau of Labor Statistics, Washington, DC, April 2003

In 1999, of the total food bill, labor costs comprised the greatest expense (39 percent). In fact, labor accounted for nearly half of all marketing costs. The farm value was the second-largest piece—20 percent of the total. Packaging was the third-largest component, accounting for 8 percent of food expenditures. (See Figure 4.9.)

## FOOD CONSUMPTION AND SPENDING TO 2020

Researchers at the Economic Research Service (ERS) of the USDA conducted a study to project future food consumption and spending ("America's Changing Appetite: Food Consumption and Spending to 2020," *FoodReview,* vol. 25, issue 1, Spring 2002). The study identified three major factors that will affect food consumption and spending over the first 20 years of the twenty-first century: age distribution of the population, changing ethnic diversity of the population, and personal income.

### Future Food Expenditures

Table 4.7 presents a summary of the report's finding on food expenditures. Total per capita expenditures for food are anticipated to increase 7.1 percent between 2000 and 2020 (seen under the column titled "Net"). This projection is primarily the result of anticipated increases in personal incomes, which are expected to cause food expenditures to rise 6.2 percent over the period. Researchers project that changes in the age distribution of the population will cause food expenditures to increase by an additional 1.0 percent. The effects of changes in the racial and ethnic composition of the population are projected to cause a slight (0.01

FIGURE 4.5

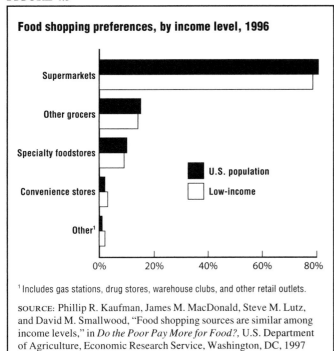

**Food shopping preferences, by income level, 1996**

Supermarkets
Other grocers
Specialty foodstores
Convenience stores
Other[1]

■ U.S. population
□ Low-income

0%   20%   40%   60%   80%

[1] Includes gas stations, drug stores, warehouse clubs, and other retail outlets.

SOURCE: Phillip R. Kaufman, James M. MacDonald, Steve M. Lutz, and David M. Smallwood, "Food shopping sources are similar among income levels," in *Do the Poor Pay More for Food?*, U.S. Department of Agriculture, Economic Research Service, Washington, DC, 1997

**TABLE 4.5**

**Food stamp redemptions by location and store type, 1996**
(Totals are in millions of dollars. Shares are in percentages.)

|  | Level of urbanization | | | |
| Redemptions | Urban | Mixed | Rural | All areas |
| --- | --- | --- | --- | --- |
| Total, all outlets | 12,912 | 6,714 | 1,317 | 20,944 |
| Share in supermarkets[1] | 74.6 | 84.1 | 58.9 | 76.7 |
| Total, low-income areas | 5,594 | 2,507 | 543 | 7,128 |
| Share in supermarkets[1] | 64.3 | 79.9 | 52.8 | 66.3 |

[1] Supermarkets are defined as outlets authorized to offer food stamps and having $2 million or more in annual sales.

SOURCE: Phillip R. Kaufman, James M. MacDonald, Steve M. Lutz, and David M. Smallwood, "Food stamp redemptions by location and store type," in *Do the Poor Pay More for Food?*, U.S. Department of Agriculture, Economic Research Service, Washington, DC, 1997

percent) decline in per capita food expenditures. This decline is based on variations in purchasing preferences by racial and ethnic group due to different dietary habits, practices, and traditions.

The decades-long trend toward more food expenditures being spent on food consumed away from home is projected to continue over the period 2000–2020. The expenditures on food at home are forecast to increase by 5.4 percent, while those for food away from home are expected to increase by 8.1 percent. (See Table 4.7.)

**Future Food Consumption**

The ERS report presents projections for food consumption, as well. Table 4.8 presents these data by specific food type. The net change in per capita beef consumption is an anticipated decline of 2.8 percent, while per capita fish consumption is projected to increase by 6.58 percent. When increases in population are calculated, these per capita figures all result in increased overall consumption, even in the cases in which per capita consumption declines, as is the case with beef. Although beef consumption per capita is expected to decline by 2.8 percent over the period 2000–2020, overall beef consumption is projected to rise by 14.65 percent as more people will be eating beef, even if at a slightly reduced rate per person.

The ERS report also highlights anticipated changes in food consumption based on increased educational level of the population as a whole. The report projects higher levels of formal educational attainment by the population by the year 2020. This higher educational attainment is expected to translate into higher consumption of fruits, vegetables, and yogurt, but lower consumption of beef, pork, eggs, and fried potatoes. (See Table 4.8.)

According to the report, increased demand for quality and variety in our food supplies is likely to outpace demand for increased quantities. During the first 20 years of the twenty-first century, average personal incomes are expected to rise and ethnic diversity of the population is projected to increase. So too, say the researchers at ERS, will our national desire for high-quality differentiated food products.

TABLE 4.6

## Weekly food cost, by type of family, 1990 and 2001

(In dollars. Assumes that food for all meals and snacks is purchased at the store and prepared at home.)

| Family type | December 1990 | | | | December 2001 | | | |
|---|---|---|---|---|---|---|---|---|
| | Thrifty-plan | Low-cost plan | Moderate-cost plan | Liberal-plan | Thrifty-plan | Low-cost plan | Moderate-cost plan | Liberal-plan |
| **Families** | | | | | | | | |
| Family of two: | | | | | | | | |
| 20–50 years | 48.10 | 60.60 | 74.70 | 92.70 | 62.60 | 80.20 | 98.70 | 122.80 |
| 51 years and over | 45.60 | 58.30 | 71.80 | 85.80 | 59.10 | 77.10 | 95.20 | 114.00 |
| Family of four: | | | | | | | | |
| Couple 20–50 years and children | | | | | | | | |
| 1–2 and 3–5 years | 70.10 | 87.30 | 106.60 | 131.00 | 91.10 | 115.30 | 141.00 | 173.40 |
| 6–8 and 9–11 years | 80.10 | 102.60 | 128.30 | 154.40 | 105.10 | 136.00 | 169.40 | 204.10 |
| **Individuals**[1] | | | | | | | | |
| Child: | | | | | | | | |
| 1–2 years | 12.70 | 15.40 | 18.00 | 21.80 | 16.40 | 20.20 | 23.80 | 28.90 |
| 3–5 years | 13.70 | 16.80 | 20.70 | 24.90 | 17.80 | 22.20 | 27.50 | 32.90 |
| 6–8 years | 16.60 | 22.20 | 27.90 | 32.50 | 22.10 | 29.60 | 36.80 | 42.80 |
| 9–11 years | 19.80 | 25.30 | 32.50 | 37.60 | 26.10 | 33.50 | 42.90 | 49.70 |
| Male: | | | | | | | | |
| 12–14 years | 20.60 | 28.60 | 35.70 | 42.00 | 27.10 | 37.90 | 47.00 | 55.30 |
| 15–19 years | 21.40 | 29.60 | 36.80 | 42.60 | 27.90 | 39.10 | 48.70 | 56.20 |
| 20–50 years | 22.90 | 29.30 | 36.60 | 44.30 | 29.80 | 38.90 | 48.40 | 58.60 |
| 51 years and over | 20.90 | 27.90 | 34.30 | 41.10 | 27.10 | 37.00 | 45.50 | 54.60 |
| Female: | | | | | | | | |
| 12–19 years | 20.80 | 24.80 | 30.10 | 36.30 | 27.10 | 32.70 | 39.60 | 47.90 |
| 20–50 years | 20.80 | 25.80 | 31.30 | 40.00 | 27.10 | 34.00 | 41.30 | 53.00 |
| 51 years and over | 20.60 | 25.10 | 31.00 | 36.90 | 26.60 | 33.10 | 41.00 | 49.00 |

[1] The costs given are for individuals in four-person families. For individuals in other size families, the following adjustments are suggested: one-person, add 20 percent; two-person, add 10 percent; three-person, add 5 percent; five- or six-person, subtract 6 percent; seven- (or more) person, subtract 10 percent.

SOURCE: "No. 694. Weekly Food Cost by Type of Family: 1990 and 2001," in *Statistical Abstract of the United States: 2002,* U.S. Census Bureau, Washington, DC, 2003

---

### FIGURE 4.6

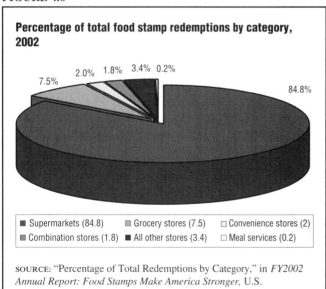

**Percentage of total food stamp redemptions by category, 2002**

- ■ Supermarkets (84.8)
- ▨ Grocery stores (7.5)
- ☐ Convenience stores (2)
- ■ Combination stores (1.8)
- ■ All other stores (3.4)
- ☐ Meal services (0.2)

SOURCE: "Percentage of Total Redemptions by Category," in *FY2002 Annual Report: Food Stamps Make America Stronger,* U.S. Department of Agriculture, Food and Nutrition Service, Benefit Redemption Division, Washington, DC, no date

### FIGURE 4.7

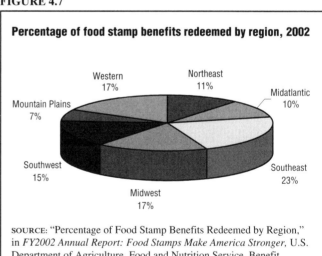

**Percentage of food stamp benefits redeemed by region, 2002**

SOURCE: "Percentage of Food Stamp Benefits Redeemed by Region," in *FY2002 Annual Report: Food Stamps Make America Stronger,* U.S. Department of Agriculture, Food and Nutrition Service, Benefit Redemption Division, Washington, DC, no date

FIGURE 4.8

## Value of food stamp benefits by region, 2002

Millions

| Region | Value |
|--------|-------|
| Northeast | $2,004,714,161 |
| Midatlantic | 1,829,001,979 |
| Southeast | 4,025,046,802 |
| Midwest | 3,003,324,389 |
| Southwest | 2,748,580,049 |
| Mountain Plains | 1,179,802,498 |
| Western | 3,083,831,502 |

SOURCE: Adapted from "Value of Food Stamp Benefits Redeemed by Region," in *FY2002 Annual Report: Food Stamps Make America Stronger,* U.S. Department of Agriculture, Food and Nutrition Service, Benefit Redemption Division, Washington, DC, no date

FIGURE 4.9

## The cost-per-dollar of marketing farm foods, 1999

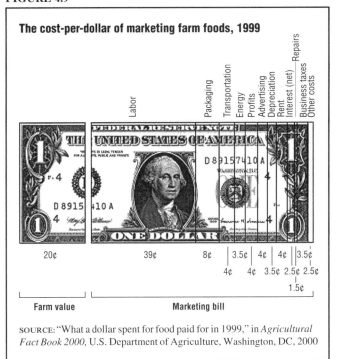

SOURCE: "What a dollar spent for food paid for in 1999," in *Agricultural Fact Book 2000,* U.S. Department of Agriculture, Washington, DC, 2000

TABLE 4.7

**Per capita effects of demographic variables on food expenditures, 2000–20**

(Percent)

| Food group | Per capita effects on food expenditures | | | | | Total effect of income, demographics, and population growth |
|---|---|---|---|---|---|---|
| | Age distribution | Regional distribution | Racial composition | Income growth | Net | |
| Total food | 1.0 | 0 | -.01 | 6.2 | 7.1 | 26.3 |
| Away from home | -1.0 | 0 | -.02 | 9.7 | 8.1 | 27.5 |
| At home | 2.2 | 0 | -.01 | 3.0 | 5.4 | 24.3 |
| Cereals and bakery products | 2.0 | 0 | .00 | 2.4 | 4.3 | 23.0 |
| Meats, poultry, fish, and eggs | 2.5 | 0 | .01 | 1.3 | 4.1 | 22.8 |
| Beef | 2.1 | 0 | .00 | 0.1 | 2.6 | 21.1 |
| Pork | 3.1 | 0 | .00 | 0.1 | 3.8 | 22.5 |
| Poultry | 0.1 | 0 | .00 | 1.6 | 3.4 | 21.9 |
| Fish | 3.1 | 0 | .00 | 1.9 | 6.2 | 25.2 |
| Dairy | 1.3 | 0 | .00 | 2.6 | 4.0 | 22.6 |
| Fruits | 3.7 | 0 | .00 | 4.2 | 8.1 | 27.5 |
| Vegetables | 3.6 | 0 | .00 | 3.3 | 7.2 | 26.5 |
| Sugars and sweets | 2.4 | 0 | .00 | 2.3 | 4.7 | 23.5 |
| Beverages | 0.4 | 0 | .00 | 2.6 | 2.7 | 21.1 |
| Fats and oils | 2.9 | 0 | .00 | 0.1 | 4.3 | 23.1 |
| Miscellaneous prepared foods | 1.1 | 0 | -.03 | 3.8 | 5.3 | 24.2 |

Note: Net effect is the combination of age, region, race, and income changes. Total effect is the net effect multiplied by changes in the U.S. population.

SOURCE: Noel Blisard et al., "Table 1—Per Capita Expenditures on Fruits and Vegetables Will Have Highest Increases as U.S. Population Ages, 2000–20," in "America's Changing Appetite: Food Consumption and Spending to 2020," *FoodReview*, vol. 25, issue 1, Spring 2002

**TABLE 4.8**

## Projected growth rate in quantities consumed per capita, 2000–20

(Percent)

| Commodity | Per capita effects on quantities consumed | | | | | | | Total effect of income, demographics, and population growth |
| | Age distribution | Regional distribution | Racial composition | Household type composition | Education distribution | Income growth | Net | |
|---|---|---|---|---|---|---|---|---|
| Meats: | | | | | | | | |
| Beef | -1.36 | -.06 | .58 | -.58 | -.48 | -.67 | -2.80 | 14.65 |
| Pork | .09 | -.50 | -.09 | -.42 | -.67 | -1.17 | -3.07 | 14.33 |
| Poultry | -1.26 | -.21 | 1.29 | -.21 | .03 | .50 | .38 | 18.41 |
| Fish | 1.76 | .30 | 2.17 | .66 | .26 | 1.11 | 6.58 | 25.71 |
| Other meat | -1.01 | -.30 | -.81 | -.36 | -.54 | -.79 | -3.76 | 13.52 |
| Eggs | 1.48 | .12 | 1.75 | -.28 | -.67 | -1.89 | .33 | 18.35 |
| Dairy: | | | | | | | | |
| Milk | -.73 | -.05 | -1.19 | .05 | .54 | -.15 | -1.19 | 16.54 |
| Cheese | -2.73 | -.01 | -1.38 | -.08 | .83 | 1.67 | -1.44 | 16.26 |
| Yogurt | .40 | -.18 | -1.56 | .50 | 1.04 | 1.39 | 2.08 | 20.41 |
| Vegetable oil | -.78 | .00 | -.19 | .21 | .29 | .77 | .40 | 18.42 |
| Fruit: | | | | | | | | |
| Citrus | .48 | -.62 | 2.48 | .60 | 2.13 | 1.87 | 7.40 | 26.68 |
| Apples | .95 | -.55 | 2.42 | .47 | 2.14 | 1.93 | 7.84 | 27.20 |
| Grapes | .59 | -.45 | 1.35 | .31 | 1.69 | 1.23 | 5.13 | 24.00 |
| Other fruit | 1.96 | .06 | 1.33 | .06 | 1.61 | 1.48 | 7.00 | 26.21 |
| Nuts and seeds | .18 | .42 | 1.67 | -.05 | .47 | .42 | 2.94 | 21.43 |
| Vegetables: | | | | | | | | |
| Fried potatoes | -5.76 | .06 | -1.72 | -.21 | -.82 | .19 | -8.60 | 7.81 |
| Other potatoes | 3.18 | -.76 | -2.19 | -.94 | .12 | -1.86 | -2.97 | 14.45 |
| Tomatoes | -.75 | .11 | .88 | -.10 | .18 | .86 | 1.25 | 19.43 |
| Lettuce | .68 | .10 | .37 | .84 | .71 | 2.12 | 5.09 | 23.96 |
| Other vegetables | 1.34 | -.04 | .54 | .41 | .57 | .65 | 3.61 | 22.21 |
| Grains | -.74 | -.04 | .88 | .16 | .45 | .63 | 1.49 | 19.72 |
| Sugar | -1.58 | -.06 | -.81 | .04 | .24 | .34 | -1.68 | 15.98 |

Note: Net effect is the combination of age, region, race, income, household type, and education. Total effect is the net effect multipied by changes in the U.S. population.

SOURCE: Noel Blisard, et. al. "Table 2–Growth in the Amount We Eat Will Be Less Than What We Spend, 2000–20," in "America's Changing Appetite: Food Consumption and Spending to 2020," *FoodReview*, vol. 25, issue 1, Spring 2002

# CHAPTER 5
# SUPERMARKET SHOPPING

The Food Marketing Institute (FMI), an association of food retailers and wholesalers, annually surveys shopping behavior. One of their publications is *Trends in the United States: Consumer Attitudes & the Supermarket, 2003* (Washington, D.C., 2003). Although designed for food retailers, the survey reveals much about American food shopping habits.

## SPENDING ON FOOD

From 1996 through 2002 grocery spending by families was fairly stable. In January 2003 the average weekly grocery bill was $91, up 5 percent from $87 in January 1999. (See Table 5.1.) Weekly grocery bills varied by the size and composition of the household, of course. While a family of five or more people spent an average of $138 per week on groceries in January 2003, a household of one spent less than half that: $52 per week. Households that earned $15,000 or less per year spent about $64 per week, while the wealthiest households, with incomes over $75,000, spent $117 a week on average. The highest rates of spending were in the East ($100), the lowest in the Midwest ($85). Suburbanites spent the most per week ($99), and those living in rural areas the least ($88).

Table 5.2 presents per-person weekly grocery expenses. In January 2003 single-person households spent more than twice as much for their groceries ($52 per person) than larger families ($24 per person in a family of five or more). This is likely because larger families can take advantage of bulk purchases. Men ($40) spent more than women ($35), although women who worked less than 20 hours a week spent slightly more ($36) than women who worked 20 or more hours a week ($34). Households without children spent more ($43) than those without children. Shoppers across the country spent about the same weekly amount per person, although shoppers in the West spent the least ($34).

## FREQUENCY OF SHOPPING AND USE OF STORE PRODUCTS AND SERVICES

In 2003 shoppers made an average of 2.2 trips per week to the supermarket. This has not changed much during the past 15 years.

FMI asked shoppers how often they used store products and services. Customers were most likely to participate in a frequent-shopper program (65 percent) or to buy private label or store brands (54 percent) at least once a week. Thirty-nine percent used the fresh-food deli, 28 percent used the in-store bakery, and 24 percent used the self-checkout/self-scanning services. (See Table 5.3.)

One in four shoppers purchased natural or organic foods, and 17 percent of shoppers bought gourmet or specialty foods, at least once a week. Thirty-four percent paid for their purchases with ATM or debit cards. With the wide use of fax machines and the Internet, people are beginning to use these conveniences to order their groceries. Ten percent of those surveyed reported ordering their groceries via the Internet. Online ordering of groceries at least once a month increased from 8 percent in January 2000 to 9 percent in January 2001, and then increased again, to 10 percent, in January 2002. (See Table 5.3.)

## EATING HOME-COOKED OR PREPARED MEALS

For the most part, the fast-food industry has remained the most popular source of takeout food eaten at home. (See Table 5.4.) While their share of the takeout food market experienced two periods of decline between 1996 and 2003 (from 48 percent in 1996 to 31 percent in 1999, and from 34 percent in 2000 to 25 percent in 2002) fast-food restaurants retained the largest share of the takeout food market in every year except 2002. In 2003 fast-food restaurants regained the lead. When shoppers bought food prepared outside the home and took it home in 2003, 33 percent reported buying it at fast-food restaurants. An

TABLE 5.1

**Average weekly family grocery expenses, by income, region, residence, and household size, 1996–2003**

Questions: About how much do you spend each week on groceries for your family across all grocery stores, not just (PRIMARY GROCERY STORE)? How much of this is spent at (STORE), your primary grocery store?

| | Jan. 2003 Base | Jan. 1996 $ | Jan. 1997 $ | Jan. 1998 $ | Jan. 1999 $ | Jan. 2000 $ | Jan. 2001 $ | Jan. 2002 $ | Jan. 2003 $ |
|---|---|---|---|---|---|---|---|---|---|
| | | | | | *Overall total* | | | | |
| **Total** | 1,000 | 82 | 83 | 87 | 87 | 85 | 91 | 88 | 91 |
| **Income** | | | | | | | | | |
| $15,000 or less | 109 | 71 | 66 | 70 | 68 | 60 | 69 | 60 | 64 |
| $15,001–$25,000 | 120 | 71 | 75 | 76 | 75 | 70 | 72 | 79 | 77 |
| $25,001–$35,000 | 124 | 76 | 79 | 80 | 81 | 75 | 87 | 82 | 92 |
| $35,001–$50,000 | 163 | 84 | 86 | 89 | 91 | 87 | 87 | 81 | 88 |
| $50,001–$75,000 | 154 | 93 | 94 | 101 | 98 | 102 | 103 | 103 | 101 |
| $75,001 or more | 157 | 113 | 107 | 117 | 118 | 123 | 119 | 111 | 117 |
| **Region** | | | | | | | | | |
| East | 190 | 91 | 87 | 88 | 93 | 89 | 90 | 96 | 100 |
| Midwest | 240 | 77 | 77 | 86 | 83 | 77 | 91 | 80 | 85 |
| South | 350 | 80 | 84 | 87 | 83 | 85 | 89 | 90 | 88 |
| West | 220 | 83 | 85 | 89 | 92 | 91 | 96 | 86 | 95 |
| **Residence** | | | | | | | | | |
| Urban | 218 | 81 | 82 | 80 | 82 | 87 | 90 | 87 | 90 |
| Suburban | 265 | 87 | 90 | 95 | 95 | 92 | 94 | 99 | 99 |
| Small town | 269 | 82 | 79 | 83 | 87 | 82 | 90 | 81 | 89 |
| Rural area | 222 | 79 | 82 | 91 | 83 | 84 | 89 | 84 | 88 |
| **Size of household** | | | | | | | | | |
| One | 195 | 47 | 48 | 51 | 51 | 49 | 55 | 52 | 52 |
| Two | 299 | 71 | 72 | 74 | 77 | 75 | 82 | 75 | 80 |
| Three-four | 362 | 93 | 97 | 100 | 102 | 101 | 105 | 101 | 104 |
| Five or more | 132 | 120 | 117 | 131 | 130 | 130 | 137 | 129 | 138 |
| | | | | | *Primary store total* | | | | |
| **Total** | 1,000 | 68 | 70 | 73 | 73 | 70 | 71 | 73 | 73 |
| **Income** | | | | | | | | | |
| $15,000 or less | 109 | 59 | 56 | 59 | 57 | 50 | 53 | 51 | 54 |
| $15,001–$25,000 | 120 | 59 | 64 | 63 | 66 | 60 | 59 | 64 | 65 |
| $25,001–$35,000 | 124 | 62 | 67 | 68 | 68 | 63 | 68 | 70 | 75 |
| $35,001–$50,000 | 163 | 71 | 73 | 75 | 75 | 72 | 68 | 68 | 73 |
| $50,001–$75,000 | 154 | 77 | 80 | 85 | 84 | 83 | 80 | 86 | 81 |
| $75,001 or more | 157 | 89 | 86 | 95 | 95 | 100 | 89 | 91 | 92 |
| **Region** | | | | | | | | | |
| East | 190 | 75 | 73 | 74 | 78 | 73 | 70 | 82 | 80 |
| Midwest | 240 | 63 | 66 | 72 | 70 | 64 | 71 | 66 | 71 |
| South | 350 | 67 | 71 | 73 | 70 | 71 | 71 | 77 | 73 |
| West | 220 | 67 | 70 | 73 | 76 | 73 | 74 | 69 | 77 |
| **Residence** | | | | | | | | | |
| Urban | 218 | 66 | 67 | 67 | 69 | 73 | 70 | 70 | 74 |
| Suburban | 265 | 71 | 75 | 79 | 79 | 75 | 73 | 83 | 84 |
| Small town | 269 | 67 | 68 | 69 | 72 | 68 | 69 | 67 | 70 |
| Rural area | 222 | 67 | 70 | 77 | 71 | 70 | 72 | 71 | 71 |
| **Size of household** | | | | | | | | | |
| One | 195 | 40 | 41 | 43 | 44 | 42 | 45 | 43 | 43 |
| Two | 299 | 59 | 60 | 61 | 64 | 63 | 66 | 64 | 67 |
| Three-four | 362 | 77 | 81 | 84 | 87 | 82 | 80 | 83 | 84 |
| Five or more | 132 | 97 | 97 | 109 | 106 | 105 | 104 | 106 | 110 |

SOURCE: "Table 12: Average weekly family grocery expenses, 1996–2003, by household size, income, region, and residence," in *Trends in the United States: Consumer Attitudes & the Supermarket, 2003,* Food Marketing Institute, Washington, DC, 2003

additional 15 percent bought takeout food from a restaurant, while 19 percent bought it in a supermarket.

Among the suppliers of takeout food eaten at home between 1996 and 2003, restaurants experienced the largest single-year decrease in market share. Between January 2001 and January 2002, the percentage of consumers using restaurants as sources of takeout food dropped 39 percent, from 23 percent to 14 percent. In comparison, eating establishments such as pizza parlors, bagel shops, and doughnut shops saw the sharpest increase in business, rising 460 percent (from 5 percent to 28 percent) during the same single-year period.

**TABLE 5.2**

## Average per person weekly grocery expenses, 1996–2003[1]

Questions: About how much do you spend each week on groceries for your family across all grocery stores, not just (PRIMARY GROCERY STORE)? How much of this is spent at (STORE), your primary grocery store?

| | Jan. 2003 Base | Jan. 1996 $ | Jan. 1997 $ | Jan. 1998 $ | Jan. 1999 $ | Jan. 2000 $ | Jan. 2001 $ | Jan. 2002 $ | Jan. 2003 $ |
|---|---|---|---|---|---|---|---|---|---|
| | | | | | *Overall total* | | | | |
| **Total** | 1,000 | 32 | 33 | 34 | 35 | 35 | 38 | 35 | 36 |
| **Gender** | | | | | | | | | |
| Men | 309 | 35 | 36 | 38 | 38 | 39 | 41 | 40 | 40 |
| Women | 691 | 31 | 32 | 33 | 35 | 33 | 37 | 32 | 35 |
| Work 20+ hrs/wk | 377 | 31 | 32 | 33 | 33 | 34 | 36 | 33 | 34 |
| Work 0-19 hrs/wk | 314 | 32 | 31 | 33 | 36 | 33 | 38 | 32 | 36 |
| **Region** | | | | | | | | | |
| East | 190 | 34 | 34 | 35 | 37 | 36 | 42 | 36 | 39 |
| Midwest | 240 | 31 | 31 | 33 | 32 | 33 | 37 | 32 | 35 |
| South | 350 | 32 | 33 | 34 | 36 | 36 | 38 | 35 | 37 |
| West | 220 | 33 | 34 | 38 | 39 | 36 | 38 | 35 | 34 |
| **Size of household** | | | | | | | | | |
| One | 195 | 47 | 48 | 51 | 50 | 49 | 55 | 52 | 52 |
| Two | 299 | 35 | 36 | 37 | 38 | 38 | 41 | 37 | 40 |
| Three-four | 362 | 27 | 28 | 29 | 29 | 29 | 30 | 29 | 30 |
| Five or more | 132 | 22 | 21 | 24 | 23 | 23 | 24 | 22 | 24 |
| **Type of household** | | | | | | | | | |
| With children | 426 | 26 | 26 | 28 | 28 | 27 | 30 | 27 | 29 |
| Aged 0 to 6 | 184 | 24 | 24 | 26 | 27 | 25 | 28 | 25 | 25 |
| Aged 7 to 17 | 334 | 27 | 29 | 30 | 28 | 27 | 29 | 27 | 29 |
| No children | 562 | 38 | 38 | 39 | 41 | 40 | 44 | 40 | 43 |
| | | | | | *Primary store total* | | | | |
| **Total** | 1,000 | 27 | 28 | 29 | 30 | 29 | 30 | 29 | 30 |
| **Gender** | | | | | | | | | |
| Men | 309 | 28 | 30 | 31 | 32 | 32 | 33 | 33 | 33 |
| Women | 691 | 26 | 27 | 28 | 30 | 28 | 30 | 27 | 29 |
| Work 20+ hrs/wk | 377 | 26 | 27 | 28 | 28 | 29 | 29 | 28 | 28 |
| Work 0-19 hrs/wk | 314 | 26 | 26 | 28 | 31 | 27 | 21 | 27 | 30 |
| **Region** | | | | | | | | | |
| East | 190 | 29 | 29 | 29 | 33 | 29 | 34 | 31 | 32 |
| Midwest | 240 | 63 | 66 | 72 | 70 | 64 | 71 | 66 | 71 |
| South | 350 | 26 | 28 | 28 | 31 | 30 | 31 | 30 | 31 |
| West | 220 | 27 | 28 | 31 | 31 | 29 | 29 | 28 | 28 |
| **Size of household** | | | | | | | | | |
| One | 195 | 40 | 41 | 43 | 43 | 42 | 45 | 43 | 44 |
| Two | 299 | 29 | 30 | 31 | 32 | 31 | 33 | 32 | 33 |
| Three-four | 362 | 22 | 24 | 24 | 25 | 24 | 23 | 24 | 25 |
| Five or more | 132 | 18 | 18 | 20 | 20 | 19 | 18 | 18 | 19 |
| **Type of household** | | | | | | | | | |
| With children | 426 | 21 | 22 | 23 | 24 | 22 | 23 | 22 | 23 |
| Aged 0 to 6 | 184 | 20 | 21 | 22 | 23 | 20 | 22 | 21 | 20 |
| Aged 7 to 17 | 334 | 22 | 24 | 25 | 24 | 22 | 23 | 22 | 23 |
| No children | 562 | 32 | 33 | 33 | 35 | 34 | 35 | 34 | 36 |

[1] Calculated from average weekly grocery expenses and household size.

Note: Respondents who couldn't provide data were omitted from the calculation.

SOURCE: "Table 13: Average per person weekly grocery expenses, 1996–2003[1]," in *Trends in the United States: Consumer Attitudes & the Supermarket, 2003,* Food Marketing Institute, Washington, DC, 2003

In 2003, 19 percent of shoppers were more likely to buy prepared meals from a supermarket than from any other food establishment. (See Table 5.5.) Single-person households (26 percent), low-income households (25 percent), persons living in the West (25 percent), and those not married (24 percent) used supermarket takeout food most often. Men (23 percent) and persons aged 50–64 (23 percent) also were more likely to use the supermarket as

a source of takeout food. In fact, men were more likely to use the supermarket for this purpose than were women for all but one year between 1996 and 2003. Families of five or more persons (23 percent) and households with incomes of $15,001–$25,000 (23 percent) also were likely to use the supermarket as their main source of takeout meals eaten at home. The survey also found that, in most of the years between 1996 and 2003, women who worked 20 hours or

**TABLE 5.3**

## Shoppers' use of store products and services, 1996–2003

Question: How often do you use/purchase (ITEM) at (STORE) your primary grocery store?

Base: Those who say their supermarkets have the product or service

| | At least once a month | | | | | | | | | Jan. 2003 | | | | |
| --- | --- | --- | --- | --- | --- | --- | --- | --- | --- | --- | --- | --- | --- | --- |
| | Jan. 2003 Base | Jan. 1996 % | Jan. 1997 % | Jan. 1998 % | Jan. 1999 % | Jan. 2000 % | Jan. 2001 % | Jan. 2002 % | Jan. 2003 % | At least once a week % | 1-3 times a month % | Less than once a month % | Never % | Not sure % |
| Private label or store brands | 901 | 88 | 86 | 86 | 84 | 85 | 82 | 87 | 87 | 54 | 33 | 7 | 5 | 0 |
| Frequent shopper program or savings club | 505 | 70 | 81 | 84 | 85 | 88 | 86 | 87 | 84 | 65 | 19 | 5 | 10 | 0 |
| Fresh-food deli or delicatessen | 895 | 75 | 76 | 77 | 72 | 73 | x | 76 | 76 | 39 | 37 | 16 | 7 | 0 |
| In-store bakery | 876 | 73 | 74 | 69 | 69 | 68 | x | 66 | 63 | 28 | 35 | 25 | 11 | 0 |
| Ethnic foods[2] | 839 | x | x | x | x | x | 57 | 60 | 62 | 23 | 39 | 22 | 17 | 0 |
| Gas pumps/gasoline | 176 | x | x | x | 53 | 44 | 50 | 54 | 60 | 26 | 34 | 12 | 29 | 0 |
| Fresh seafood section | 746 | 48 | 50 | 49 | 49 | 51 | x | 51 | 55 | 22 | 33 | 22 | 23 | 0 |
| Accepts ATM or debit cards for purchases | 845 | 35 | 39 | 37 | 42 | 40 | 49 | 50 | 54 | 34 | 20 | 7 | 40 | 0 |
| Self-checkout/self-scanning | 288 | x | x | x | 63 | 63 | 53 | 49 | 53 | 24 | 29 | 12 | 35 | 0 |
| Natural or organic foods | 698 | 58 | 58 | 59 | 54 | 54 | 48 | 47 | 48 | 25 | 23 | 21 | 31 | 0 |
| Gourmet or specialty foods[2] | 771 | x | x | x | x | x | 46 | 49 | 45 | 17 | 28 | 27 | 27 | 1 |
| In-store pharmacy that fills prescriptions | 570 | 28 | 28 | 25 | 26 | 23 | 21 | 28 | 29 | 6 | 23 | 19 | 51 | 0 |
| Video rental[1] | 238 | 36 | 32 | 29 | 24 | 20 | 20 | 24 | 24 | 5 | 18 | 11 | 66 | 0 |
| In-store bank with a teller | 420 | 30 | 33 | 26 | 29 | 22 | 22 | 24 | 19 | 7 | 12 | 9 | 72 | 0 |
| Sit down eating area | 411 | x | x | x | x | x | 18 | 15 | 17 | 5 | 12 | 23 | 59 | 1 |
| Coffee bar[1] | 329 | 32 | 33 | 36 | 24 | 21 | 20 | 21 | 16 | 11 | 15 | 9 | 64 | NA |
| Child care | 50 | 24 | 21 | 20 | 15 | 3 | 11 | 13 | 11 | 6 | 5 | 4 | 86 | NA |
| Online ordering | 143 | x | x | x | x | 8 | 9 | 10 | 10 | 5 | 5 | 6 | 85 | 0 |
| Home delivery | 111 | 2 | 7 | 3 | 12 | 7 | 7 | 10 | 10 | 5 | 5 | 1 | 88 | NA |
| Juice bar | x | x | x | x | x | 42 | x | 20 | x | x | x | x | x | x |
| Accepts credit cards for purchases | x | 19 | 23 | 22 | 27 | 27 | x | x | x | x | x | x | x | x |
| Dry cleaner | x | 10 | 8 | 15 | 12 | 8 | x | x | x | x | x | x | x | x |
| Floral department | x | 20 | 22 | 20 | 17 | 18 | x | x | x | x | x | x | x | x |
| Gourmet, specialty or ethnic foods[2] | x | 47 | 53 | 53 | 54 | 52 | x | x | x | x | x | x | x | x |
| In-store restaurant | x | x | 32 | 30 | 21 | 28 | x | x | x | x | x | x | x | x |
| Nutrition and health information for shoppers | x | 58 | 58 | 63 | 63 | 57 | x | x | x | x | x | x | x | x |
| Photo finishing department | x | 21 | 27 | 20 | 20 | 18 | x | x | x | x | x | x | x | x |

NOTE: May not add to 100 percent due to rounding.

x = Not reported as a category that year.

* = Less than 0.5 percent.

[1] Change in question wording in 2001.

[2] Change in question working in 2002.

SOURCE: "Table 15: Shoppers' use of store products and services, 1996-2003," in *Trends in the United States: Consumer Attitudes & the Supermarket, 2003*, Food Marketing Institute, Washington, DC, 2003

more per week were less likely to use the supermarket as a source of takeout meals eaten at home than were women who worked fewer hours.

## CONCERN ABOUT NUTRITION

The 2003 *Trends* survey found a steady decline during the late 1990s in the number of people who were concerned about the nutritional content of their diet, a decline that began to reverse after reaching a low of 46 percent in 2000. By 2003 more than half of respondents (53 percent) reported such a concern.

The survey also found that, while concern about some aspects of the nutritional content of food dropped in the one-year period from January 2002 to January 2003 (concern about cholesterol content dropped from 16 percent to 13 percent; about nutritional value, from 15 percent to 12

percent; and about chemical additives, from 9 percent to 7 percent), concern about most aspects of the nutritional content of food remained unchanged. (See Table 5.6.) There was a slight increase in concern about calorie content, from 13 percent to 14 percent.

Among shoppers who were very or somewhat concerned about the nutritional content of their foods, 49 percent were concerned about fat content, the same percentage as in 2002, but up 3 percentage points from 2000. (Concern about the fat content of food fluctuated between 1996 and 2003, with a high of 60 percent in 1996 and a low of 46 percent in 2000.) Concern about the sugar content of foods, however, has doubled since 1999, when 9 percent of shoppers surveyed expressed concern, to 18 percent in 2003, an increase likely prompted by awareness of the growing prevalence of obesity. Concern about the calorie

TABLE 5.4

**Sources of takeout food, 1996–2003**

Question: Now I would like you to think about all meals that are eaten at home, but not prepared at home, are they purchased most often from a fast-food restaurant, a restaurant, a supermarket, convenience store, gourmet or specialty store, or from some other place? (Single answer accepted.)

| | Jan. 1996 % | Jan. 1997 % | Jan. 1998 % | Jan. 1999 % | Jan. 2000 % | Jan. 2001 % | Jan. 2002 % | Jan. 2003 % |
|---|---|---|---|---|---|---|---|---|
| Base | 1,001 | 1,018 | 1,002 | 1,002 | 1,000 | 1,000 | 1,001 | 1,000 |
| Fast-food restaurant | 48 | 41 | 37 | 31 | 34 | 32 | 25 | 33 |
| Restaurant | 25 | 21 | 20 | 21 | 22 | 23 | 14 | 15 |
| Supermarket | 12 | 22 | 20 | 20 | 18 | 20 | 17 | 19 |
| Deli/pizza parlor/bagel shop/coffee shop/donut shop | 4 | 5 | 7 | 11 | 7 | 5 | 28 | 12 |
| Some other place | 2 | 0 | 4 | 2 | 2 | 5 | 6 | 3 |
| Gourmet or specialty store | 3 | 7 | 4 | 5 | 5 | 3 | 3 | 7 |
| Convenience store | 1 | 1 | 1 | 1 | 1 | 1 | 1 | 1 |
| None | 2 | 3 | 5 | 8 | 10 | 8 | 3 | 0 |
| Don't know | 2 | 0 | 2 | 1 | 2 | 4 | 4 | 7 |

NOTE: Modifications to question wording occurred year to year. Deli/pizza parlor/bagel shop/donut shop, etc. was an unaided response, in years other than 2002. However, in 2002 these venues were probed specifically. For trending purposes, 2003 should be compared with 2001.

SOURCE: "Table 33: Sources of Takeout Food, 1996–2003," in *Trends in the United States: Consumer Attitudes & the Supermarket, 2003*, Food Marketing Institute, Washington, DC, 2003

content of foods has increased 75 percent, from 8 percent in 1999 to 14 percent in 2003.

The number of surveyed shoppers who felt that their diets could be a lot healthier or somewhat healthier than their present diet ranged from 68 percent to 70 percent between 1999 and 2003, according to the *Trends* survey. In January 2003 most shoppers (98 percent) claimed they were taking actions to ensure that their diet was healthy. Somewhat under three-quarters (71 percent) reported eating more fruits and vegetables. (See Table 5.7.) Nearly a quarter said they ate less fats and oils (24 percent) and 18 percent said they ate less meat. Other dietary initiatives included eating fewer snacks or junk foods and less sugar and salt.

TABLE 5.5

## Use of supermarket as a source of meals eaten at home but not prepared at home, 1996–2003

Question: Now I would like you to think about all the meals that are eaten at home, but not prepared at home, are they purchased most often from a fast-food restaurant, a restaurant, a supermarket, convenience store, gourmet or specialty store, or from some other place?

| | | | | | Use supermarket most often for takeout food | | | | |
|---|---|---|---|---|---|---|---|---|---|
| | Jan. 2003 Base | Jan. 1996 % | Jan. 1997 % | Jan. 1998 % | Jan. 1999 % | Jan. 2000 % | Jan. 2001 % | Jan. 2002 % | Jan. 2003 % |
| **Total** | 1,000 | 12 | 22 | 20 | 20 | 18 | 20 | 17 | 19 |
| **Gender** | | | | | | | | | |
| Men | 309 | 13 | 28 | 23 | 24 | 14 | 21 | 19 | 23 |
| Women | 691 | 12 | 19 | 19 | 17 | 19 | 20 | 16 | 18 |
| Work 20+ hrs/wk | 377 | 8 | 18 | 18 | 15 | 19 | 18 | 14 | 19 |
| Work 0-19 hrs/wk | 314 | 17 | 21 | 19 | 20 | 19 | 23 | 17 | 16 |
| **Age** | | | | | | | | | |
| 15 to 24[1] | 95 | 16 | 29 | 21 | 21 | 15 | 19 | 18 | 17 |
| 25 to 39 | 250 | 8 | 18 | 21 | 19 | 16 | 20 | 13 | 15 |
| 40 to 49 | 257 | 10 | 18 | 16 | 19 | 14 | 17 | 14 | 19 |
| 50 to 64 | 256 | 14 | 22 | 19 | 19 | 20 | 20 | 20 | 23 |
| 65 and older | 104 | 25 | 32 | 26 | 21 | 25 | 23 | 18 | 21 |
| **Income** | | | | | | | | | |
| $15,000 or less | 109 | 18 | 24 | 22 | 30 | 23 | 28 | 17 | 25 |
| $15,001-$25,000 | 120 | 12 | 21 | 29 | 20 | 14 | 23 | 23 | 23 |
| $25,001-$35,000 | 124 | 14 | 23 | 22 | 19 | 19 | 17 | 22 | 20 |
| $35,001-$50,000 | 163 | 12 | 19 | 19 | 15 | 20 | 19 | 11 | 15 |
| $50,001-$75,000 | 154 | 10 | 18 | 17 | 19 | 11 | 23 | 15 | 16 |
| $75,001 or more | 157 | 5 | 21 | 14 | 16 | 13 | 15 | 14 | 15 |
| **Region** | | | | | | | | | |
| East | 190 | x | 22 | 16 | 19 | 17 | 19 | 19 | 16 |
| Midwest | 240 | x | 25 | 22 | 19 | 17 | 17 | 15 | 20 |
| South | 350 | x | 18 | 19 | 19 | 16 | 20 | 14 | 17 |
| West | 220 | x | 22 | 23 | 21 | 21 | 24 | 20 | 25 |
| **Marital status** | | | | | | | | | |
| Married | 579 | 12 | 19 | 19 | 17 | 16 | 18 | 15 | 17 |
| Not married | 405 | 14 | 25 | 22 | 24 | 20 | 22 | 18 | 24 |
| **Size of household** | | | | | | | | | |
| One | 195 | 14 | 32 | 25 | 25 | 23 | 23 | 20 | 26 |
| Two | 299 | 15 | 22 | 19 | 18 | 16 | 20 | 17 | 18 |
| Three–four | 362 | 10 | 18 | 18 | 21 | 18 | 18 | 13 | 17 |
| Five or more | 132 | 10 | 18 | 20 | 9 | 15 | 22 | 20 | 23 |

Note: Modifications to question wording occurred year to year. Deli/pizza parlor/bagel shop/coffee shop/donut shop, etc. was an unaided response in years other than 2002. However, in 2002 these venues were probed specifically. For trending purposes, 2003 should be compared with 2001.

x = Not reported as a category in that year.

[1] Prior to 2000, the youngest age category was 18-24 years.

SOURCE: "Table 34: Use of supermarket as a source of meals eaten at home but not prepared at home, 1996-2003," in *Trends in the United States: Consumer Attitudes & the Supermarket, 2003,* Food Marketing Institute, Washington, DC, 2003

TABLE 5.6

## Nature of concern about nutritional content, 1996–2003

Question: What is it about the nutritional content of what you eat that concerns you most? What other concerns do you have? (Verbatim responses coded to categories listed below; multiple answers accepted.)

Base: 870 shoppers who are very or somewhat concerned about the nutritional content of the food they eat.

| | Jan. 1996 | Jan. 1997 | Jan. 1998 | Jan. 1999 | Jan. 2000 | Jan. 2002 | Jan. 2003 |
| --- | --- | --- | --- | --- | --- | --- | --- |
| | % | % | % | % | % | % | % |
| Fat content, low fat | 60 | 56 | 59 | 50 | 46 | 49 | 49 |
| Sugar content/less sugar | 12 | 11 | 12 | 9 | 13 | 18 | 18 |
| Salt/sodium content, less salt | 28 | 23 | 24 | 16 | 17 | 17 | 17 |
| Calories/low calorie | 12 | 10 | 11 | 8 | 9 | 13 | 14 |
| Cholesterol levels | 26 | 20 | 20 | 18 | 17 | 16 | 13 |
| Food/nutritional value | 6 | 11 | 12 | 17 | 12 | 15 | 12 |
| Chemical additives | 7 | 6 | 6 | 8 | 7 | 9 | 7 |
| Preservatives | 8 | 7 | 5 | 6 | 4 | 7 | 7 |
| Desire to be healthy/eat what's good for us | 5 | 3 | 3 | 3 | 6 | x | x |
| Vitamin/mineral content | 12 | 5 | x | 2 | 3 | x | x |
| Balanced diet | 3 | 3 | 1 | 1 | 2 | x | x |
| Carbohydrate content | 1 | 1 | 2 | 1 | 2 | x | x |
| Freshness/purity/no spoilage | 5 | 4 | 4 | 3 | 3 | x | x |
| Protein value | 1 | 1 | 1 | 2 | 1 | x | x |
| Fiber content | 2 | 1 | 2 | 1 | 1 | x | x |
| Nothing | 1 | 1 | 1 | 3 | 3 | 3 | 3 |
| Other | 5 | 6 | 1 | 5 | 6 | 16 | 18 |
| Don't know/no answer | 4 | 4 | 3 | 4 | 7 | 5 | 4 |

x = Not reported as a category in that year.

SOURCE: "Table 38: Nature of concern about nutritional content, 1996-2003," in *Trends in the United States: Consumer Attitudes & the Supermarket, 2003*, Food Marketing Institute, Washington, DC, 2003

TABLE 5.7

## Changes for healthier diet, 1996–2003

Question: What, if anything, are you eating more of to ensure that your diet is healthy? What, if anything, are you eating less of to ensure that your diet is healthy? (Verbatim responses coded to categories listed below; multiple responses accepted.)

| | Jan. 1996 % | Jan. 1997 % | Jan. 1998 % | Jan. 1999 % | Jan. 2000 % | Jan. 2002 % | Jan. 2003 % |
|---|---|---|---|---|---|---|---|
| Base | 1,007 | 1,011 | 1,000 | 1,004 | 1,000 | 1,001 | 1,001 |
| Any dietary change (NET) | 97 | 93 | 90 | 95 | 93 | 96 | 98 |
| More fruits/vegetables | 77 | 78 | 78 | 71 | 68 | 68 | 71 |
| Less fats/oils | 42 | 35 | 32 | 28 | 23 | 21 | 24 |
| Less junk food/snack food | 18 | 24 | 25 | 22 | 18 | 19 | 23 |
| Less sugar | 20 | 16 | 18 | 14 | 17 | 24 | 23 |
| Less meats/red meats | 32 | 35 | 33 | 27 | 22 | 20 | 18 |
| More chicken/turkey/white meat | 12 | 13 | 12 | 10 | 9 | 10 | 11 |
| More whole grains | x | x | x | 4 | 4 | 12 | 9 |
| More fiber | x | x | x | 4 | 3 | -- | -- |
| Less fried foods | x | x | x | 6 | 7 | 8 | 9 |
| More fish | x | x | x | 5 | 7 | 6 | 7 |
| Less bread | 2 | 1 | 5 | 3 | 3 | 6 | 7 |
| More water/bottled water | * | 2 | 3 | 2 | 2 | 5 | 6 |
| Less salt/sodium/food low in salt/sodium | 13 | 11 | 10 | 9 | 8 | 6 | 6 |
| More low fat or skim milk products | x | x | x | 5 | 5 | 5 | 5 |
| Less soda | 2 | 2 | 2 | 2 | 3 | 5 | 4 |
| More vitamin/mineral supplements/pills | 2 | 2 | 2 | 2 | 2 | 5 | 4 |
| More protein | 2 | 1 | 2 | 2 | 3 | 4 | 4 |
| Less dairy products | x | x | x | 7 | 5 | 6 | 4 |
| More starches (pasta, beans, rice) | 6 | 3 | 3 | 4 | 2 | 2 | 3 |
| More fresh foods | 3 | 2 | 2 | 2 | 1 | 3 | 3 |
| More calcium | 2 | 1 | 2 | 1 | 1 | 2 | 3 |
| Less cholesterol/food low in cholesterol | 6 | 4 | 4 | 4 | 3 | 3 | 3 |
| Less prepared/processed foods | 3 | 3 | 4 | 1 | 3 | 2 | 3 |
| Less calories/food low in calories | 1 | 1 | 1 | 1 | 1 | 1 | 2 |
| More juices | 2 | 1 | 3 | 2 | 3 | 4 | 2 |
| More balanced diet/more variety | 1 | 3 | 3 | 3 | 1 | 2 | 2 |
| More organically grown/natural foods | 1 | 1 | * | 1 | 1 | 1 | 1 |
| More foods high in vitamins/minerals | 1 | 1 | 1 | * | 1 | 1 | 1 |
| More salads | x | x | x | x | 2 | x | x |
| More meat | x | x | x | 1 | 1 | x | x |
| Less carbohydrates | x | x | x | 1 | 1 | x | x |

x = Not reported as a category in that year.
* = Less than 0.5 percent.
-- = Blank in the source table without explanation.
Note: More fiber/whole grains combined into one category in 2002.

SOURCE: "Table 43: Changes for healthier diet, 1996-2003," in *Trends in the United States: Consumer Attitudes & the Supermarket, 2003*, Food Marketing Institute, Washington, DC, 2003

CHAPTER 6

# FOOD LABELING

## HISTORY

In 1938 Congress enacted the Federal Food, Drug, and Cosmetic Act (52 Stat 1040), at a time when illnesses caused by nutritional deficiencies (for example, rickets, a bone disease caused by inadequate intake of vitamin D) were a common problem for the American people. The act required that the label of every processed, packaged food contain the name of the food, its net weight, and the name and address of the manufacturer or distributor. Certain products also had to carry a list of ingredients. The law further prohibited false or misleading statements in food labeling. In 1957, under the Poultry Products Inspection Act (PL 85-172), the U.S. Department of Agriculture (USDA) began regulating the labeling of poultry products.

Although some scientific evidence pointed to the possible link between blood cholesterol and heart disease during the 1950s, it was not until 1965 that the Food and Drug Administration (FDA) permitted fat and cholesterol statements on food labels. Products could carry the statement "Information on fat and cholesterol is provided for individuals who, on the advice of a physician, are modifying their dietary intake of fat and cholesterol."

In 1969 the White House Conference on Food, Nutrition, and Health studied the American diet to determine deficiencies. The conference recommended that the federal government establish a system for providing nutrient content information on food labels to promote public awareness of proper nutrition. In 1973, the FDA, for the first time, ordered that fortified foods (foods with one or more added nutrients) and those making a health claim had to carry nutrition labeling. For all other food products, nutrition labeling was voluntary. Manufacturers that provided nutrient content information on their food labels were required to list the calorie content as well as the grams of protein, carbohydrate, and fat in a single serving. The FDA

**FIGURE 6.1**

**A revised nutrition facts label**

**Nutrition Facts**

Serving Size 1 cup (228g)
Servings Per Container 2

| **Amount Per Serving** | |
|---|---|
| **Calories** 260 | Calories from Fat 120 |
| | **% Daily Value*** |
| **Total Fat** 13g | **20%** |
| Saturated Fat 5g | **25%** |
| *Trans* Fat 2g | |
| **Cholesterol** 30mg | **10%** |
| **Sodium** 660mg | **28%** |
| **Total Carbohydrate** 31g | **10%** |
| Dietary Fiber 0g | **0%** |
| Sugars 5g | |
| **Protein** 5g | |

| | | |
|---|---|---|
| Vitamin A 4% | * | Vitamin C 2% |
| Calcium 20% | * | Iron 4% |

* Percent Daily Values are based on a 2,000 calorie diet. Your daily values may be higher or lower depending on your calorie needs:

| | Calories: | 2,000 | 2,500 |
|---|---|---|---|
| Total Fat | Less than | 65g | 80g |
| Sat Fat | Less than | 20g | 25g |
| Cholesterol | Less than | 300mg | 300mg |
| Sodium | Less than | 2,400mg | 2,400mg |
| Total Carbohydrate | | 300g | 375g |
| Dietary Fiber | | 25g | 30g |

Calories per gram:
Fat 9 * Carbohydrate 4 * Protein 4

SOURCE: "Examples of Revised Nutrition Facts Panel Listing Trans Fat," U.S. Food and Drug Administration, Center for Food Safety and Applied Nutrition, Office of Nutritional Products, Labeling and Dietary Supplements, Washington, DC, July 9, 2003

also required a list of seven vitamins and minerals. See Figure 6.1 for a sample FDA nutrition label.

In the late 1970s nutritionists and other experts who recognized the relationship between dietary practices and

FIGURE 6.2

**How to read a nutrition facts label**

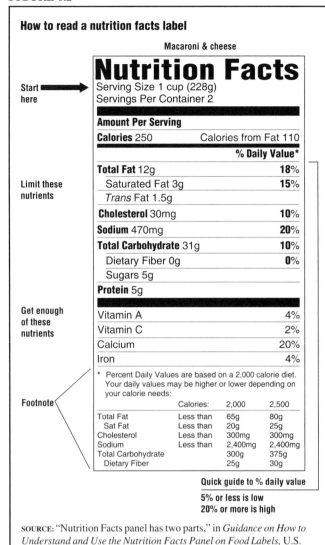

SOURCE: "Nutrition Facts panel has two parts," in *Guidance on How to Understand and Use the Nutrition Facts Panel on Food Labels*, U.S. Food and Drug Administration, Center for Food Safety and Applied Nutrition, Washington, DC, June 2000, updated July 2003 [Online] http://vm.cfsan.fda.gov/~dms/foodlab.html [accessed August 1, 2003]

TABLE 6.1

**The nutritional information panel**

Under the label's "Nutrition Facts" panel, manufacturers are required to provide information on certain nutrients. The mandatory (underlined) and voluntary components and the order in which they must appear are:

• total calories
• calories from fat
• calories from saturated fat
• total fat
• saturated fat
• trans fat
• polyunsaturated fat
• monounsaturated fat
• cholesterol
• sodium
• potassium
• total carbohydrate
• dietary fiber
• souble fiber
• insoluble fiber
• sugars
• sugar alcohol (for example, the sugar substitutes xylitol, mannitol, and sorbitol)
• other carbohydrate (the difference between total carbohydrate and the sum of dietary fiber, sugars, and sugar alcohol if declared)
• protein
• vitamin A
• percent of vitamin A present as beta–carotene
• vitamin C
• calcium
• iron
• other essential vitamins and minerals

SOURCE: Adapted from "Nutritional information panel" in "The Food Label," *FDA Backgrounder,* U.S. Food and Drug Administration, Washington, DC, May 1999 [Online] http://vm.cfsan.fda.gov/~dms/fdnewlab.html [accessed August 8, 2003]

*Disease* (Washington, DC) offered scientific evidence of the growing acceptance of this relationship.

In 1990 Congress passed the Nutrition Labeling and Education Act (NLEA; PL 101-535), which authorized the FDA to require all packaged foods to carry nutrition labeling. The NLEA is intended to provide consumers with uniform and accurate nutrition information about the foods they eat.

Although under no congressional mandate, the Food Safety and Inspection Service (FSIS) of the USDA has coordinated efforts with the FDA by requiring meat and poultry labeling. While the FSIS is responsible for nutrition labels on raw meat and poultry products, the FDA is responsible for food labels on all other food products. Final implementation of the new rules became effective in 1994.

**THE NUTRITION LABEL**

Previously referred to as "Nutrition Information per Serving," since May 8, 1994, the nutrition label has been called "Nutrition Facts." The Nutrition Facts label provides more complete, useful, and accurate nutrition information. (See Figure 6.2.) Manufacturers who wish to present

long-term health pushed for food-labeling reforms. In 1980, in response to the public's desire for authoritative, consistent guidelines on diet and health, the USDA and the Department of Health and Human Services (HHS) first published *Nutrition and Your Health: Dietary Guidelines for Americans* (Washington, DC).

In 1984 the FDA added sodium to the list of required nutrients on food labels. The addition of potassium to the nutrient list was optional. The following year, the agency allowed such terms as "low sodium" to be added as nutrient claims.

The federal government formally acknowledged the role of diet in such major chronic diseases as heart disease and cancer in the 1988 *Surgeon General's Report on Nutrition and Health.* The 1989 National Research Council report *Diet and Health: Implications for Reducing Chronic*

FIGURE 6.3

## A comparison of reduced and nonfat milk

**Reduced Fat Milk**
**2% Milkfat**

**Chocolate Nonfat Milk**

| **Nutrition Facts** | |
|---|---|
| Serving Size 1 cup (236ml) | |
| Servings Per Container 1 | |
| **Amount Per Serving** | |
| **Calories** 120 | Calories from Fat 45 |
| | **% Daily Value\*** |
| **Total Fat** 5g | 8% |
| Saturated Fat 3g | 15% |
| *Trans* Fat 0g | |
| **Cholesterol** 20mg | 7% |
| **Sodium** 120mg | 5% |
| **Total Carbohydrate** 11g | 4% |
| Dietary Fiber 0g | 0% |
| Sugars 11g | |
| **Protein** 9g | 17% |
| Vitamin A 10% • Vitamin C 4% | |
| Calcium 30% • Iron 0% • Vitamin D 25% | |
| \* Percent Daily Values are based on a 2,000 calorie diet. Your daily values may be higher or lower depending on your calorie needs. | |

| **Nutrition Facts** | |
|---|---|
| Serving Size 1 cup (236ml) | |
| Servings Per Container 1 | |
| **Amount Per Serving** | |
| **Calories** 80 | Calories from Fat 0 |
| | **% Daily Value\*** |
| **Total Fat** 0g | 0% |
| Saturated Fat 0g | 0% |
| *Trans* Fat 0g | |
| **Cholesterol** Less than 5mg | 0% |
| **Sodium** 120mg | 5% |
| **Total Carbohydrate** 11g | 4% |
| Dietary Fiber 0g | 0% |
| Sugars 11g | |
| **Protein** 9g | 17% |
| Vitamin A 10% • Vitamin C 4% | |
| Calcium 30% • Iron 0% • Vitamin D 25% | |
| \* Percent Daily Values are based on a 2,000 calorie diet. Your daily values may be higher or lower depending on your calorie needs. | |

SOURCE: "Comparison Example #2" in *Guidance on How to Understand and Use the Nutrition Facts Panel on Food Labels,* Center for Food Safety and Applied Nutrition, U.S. Food and Drug Administration, June 2000, updated July 2003 [Online] http://vm.cfsan.fda.gov/~dms/foodlab.html [accessed August 1, 2003]

nutrition labeling in a second language may do so either on a separate label or on the same label.

The FDA requires that the following nutrients be listed in order on the food label: total calories, calories from fat, total fat, saturated fat, cholesterol, sodium, total carbohydrate, dietary fiber, sugars, protein, vitamin A, vitamin C, calcium, and iron. In addition, manufacturers may choose to include several additional nutrients. (See Table 6.1.) If the food manufacturer makes a claim about an optional component, or if the food is fortified or enriched, the relevant nutrition information for these components becomes mandatory.

According to the FDA, the addition of trans fat to the Nutrition Facts panel effective January 1, 2006, "is the first significant change to the Nutrition Facts panel since the regulations implementing the Nutrition Labeling and Education Act were finalized in 1993." Under the new regulation, food manufacturers are required to list trans fatty acids, or trans fat, to the label on foods and some dietary supplements ("FDA Acts to Provide Better Information to Consumers on Trans Fats," *FDA Backgrounder,* July 9, 2003). (See Figure 6.1 and Figure 6.2.) The new requirement applies to any food with a level of at least 0.5 grams of trans fat. After a review of scientific evidence submitted to it by health experts, including the Institute of Medicine and the National Cholesterol Education Program of the National Institutes of Health (NIH), the FDA was persuaded that consumption of trans fat contributes to high cholesterol and, by extension, the risk of heart disease.

TABLE 6.2

## Daily reference values recommended by the U.S. Food and Drug Administration, 1999

(Based on a 2000 calorie intake; for adults and children 4 or more years of age.)

| Nutrient | Unit of measure | Daily values |
|---|---|---|
| Total fat | grams (g) | 65 |
| Saturated fatty acids | grams (g) | 20 |
| Cholesterol | milligrams (mg) | 300 |
| Sodium | milligrams (mg) | 2400 |
| Potassium | milligrams (mg) | 3500 |
| Total carbohydrate | grams (g) | 300 |
| Fiber | grams (g) | 25 |
| Protein | grams (g) | 50 |
| Vitamin A | International Unit (IU) | 5000 |
| Vitamin C | milligrams (mg) | 60 |
| Calcium | milligrams (mg) | 1000 |
| Iron | milligrams (mg) | 18 |
| Vitamin D | International Unit (IU) | 400 |
| Vitamin E | International Unit (IU) | 30 |
| Vitamin K | micrograms (μg) | 80 |
| Thiamine | milligrams (mg) | 1.5 |
| Riboflavin | milligrams (mg) | 1.7 |
| Niacin | milligrams (mg) | 20 |
| Vitamin $B_6$ | milligrams (mg) | 2.0 |
| Folate | micrograms (μg) | 400 |
| Vitamin $B_{12}$ | micrograms (μg) | 6.0 |
| Biotin | micrograms (μg) | 300 |
| Pantothenic acid | milligrams (mg) | 10 |
| Phosphorus | milligrams (mg) | 1000 |
| Iodine | micrograms (μg) | 150 |
| Magnesium | milligrams (mg) | 400 |
| Zinc | milligrams (mg) | 15 |
| Selenium | micrograms (μg) | 70 |
| Copper | milligrams (mg) | 2.0 |
| Manganese | milligrams (mg) | 2.0 |
| Chromium | micrograms (μg) | 120 |
| Molybdenum | micrograms (μg) | 7.5 |
| Chloride | milligrams (mg) | 3400 |

Notes: Nutrients in this table are listed in the order in which they are required to appear on a label in accordance with 101.9(c). This list includes only those nutrients for which a Daily Reference Value (DRV) has been established in 101.9(c)(9) or a Reference Daily Intake (RDI) in 101.9(c)(8)(iv).

SOURCE: "Reference Values for Nutrition Labeling," in *A Food Labeling Guide,* U.S. Food and Drug Administration, Center for Food Safety and Applied Nutrition, September 1994, revised June 1999 [Online] http://www.cfsan.fda.gov/~dms/flg-7a.html [accessed August 1, 2003]

Despite the conclusion that intake of trans fat may lead to increased risk of heart disease, health experts warn against completely eliminating trans fat from the diet, because to do so could lead to insufficient intake of important proteins and other nutrients.

Since 1997 the FDA has required that dietary supplements carry a "Supplement Facts" panel with information similar to the food Nutrition Facts panel. Dietary supplement manufacturers must also list trans fat on the Supplement Facts panel when their products contain a minimum of 0.5 grams of trans fat per serving. Examples of dietary supplements with trans fat include energy bars and nutrition bars.

According to the FDA, no scientific reports have provided a reference value for trans fat or any other information the FDA believes is sufficient to establish a

TABLE 6.3

**Recommended energy intake by age, sex, and activity level**

| Category | Age | Calories Per Day | | |
|---|---|---|---|---|
| | | Light activity | Moderate activity | Heavy activity |
| Children | 4-6 | | 1,800 | |
| | 7-10 | | 2,000 | |
| Males | 11-14 | | 2,500 | |
| | 15-18 | | 3,000 | |
| | 19-24 | 2,700 | 3,000 | 3,600 |
| | 25-50 | 3,000 | 3,200 | 4,000 |
| | 51+ | | 2,300* | |
| Females | 11-18 | | 2,200 | |
| | 19-24 | 2,000 | 2,100 | 2,600 |
| | 25-50 | 2,200 | 2,300 | 2,800 |
| | 51+ | | 1,900* | |

Pregnant women in their second and third trimesters should add 300 calories to the figure the table indicates for their age. Nursing mothers should add 500.
* based on light to moderate activity

**Activity Levels**
**Very Light:** Driving, typing, painting, laboratory work, ironing, sewing, cooking, playing cards, playing a musical instrument, other seated or standing activities
**Light:** Housecleaning, child care, garage work, electrical trade work, carpentry, restaurant work, golf, sailing, table tennis, walking on a level surface at 2.5 to 3 miles per hour
**Moderate:** Weeding, hoeing, carrying a load, cycling, skiing, tennis, dancing, walking 3.5 to 4 miles per hour
**Heavy:** Heavy manual digging, tree felling, basketball, climbing, football, soccer, carrying a load uphill

SOURCE: "Recommended Energy Intake" in "Recommended Daily Allowances," National Academy of Sciences, Washington, DC, no date

Daily Reference Value (DRV). For the time being, therefore, a Daily Value (% Daily Value) will not be listed on the label.

Food manufacturers have until January 1, 2006, to add the new listing to their labels. In keeping with the FDA's requirements as to the order in which ingredients must be listed, the listing for trans fat must be placed immediately after that for saturated fat.

The FDA selects nutrients for listing based on current health concerns, and the order in which they must be listed reflects their importance. Such nutrients as thiamine, riboflavin, and niacin are no longer required on the label because deficiencies of these B vitamins are no longer considered public health problems.

### Serving Sizes

With the passage of the NLEA, the FDA requires that a serving size reflect the amount of food a person actually eats at one time. This is determined primarily by nutritional food consumption surveys. Serving sizes must be stated in terms of both household and metric measurements.

### Percent Daily Value

A dietary reference term called "Percent Daily Value" shows how a food fits into a person's daily diet. According to the FDA, consumers should keep in mind that the listed Daily Value is not a recommended intake of a particular nutrient. Rather, the Percent Daily Value enables the consumer to see what proportion of the Daily Value

for each nutrient a serving of a particular food offers. (See Figure 6.2.)

For example, a food label may state that a certain food contains 5 grams of saturated fat per serving. As of 2003 the FDA recommendation for daily saturated fat was 20 grams or less. Although 5 grams of saturated fat may seem like a small amount, the Percent Daily Value shows that 5 grams of fat actually constitutes 25 percent of the total Daily Value for saturated fat.

Food labels also allow for comparisons between foods. Figure 6.3 presents labels for two food items: reduced fat milk and chocolate nonfat milk. The reduced fat milk contains 15 percent of the Daily Value for saturated fat and 8 percent of the total fat Daily Value, compared with the nonfat milk's 0 percent. Both provide the same percent Daily Values for total carbohydrate, protein, calcium, and the vitamins listed. The reduced fat milk contains 50 percent more calories than the nonfat milk.

Daily Values are derived from two sets of dietary standards: Daily Reference Values (DRVs) and Reference Daily Intakes (RDIs). Although these two dietary references serve as the basis for calculating Daily Values, only the term Daily Value is used for food labeling.

DRVs are dietary references for macronutrients that are sources of energy (fat, saturated fat, protein, and total carbohydrates, including fiber) and for cholesterol, sodium, and potassium that do not contribute calories. (See Table 6.2.) DRVs for the energy sources are based on the number of calories consumed each day.

**TABLE 6.4**

## Reference daily intakes (RDIs) for vitamins and nutrients

| Nutrient | Amount | DRV or RDI[1] | Amount per 100 calories |
|---|---|---|---|
| Protein | grams (g) | 50 | 2.5 |
| Vitamin A | International Units (IU) | 5,000 | 250 |
| Vitamin C | milligrams (mg) | 60 | 3 |
| Calcium | g | 1 | 0.05 |
| Iron | mg | 18 | 0.9 |
| Vitamin D | IU | 400 | 20 |
| Vitamin E | do | 30 | 1.5 |
| Thiamine | mg | 1.5 | 0.08 |
| Riboflavin | do | 1.7 | 0.09 |
| Niacin | do | 20 | 1 |
| Vitamin B6 | do | 2.0 | 0.1 |
| Folate | micrograms ([mu]g) | 400 | 20 |
| Vitamin B12 | do | 6.0 | 0.3 |
| Biotin | mg | 0.3 | 0.015 |
| Pantothenic acid | do | 10 | 0.5 |
| Phosphorus | g | 1.0 | 0.05 |
| Magnesium | mg | 400 | 20 |
| Zinc | do | 15 | 0.8 |
| Iodine | [mu]g | 150 | 7.5 |
| Copper | mg | 2.0 | 0.1 |
| Potassium | do | 3,500 | 175 |

[1] RDI's for adults and children 4 or more years of age.

Selected paragraphs within the Code of Federal Regulations Title 21, Chapter I, Part 104–Nutritional Quality Guidelines for Foods:

(e) A nutrient(s) may appropriately be added to a food that replaces traditional food in the diet to avoid nutritional inferiority in accordance with Sec. 101.3(e)(2) of this chapter.

(f) Nutrient(s) may be added to foods as permitted or required by applicable regulations established elsewhere in this chapter.

(g) A nutrient added to a food is appropriate only when the nutrient:

(1) Is stable in the food under customary conditions of storage, distribution, and use;

(2) Is physiologically available from the food;

(3) Is present at a level at which there is a reasonable assurance that consumption of the food containing the added nutrient will not result in an excessive intake of the nutrient, considering cumulative amounts from other sources in the diet; and

(4) Is suitable for its intended purpose and is in compliance with applicable provisions of the act and regulations governing the safety of substance in food.

(h) Any claims or statements in the labeling of food about the addition of a vitamin, mineral, or protein to a food shall be made only if the claim or statement is not false or misleading and otherwise complies with the act and any applicable regulations. The following label claims are acceptable:

(1) The labeling claim "fully restored with vitamins and minerals" or "fully restored with vitamins and minerals to the level of unprocessed ——" (the blank to be filled in with the common or usual name of the food) may be used to describe foods fortified in accordance with the principles established in paragraph (c) of this section.

(2) The labeling claim, "vitamins and minerals (and "protein" when appropriate) added are in proportion to caloric content" may be used to describe food fortified in accordance with the principles established in paragraph (d) of this section.

(3) When labeling claims are permitted, the term "enriched," "fortified," "added," or similar terms may be used interchangeably to indicate the addition of one or more vitamins or minerals or protein to a food, unless an applicable Federal regulation requires the use of specific words or statements.

(i) It is inappropriate to make any claim or statement on a label or in labeling, other than in a listing of the nutrient ingredients as part of the ingredient statement, that any vitamin, mineral, or protein has been added to a food to which nutrients have been added pursuant to paragraph (e) of this section.

[45 FR 6323, Jan. 25, 1980, as amended at 58 FR 2228, Jan. 6, 1993]

SOURCE: "Title 21–Food and Drugs," in *Code of Federal Regulations*, U.S. Food and Drug Administration, Center for Devices and Radiological Health, Washington, DC, revised as of April 1, 2003

For the purpose of food labeling, the FDA and the USDA base the DRVs and, consequently, the Percent Daily Values on a 2,000-calorie-a-day diet. The number of calories a person needs is based on body size, age, height, weight, activity level, and metabolism. The National Academy of Sciences has prepared recommendations for daily caloric intake based on these factors. (See Table 6.3.) Although many consumers require more than 2,000 calories a day, health experts agree that 2,000 calories represents the caloric requirement for postmenopausal women—the group with the highest risk for excessive intake of calories and fat. However, manufacturers may include Daily Values for other calorie levels if they so desire. Many food packages include Daily Values for a 2,500-calorie diet.

Regardless of a person's recommended calorie intake, the DRVs are calculated as follows:

- Fat: no more than 30 percent of calories.

- Saturated fat: no more than 10 percent of calories.

- Carbohydrate: no more than 60 percent of calories.

- Fiber: no more than 11.5 grams (g) of fiber per 1,000 calories.

- Protein: no more than 10 percent of calories. (The DRV for protein applies only to adults and children over age 4. RDIs for protein have been established for other groups—children ages 1–4, 14 g; pregnant women, 60 g; and nursing mothers, 65 g.)

Let's assume, for example, that a person's daily caloric intake is 2,000. The recommended DRV for saturated fat is no more than 10 percent of the total daily caloric intake. The person should, therefore, limit his or her calories from saturated fat to 200. A gram of fat has 9 calories, which means that the person should consume no more than 22 grams of saturated fat.

Based on scientific evidence that links certain nutrients and diseases, the federal government has established DRV parameters for these nutrients:

- Total fat: less than 65 g.

- Saturated fat: less than 20 g.

- Cholesterol: less than 300 milligrams (mg).

- Sodium: less than 2,400 mg.

Pursuant to the NLEA, RDIs (see Table 6.4) replaced the term U.S. RDAs (U.S. Recommended Daily Allowances), which was introduced in 1973 by the FDA as a label reference value for vitamins, minerals, and protein in voluntary nutrition labeling. RDIs also are used in calculating Daily Values for food labels.

### Nutrition Labeling for Children's Food

Food labels for children under 2 years of age cannot carry information on calories from fat and saturated fat. In addition, labels cannot have quantitative amounts for saturated fat, polyunsaturated fat, monounsaturated fat,

FIGURE 6.4

**Food label for fruit dessert for children less than two years old**

# Nutrition Facts
Serving Size 1 jar (140g)

**Amount Per Serving**

**Calories** 110

| | |
|---|---|
| **Total Fat** | 0g |
| **Sodium** | 10mg |
| **Total Carbohydrate** | 27mg |
| Dietary Fiber | 4g |
| Sugars | 0g |
| **Protein** | 0g |

% Daily Value

| Protein 0% | • | Vitamin A 6% |
|---|---|---|
| Vitamin C 45% | • | Calcium 2% |
| Iron 2% | | |

SOURCE: *A Food Labeling Guide,* U.S. Food and Drug Administration, Washington, DC, 1999

FIGURE 6.5

**Food label for fruit dessert for children aged two years to four years**

# Nutrition Facts
Serving Size 1 jar (140g)

**Amount Per Serving**

| **Calories** 110 | Calories from Fat 0 |
|---|---|
| **Total Fat** | 0g |
| Saturated Fat | 0g |
| **Cholesterol** | 0mg |
| **Sodium** | 10mg |
| **Total Carbohydrate** | 27mg |
| Dietary Fiber | 4g |
| Sugars | 0g |
| **Protein** | 0g |

% Daily Value

| Protein 0% | • | Vitamin A 6% |
|---|---|---|
| Vitamin C 45% | • | Calcium 2% |
| Iron 2% | | |

SOURCE: *A Food Labeling Guide,* U.S. Food and Drug Administration, Washington, DC, 1999

and cholesterol. (See Figure 6.4.) This is to prevent parents from thinking that infants and toddlers should limit their fat intake, when, in fact, fat is necessary for healthy growth and development at this stage of life. Food labels for children ages 2–4 cannot include Percent Daily Values for macronutrients such as carbohydrates and fiber because the FDA has not determined Daily Values for this age group. (See Figure 6.5.)

## NUTRIENT CONTENT CLAIMS IN FOOD LABELS

The NLEA also specifies what terms may be used to describe the level of a nutrient in a food and how the terms can be used. Table 6.5 explains the criteria for the following nutrient content claims permitted by the NLEA:

- Free
- Low
- Very Low
- Percent fat free
- Substantially less
- No added sugars
- Without added sugars
- Reduced/less
- Light or lite
- Fewer

The term "free" means that a product contains no amount of, or only trivial or "physiologically inconsequential" amounts of, the nutrient. "Low" can be used on foods that can be eaten frequently without exceeding the Daily Value for that nutrient. (See Table 6.5 for synonyms for the terms "free" and "low.")

Manufacturers are allowed to use alternative spellings of these terms and their synonyms—for example, lite (light) or lo (low)—as long as the alternative word is not misleading.

### Nutritionally Altered Products

The NLEA allows manufacturers to compare nutritionally altered products with regular products (referred to as reference foods) by making a relative claim, using such terms as reduced, less, light, fewer, and more. The regular product may be an individual food or a group of foods representative of the type of food. A relative claim must include the percent difference and the identity of the regular food.

The term "reduced" means that a nutritionally altered product contains at least 25 percent less of a nutrient, or of calories, than the reference food. The terms "less" or "fewer" mean that a food, whether or not it has been altered, contains 25 percent less of a particular nutrient, or 25 percent fewer calories, than the reference food.

TABLE 6.5

## U.S. Food and Drug Administration definitions for nutrient content claims

| Nutrient | Free | Low | Reduced/Less | Comments |
|---|---|---|---|---|
| | Synonyms for "Free" : "Zero", "No", "Without", "Trivial Source of", "Negligible Source of", "Dietarily Insignificant Source of." Definitions for "Free" for meals and main dishes are the stated values per labeled serving. | Synonyms for "Low": "Little", ("Few" for Calories), "Contains a Small Amount of", "Low Source of." | Synonyms for "Reduced/Less": "Lower" ("Fewer" for Calories). "Modified" may be used in statement of identity. Definitions for meals and main dishes are same as for individual foods on a per 100 g basis. | For "Free", "Very Low", or "Low", must indicate if food meets a definition without benefit of special processing, alteration, formulation or reformulation; e.g., "broccoli, a fat-free food" or "celery, a low calorie food." |
| **Calories** 21 CFR 101.60(b) | Less than 5 cal per reference amount and per labeled serving. | 40 cal or less per reference amount (and per 50 g if reference amount is small). Meals and main dishes: 120 cal or less per 100 g. | At least 25% fewer calories per reference amount than an appropriate reference food. Reference food may not be "Low Calorie". Uses term "Fewer" rather than "Less." | "Light" or "Lite": If 50% or more of the calories are from fat, fat must be reduced by at least 50% per reference amount. If less than 50% of calories are from fat, fat must be reduced at least 50% or calories reduced at least 1/3 per reference amount. "Light" or "Lite" meal or main dish product meets definition for "Low Calorie" or "Low Fat" meal and is labeled to indicate which definition is met. For dietary supplements: Calorie claims can only be made when the reference product is greater than 40 calories per serving. |
| **Total Fat** 21 CFR 101.62(b) | Less than 0.5 g per reference amount and per labeled serving (or for meals and main dishes, less than 0.5 g per labeled serving). Not defined for meals or main dishes. | 3 g or less per reference amount (and per 50 g if reference amount is small). Meals and main dishes: 3 g or less per 100 g and not more than 30% of calories from fat. | At least 25% less saturated fat per reference amount than an appropriate reference food. Reference food may not be "Low Fat." | "__% Fat Free": OK if meets the require-ments for "Low Fat". 100% Fat Free: Food must be "Fat Free". "Light"—see above. For dietary supplements: Calorie claims cannot be made for products that are 40 calories or less per serving. |
| **Saturated Fat** 21 CFR 101.62(c) | Less than 0.5 g saturated fat and less than 0.5 g trans fatty acids per reference amount and per labeled serving (or for meals and main dishes, less than 0.5 g saturated fat and less than 0.5 g trans fatty acids per labeled serving). No ingredient that is understood to contain saturated fat except as noted below(*). | 1 g or less per reference amount and 15% or less of calories from saturated fat. Meals and main dishes: 1 g or less per 100 g and less than 10% of calories from saturated fat. | At least 25% less saturated fat per reference amount than an appropriate reference food. Reference food may not be "Low Saturated Fat." | Next to all saturated fat claims, must declare the amount of cholesterol if 2 mg or more per reference amount; and the amount of total fat if more than 3 g per reference amount (or 0.5 g or more of total fat for "Saturated Fat Free"). For dietary supplements: saturated fat claims cannot be made for products that are 40 calories or less per serving. |
| **Cholesterol** 21 CFR 101.62(d) | Less than 2 mg per reference amount and per labeled serving (or for meals and main dishes, less than 2 mg per labeled serving). No ingredient that contains cholesterol except as noted below(*). If less than 2 mg per reference amount by special processing and total fat exceeds 13 g per reference amount and labeled serving, the amount of cholesterol must be "Substantially Less" (25%) than in a reference food with significant market share (5% of market). | 20 mg or less per reference amount (and per 50 g of food if reference amount is small). If qualifies by special processing and total fat exceeds 13 g per reference and labeled serving, the amount of cholesterol must be "Substantially Less" (25%) than in a reference food with significant market share (5% of market). Meals and main dishes: 20 mg or less per 100 g. | At least 25% less cholesterol per reference amount than an appropriate reference food. Reference food may not be "Low Cholesterol." | Cholesterol claims only allowed when food contains 2 g or less saturated fat per reference amount; or for meals and main dish products—per labeled serving size for "Free" claims or per 100 g for "Low" and "Reduced/Less" claims. Must declare the amount of total fat next to cholesterol claim when fat exceeds 13 g per reference amount and labeled serving (or per 50 g of food if reference amount is small), or when the fat exceeds 19.5 g per labeled serving for main dishes or 26 g for meal products. For dietary supplements: Cholesterol claims cannot be made for products that are 40 calories or less per serving. |
| **Sodium** 21 CFR 101.61 | Less than 5 mg per reference amount and per labeled serving (or for meals and main dishes, less than 5 mg per labeled serving). No ingredient that is sodium chloride or generally understood to contain sodium except as noted below(*). | 140 mg or less per reference amount (and per 50 g if reference amount is small). Meals and main dishes: 140 mg or less per 100 g. | At least 25% less sodium per reference amount than an appropriate reference food. Reference food may not be "Low Sodium." | "Light" (for sodium reduced products): If food is "Low Calorie" and "Low Fat" and sodium is reduced by at least 50%. "Light in Sodium": If sodium is reduced by at least 50% per reference amount. Entire term "Light in Sodium" must be used in same type, size, color & prominence. "Light in Sodium" for meals = "Low in Sodium." |

The term "light" or "lite" can be used in a variety of ways. Two of the most frequently used examples are used to describe one of two different things:

- A nutritionally altered product that contains one-third fewer calories or half the fat of the reference food. If the food derives 50 percent or more of its

| Nutrient | Free | Low | Reduced/Less | Comments |
|---|---|---|---|---|
| | | | | "Very Low Sodium": 35 mg or less per reference amount (and per 50 g if reference amount is small). For meals and main dishes: 35 mg or less per 100 g.<br>"Salt Free" must meet criterion for "Sodium Free".<br>"No Salt Added" and "Unsalted" must note conditions of use and must declare "This is Not A Sodium Free Food" on information panel if food is not "Sodium Free".<br>"Lightly Salted": 50% less sodium than normally added to reference food and if not "Low Sodium", so labeled on information panel. |
| **Sugars**<br>21 CFR 101.60(c) | "Sugar Free": Less than 0.5 g sugars per reference amount and per labeled serving (or for meals and main dishes, less than 0.5 g per labeled serving).<br>No ingredient that is a sugar or generally understood to contain sugars except as noted below(*).<br>Disclose calorie profile (e.g., "Low Calorie"). | Not Defined. No basis for recommended intake. | At least 25% less sugars per reference amount than an appropriate reference food. May not use this claim on dietary supplements of vitamins and minerals. | "No Added Sugar" and "Without Added Sugars" are allowed if no sugar or sugar containing ingredient is added during processing.<br>State if food is not "Low" or "Reduced Calorie".<br>The terms "Unsweetened" and "Added Sweeteners" remain as factual statements. Claims about reducing dental caries are implied health claims.<br>Does not include sugar alcohols. |

Notes: * Except if the ingredient listed in the ingredient statement has an asterisk that refers to footnote (e.g., "* adds a trivial amount of fat").
• "Reference Amount" = serving, or amount customarily consumed.
• "Small Reference Amount" = reference amount of 30 g or less or 2 tablespoons or less (for dehydrated foods that are typically consumed when rehydrated with water or a diluent containing an insignificant amount, as defined in 21 CFR 101.9(f)(1), of all nutrients per reference amount, the per 50 g criterion refers to the prepared form of the food).
• When levels exceed: 13 g Fat, 4 g Saturated Fat, 60 mg Cholesterol, and 480 mg Sodium per reference amount, per labeled serving or, for foods with small reference amounts, per 50 g, a disclosure statement is required as part of claim (e.g., "See nutrition information for___content" with the blank filled in with nutrient(s) that exceed the prescribed levels).

SOURCE: *A Food Labeling Guide*, U.S. Food and Drug Administration, Washington, DC, 1999

calories from fat, the reduction must be 50 percent of the fat.

• A low-calorie, low-fat food in which the sodium content has been reduced by 50 percent. The description "light in sodium" may be used if the food has at least 50 percent less sodium than a reference food.

In addition, the term "light" can be used to describe such properties as color and texture, as long as the label explains the intended use of the term—for example, "light brown sugar" and "light and fluffy."

A serving of food bearing the "more" claim must contain at least 10 percent more of the Daily Value for the particular nutrient than a similar reference food. The 10 percent of Daily Value also applies to such nutrient claims as "fortified," "enriched," "added," "extra," and "plus," but in those cases the food must be nutritionally altered.

## HEALTH CLAIMS

The FDA also allows health claims on food labels. Health claims are different from "structure/function" claims found on labels of conventional food and dietary supplements. While manufacturers use health claims primarily to sell their products, the FDA believes that "these claims alert shoppers to a product's health potential by stating that certain foods or food substances—as part of an overall healthy diet—may reduce the risk of certain diseases."

Claims can be made in several ways: through third party references, such as the National Cancer Institute; via statements; by using symbols, such as a heart; and by descriptions. A health claim can use only the terms "may" or "might" in discussing the link between the nutrient and the disease; in addition, it cannot state any degree of risk reduction. Moreover, the claim must state that other factors play a role in the disease. Finally, health claims cannot be made for infants and toddlers under 2 years old.

## Food and Drug Administration Modernization Act of 1997

In 1993 seven health claims were authorized under the 1990 NLEA. As of July 2003 the FDA has allowed 14 health claims. The Food and Drug Administration Modernization Act of 1997 (PL 105-115) provides that the lengthy process needed for establishing the scientific basis for health claims be expedited. Prior to 1997 it took on average more than a year to complete the process of approving a health claim. In part this was the result of the

**TABLE 6.6**

**Guide to U.S. Food and Drug Administration requirements for claiming certain health benefits on food labels**

| Approved claims | Food requirements | Label requirements | Model claim statements |
|---|---|---|---|
| Calcium and Osteoporosis—21 CFR 101.72 | - High in calcium,<br>- Assimilable (Bioavailable),<br>- Supplements must disintegrate and dissolve, and<br>- Phosphorus content cannot exceed calcium content | Indicates disease depends on many factors by listing risk factors of the disease: Gender—Female. Race—Caucasian and Asian. Age—Growing older.<br><br>Primary target population: Females, Caucasian and Asian races, and teens and young adults in their bone-forming years.<br><br>Additional factors necessary to reduce risk: Eating healthful meals, regular exercise.<br><br>Mechanism relating calcium to osteoporosis: Optimizes peak bone mass.<br><br>Foods or supplements containing more than 400 mg calcium must state that total intakes of greater than 2,000 mg calcium provide no added benefit to bone health. | Regular exercise and a healthy diet with enough calcium helps teens and young adult white and Asian women maintain good bone health and may reduce their high risk of osteoporosis later in life. |
| Sodium and Hypertension—21 CFR 101.74 | - Low sodium | Required terms: "Sodium", "High blood pressure"<br><br>Includes physician statement (Individuals with high blood pressure should consult their physicians) if claim defines high or normal blood pressure. | Diets low in sodium may reduce the risk of high blood pressure, a disease associated with many factors. |
| Dietary Fat and Cancer—21 CFR 101.73 | - Low fat (Fish & game meats: "Extra lean") | Required terms: "Total fat" or "Fat", "Some types of cancers" or "Some cancers"<br><br>Does not specify types of fats or fatty acids that may be related to risk of cancer. | Development of cancer depends on many factors. A diet low in total fat may reduce the risk of some cancers. |
| Dietary Saturated Fat and Cholesterol and Risk of Coronary Heart Disease—21 CFR 101.75 | - Low saturated fat,<br>- Low cholesterol, and<br>- Low fat (Fish & game meats: "Extra lean") | Required terms: "Saturated fat and cholesterol", "Coronary heart disease" or "Heart disease"<br><br>Includes physician statement (individuals with elevated blood total —or LDL—cholesterol should consult their physicians) if claim defines high or normal blood total—and LDL— cholesterol. | While many factors affect heart disease, diets low in saturated fat and cholesterol may reduce the risk of this disease. |
| Fiber-Containing Grain Products, Fruits, and Vegetables and Cancer—21 CFR 101.76 | - A grain product, fruit, or vegetable that contains dietary fiber,<br>- Low fat, and<br>- Good source of dietary fiber (without fortification) | Required terms: "Fiber", "Dietary fiber", or "Total dietary fiber"; "Some types of cancer" or "Some cancers"<br><br>Does not specify types of dietary fiber that may be related to risk of cancer. | Low fat diets rich in fiber-containing grain products, fruits, and vegetables may reduce the risk of some types of cancer, a disease associated with many factors. |
| Fruits, Vegetables and Grain Products that contain Fiber, particularly Soluble Fiber, and Risk of Coronary Heart Disease—21 CFR 101.77 | - A fruit, vegetable, or grain product that contains fiber,<br>- Low saturated fat,<br>- Low cholesterol,<br>- Low fat,<br>- At least 0.6 grams of soluble fiber per RA (without fortification), and<br>- Soluble fiber content provided on label | Required terms: "Fiber", "Dietary fiber", "Some types of dietary fiber", "Some dietary fibers", or "Some fibers"; "Saturated fat" and "Cholesterol"; "Heart disease" or "Coronary heart disease"<br><br>Includes physician statement ("Individuals with elevated blood total—or LDL—cholesterol should consult their physicians") if claim defines high or normal blood total —and LDL—cholesterol. | Diets low in saturated fat and cholesterol and rich in fruits, vegetables, and grain products that contain some types of dietary fiber, particularly soluble fiber, may reduce the risk of heart disease, a disease associated with many factors. |

lengthy time period needed in order to carry out the required scientific review and the additional time necessary for the issuance of a proposed rule.

The new law allows a manufacturer to notify the FDA that it intends to use a new health claim based on an authoritative statement of one or more federal scientific bodies (for example, the National Academy of Sciences, USDA, or Institute of Medicine). The FDA has 120 days to act or make changes to the claim, after which the claim can be used.

TABLE 6.6

## Guide to U.S. Food and Drug Administration requirements for claiming certain health benefits on food labels [CONTINUED]

| Approved claims | Food requirements | Label requirements | Model claim statements |
|---|---|---|---|
| Fruits and Vegetables and Cancer—21 CFR 101.78 | - A fruit or vegetable,<br>- Low fat, and<br>- Good source (without fortification) of at least one of the following:<br>Vitamin A,<br>Vitamin C, or<br>Dietary fiber | Required terms: "Fiber", "Dietary fiber", or "Total dietary fiber"; "Total fat" or "Fat"; "Some types of cancer" or "Some cancers"<br><br>Characterizes fruits and vegetables as "Foods that are low in fat and may contain Vitamin A, Vitamin C, and dietary fiber." Characterizes specific food as a "Good source" of one or more of the following: Dietary fiber, Vitamin A, or Vitamin C. Does not specify types of fats or fatty acids or types of dietary fiber that may be related to risk of cancer. | Low fat diets rich in fruits and vegetables (foods that are low in fat and may contain dietary fiber, Vitamin A, or Vitamin C) may reduce the risk of some types of cancer, a disease associated with many factors. Broccoli is high in vitamin A and C, and it is a good source of dietary fiber. |
| Folate and Neural Tube Defects—21 CFR 101.79 | -"Good source" of folate (at least 40 mg folate per serving)<br>- Dietary supplements, or foods in conventional food form that are naturally good sources of folate (i.e., only non-fortified food in conventional food form)<br>- The claim shall not be made on products that contain more than 100% of the RDI for vitamin A as retinol or preformed vitamin A or vitamin D.<br>- Dietary supplements shall meet USP standards for disintegration and dissolution or otherwise bioavailable.<br>-Amount of folate required in N.L. | Required terms: Terms that specify the relationship (e.g., women who are capable of becoming pregnant and who consume adequate amounts of folate) "Folate", "folic acid", "folacin","folate, a B vitamin", "folic acid, a B vitamin," "folacin, a B vitamin," "neural tube defects", "birth defects, spinal bifida, or anencephaly", "birth defects of the brain or spinal cord—anencephaly or spinal bifida", "spinal bifida or anencephaly, birth defects of the brain or spinal cord."<br><br>Must also include information on the multifactorial nature of neural tube defects, and the safe upper limit of daily intake. | Healthful diets with adequate folate may reduce a woman's risk of having a child with a brain or spinal cord defect. |
| Dietary Sugar Alcohol and Dental Caries—21 CFR 101.80 | - Sugar free.<br>- The sugar alcohol must be xylitol, sorbitol, mannitol, maltitol, isomalt, lactitol, hydrogenated starch hydrolysates, hydrogenated glucose syrups, erythritol, or a combination.<br>- When a fermentable carbohydrate is present, the food must not lower plaque pH below 5.7. | Required terms: "does not promote," "may reduce the risk of", "useful [or is useful] in not promoting" or "expressly [or is expressly] for not promoting" dental caries; "sugar alcohol" or "sugar alcohols" or the name or names of the sugar alcohols, e.g., sorbitol; "dental caries" or "tooth decay."<br><br>Includes statement that frequent between meal consumption of foods high in sugars and starches can promote tooth decay.<br><br>Packages with less than 15 square inches of surface area available for labeling may use a shortened claim. | **Full claim:** Frequent between-meal consumption of foods high in sugars and starches promotes tooth decay. The sugar alcohols in [name of food] do not promote tooth decay.<br><br>**Shortened claim (on small packages only):** Does not promote tooth decay. |
| Soluble Fiber from Certain Foods and Risk of Coronary Heart Disease—21 CFR 101.81 | - Low saturated fat,<br>- Low cholesterol,<br>- Low fat,<br>- Include either (1) one or more eligible sources of whole oats, containing at least 0.75 g whole oat soluble fiber per RA; or (2) psyllium seed husk containing at least 1.7 g of psyllium husk soluble fiber per RA, and<br>- Amount of soluble fiber per RA declared in nutrition label.<br><br>**Eligible Source of Soluble Fiber:**<br>Beta glucan soluble fiber from oat bran, rolled oats (or oatmeal), and whole oat flour. Oat bran must provide at least 5.5% glucan soluble fiber, rolled oats must provide at least 4% glucan soluble fiber, and whole oat flour must provide at least 4% glucan soluble fiber or psyllium husk with purity of no less than 95%. | Required terms: "Heart disease" or "coronary heart disease"; "Soluble fiber" qualified by either "psyllium seed husk" or the name of the eligible source of whole oat soluble fiber; "saturated fat" and "cholesterol." Daily dietary intake of the soluble fiber source necessary to reduce the risk of CHD and the contribution one serving of the product makes to this level of intake.<br><br>**Additional Required Label Statement:**<br>Foods bearing a psyllium seed husk health claim must also bear a label statement concerning the need to consume them with adequate amounts of fluids; e.g., "NOTICE: This food should be eaten with at least a full glass of liquid. Eating this product without enough liquid may cause choking. Do not eat this product if you have difficulty in swallowing." (21 CFR 101.17(f)) | Soluble fiber from foods such as [name of soluble fiber source, and, if desired, name of food product], as part of a diet low in saturated fat and cholesterol, may reduce the risk of heart disease. A serving of [name of food product] supplies __ grams of the [necessary daily dietary intake for the benefit] soluble fiber from [name of soluble fiber source] necessary per day to have this effect. |

**TABLE 6.6**

**Guide to U.S. Food and Drug Administration requirements for claiming certain health benefits on food labels** [CONTINUED]

| Approved claims | Food requirements | Label requirements | Model claim statements |
|---|---|---|---|
| Soy Protein and Risk of Coronary Heart Disease—21 CFR 101.82 | - At least 6.25 g soy protein per RA,<br>- Low saturated fat,<br>- Low cholesterol, and<br>- Low fat (except that foods made from whole soybeans that contain no fat in addition to that inherent in the whole soybean are exempt from the "low fat" requirement) | Required terms: "Heart disease"or "coronary heart disease"; "Soy protein"; "Saturated fat" and "cholesterol"<br><br>Claim specifies daily dietary intake levels of soy protein associated with reduced risk.<br><br>Claim specifies amount of soy protein in a serving of food. | (1) 25 grams of soy protein a day, as part of a diet low in saturated fat and cholesterol, may reduce the risk of heart disease. A serving of [name of food] supplies ___ grams of soy protein.<br><br>(2) Diets low in saturated fat and cholesterol that include 25 grams of soy protein a day may reduce the risk of heart disease. One serving of [name of food] provides ___ grams of soy protein. |
| Plant Sterol/Stanol Esters and Risk of Coronary Heart Disease—21 CFR 101.83 | - At least 0.65 g plant sterol esters per RA of spreads and salad dressing, or<br>- At least 1.7 g plant stanol esters per RA of spreads, salad dressings, snack bars, and dietary supplements.<br>- Low saturated fat,<br>- Low cholesterol, and<br>- Spreads and salad dressings that exceed 13 g fat per 50 g must bear the statement "see nutrition information for fat content"<br><br>Salad dressings are exempted from the minimum 10% DV nutrient requirement (see General Criteria below) | Required terms: "May" or "might" reduce the risk of CHD; "Heart disease" or "coronary heart disease"; "Plant sterol esters" or "plant stanol esters"; except "vegetable oil" may replace the term "plant" if vegetable oil is the sole source of the sterol/stanol ester.<br><br>Claim specifies plant sterol/stanol esters are part of a diet low in saturated fat and cholesterol.<br><br>Claim does not attribute any degree of CHD risk reduction.<br><br>Claim specifies the daily dietary intake of plant sterol or stanol esters necessary to reduce CHD risk, and the amount provided per serving.<br><br>Claim specifies that plant sterol or stanol esters should be consumed with two different meals each a day. | (1) Foods containing at least 0.65 gram per serving of vegetable oil sterol esters, eaten twice a day with meals for a daily total intake of at least 1.3 grams, as part of a diet low in saturated fat and cholesterol, may reduce the risk of heart disease. A serving of [name of food] supplies ___ grams of vegetable oil sterol esters.<br><br>(2) Diets low in saturated fat and cholesterol that include two servings of foods that provide a daily total of at least 3.4 grams of plant stanol esters in two meals may reduce the risk of heart disease. A serving of [name of food] supplies ___ grams of plant stanol esters. |

**CLAIMS AUTHORIZED BASED ON AUTHORITATIVE STATEMENTS BY FEDERAL SCIENTIFIC BODIES**

| | | | |
|---|---|---|---|
| Whole Grain Foods and Risk of Heart Disease and Certain Cancers—Docket No. 99P-2209 | - Contains 51 percent or more whole grain ingredients by weight per RA, and<br>- Dietary fiber content at least:<br>  • 3.0 g per RA of 55 g<br>  • 2.8 g per RA of 50 g<br>  • 2.5 g per RA of 45 g<br>  • 1.7 g per RA of 35 g<br>- Low fat | Required wording of the claim: "Diets rich in whole grain foods and other plant foods and low in total fat, saturated fat, and cholesterol may reduce the risk of heart disease and some cancers." | NA |
| Potassium and the Risk of High Blood Pressure and Stroke—Docket No. 00Q-1582 | - Good source of potassium,<br>- Low sodium,<br>- Low total fat,<br>- Low saturated fat, and<br>- Low cholesterol | Required wording of the claim: "Diets containing foods that are a good source of potassium and that are low in sodium may reduce the risk of high blood pressure and stroke." | NA |

**GENERAL CRITERIA ALL CLAIMS MUST MEET**

All information must appear in one place without intervening material (reference statement permitted). Only information on the value that intake or reduced intake, as part of a total dietary pattern, may have on a disease or health-related condition is permitted. Enables public to understand information provided and significance of information in the context of a total daily diet. Must be complete, truthful, and not misleading. Food contains, without fortification, 10% or more of the Daily Value for one of six nutrients (dietary supplements excepted):

Vitamin A 500 IU     Calcium 100 mg
Vitamin C 6 mg     Protein 5 g
Iron 1.8 mg     Fiber 2.5 g

Not represented for infants or toddlers less than 2 years of age. Uses "may" or "might" to express relationship between substance and disease. Does not quantify any degree of risk reduction. Indicates disease depends on many factors.

Food contains less than the specified levels of four disqualifying nutrients:

| Disqualifying Nutrients | Foods | Main Dishes | Meal Products |
|---|---|---|---|
| Fat | 13 g | 19.5 g | 26 g |
| Saturated Fat | 4 g | 6 g | 8 g |
| Cholesterol | 60 mg | 90 mg | 120 mg |
| Sodium | 480 mg | 720 mg | 960 mg |

Abbreviations: RA = reference amount, IU = International Units

SOURCE: *A Food Labeling Guide*, U.S. Food and Drug Administration, Washington, DC, 1999

## Current Health Claims

As of June 2003 the health claims (see Table 6.6) permitted by the FDA may show a link between:

* A diet with enough calcium and a lower risk of osteoporosis.

* A diet low in sodium and a reduced risk of high blood pressure.

* A diet low in total fat and a reduced risk of some cancers.

* A diet low in saturated fat and cholesterol and a reduced risk of coronary heart disease.

* A diet rich in fiber-containing grain products, fruits, and vegetables and a reduced risk of some cancers.

* A diet rich in fruits, vegetables, and grain products that contain fiber, especially soluble fiber, and a reduced risk of coronary heart disease.

* A diet rich in fruits and vegetables and a reduced risk of some cancers.

* Folic acid and a decreased risk of neural tube defect during pregnancy.

* Dietary sugar alcohols and a reduced risk of dental caries.

* Soluble fiber from certain foods, such as whole oats and psyllium seed husk, as part of a diet low in saturated fat and cholesterol, and a reduced risk of heart disease.

* Soy protein and the risk of coronary heart disease.

* Plant sterol/stanol esters and the risk of coronary heart disease.

* Whole grain foods and the risk of heart disease and certain cancers.

* Potassium and the risk of high blood pressure and stroke.

In addition, the FDA identified fat, saturated fat, cholesterol, and sodium as risk nutrients and set specific levels per serving of these "disqualifying nutrients." Single-item foods bearing a health claim must contain 20 percent or less of the Daily Value of fat (13 g), saturated fat (4 g), cholesterol (60 mg), and sodium (480 mg). For example, whole milk, which it is rich in calcium, is not permitted to bear a calcium-osteoporosis claim on its nutrition label because its fat content exceeds the disqualifying levels. (See Table 6.6 footnotes for other FDA-specified levels of disqualifying nutrients for main dishes and meal products.)

In July 2003, based on its review of scientific evidence submitted to it by health experts, the FDA added oatrim, the soluble portion of oat bran or whole oat flour, to the health claim linking consumption of soluble dietary fiber from certain foods to a reduced risk of coronary heart disease (CHD) (*Federal Register,* July 28, 2003 [vol. 68, no. 144]).

## Qualified Health Claims

As a consequence of a 1999 ruling by the U.S. Court of Appeals for the D.C. Circuit in the case of *Pearson v. Shalala* (64 F.3d 6 50 [D.C. Cir. 1999]), the FDA now permits the use of qualified health claims on nutrition labels ("Claims That Can Be Made for Conventional Foods and Dietary Supplements," FDA, March 20, 2001). (Recent announcements of new qualified health claims can be found on the FDA Web site [Online] http://www.cfsan.fda.gov/label.html.) Such claims are those that may not meet the standard known as "scientific agreement," but may instead have more scientific evidence to support them than evidence that would refute them. Although the court ruling involved health claims made for dietary supplements, the FDA decided in December 2002 to allow some foods to make qualified health claims.

On January 16, 2003, the FDA announced the establishment of its Task Force on Consumer Health Information for Better Nutrition. The task force is made up of health and science experts from the FDA, the National Institutes of Health (NIH), and others. The task force will evaluate several nutrition initiatives, among them the new standard for qualified health claims.

The task force may evaluate the use on food labels of a dietary guidance message from the National Cancer Institute (NCI) on the potential health benefits of a diet filled with fruits and vegetables: "Diets rich in fruits and vegetables may reduce the risk of some types of cancer and other chronic diseases." There are specific requirements, however, for inclusion of the dietary guidance message and/or use of the NCI's new "5-to-9-a-Day" logo.

## OTHER LABEL CLAIMS

According to the NLEA, in order to use the claim "percent fat free," a product also must be a low-fat or a fat-free food. The claim also must accurately reflect the amount of fat present in 100 grams of the food. In other words, if a food contains 2.5 grams of fat per 50 grams, the product claim must be "95 percent fat free."

A "healthy" food must be low in total fat and saturated fat and contain limited amounts of sodium and cholesterol. If it is a single-serving food, it must provide at least 10 percent of one or more of vitamins A or C, iron, calcium, protein, or fiber. "Healthy" meal-type products, such as frozen dinners, must provide 10 percent of two or three of these nutrients. These nutrients would have to occur naturally in the food; they cannot be added. Moreover, the sodium content cannot exceed 360 mg per serving for single-serving foods and 480 mg for meal-type foods.

The NLEA allows manufacturers to reduce the fat content of certain foods and call them "low fat" or "light" as long as those foods are still nutritionally equivalent to the original product. For example, sour cream can be called "light" if the fat content is reduced to 9 percent (from the regular 18 percent) and has vitamin A added to replace the amount lost when the fat was removed. If the manufacturer does not replace the vitamin A, the product must be labeled "imitation light sour cream."

## "IMPLIED" CLAIMS ARE PROHIBITED

An implied claim occurs when a product label appears to confer a certain health benefit through a nutrition claim. The FDA prohibits this. For example, if a product advertises that it is "made with canola oil," it is implying that the product is low in saturated fat. To carry that claim, however, the food itself, not just the canola oil that went into the recipe, must actually be low in saturated fat.

### Exceptions

Certain statements that do not fall under the "implied" claim prohibition, and therefore are allowed, include:

- Avoidance claims for religious or food-intolerance reasons, such as the term "milk/dairy-free."

- Statements about non-nutritive ingredients, such as "no preservatives" or "no artificial colors."

- Added-value statements, such as "contains real fruit" or "made with real butter."

- Statements of identity, such as "corn oil margarine" or "Colombian coffee."

## LABELING FOR FAT-REDUCED MILK

Milk occupies a significant place in the American diet, providing a large portion of saturated fat (after cheese and beef). Replacing full-fat (whole) milk with lower-fat or skim milk could significantly lower an individual's saturated-fat intake. Eight ounces of full-fat milk provides 26 percent of the Daily Value for saturated fat, compared with skim milk, which provides none.

In January 1998 the FDA ruled that the labeling of fat-reduced milk and milk products must follow the same specifications applicable to other foods reduced in fat. In making milk labeling consistent with that of other food products, the FDA aimed to give consumers more accurate, consistent information. For example, low-fat milk, or 1 percent milk, is required to have the same fat content as any low-fat dessert. The FDA allows these low-fat food items to provide no more than three grams of fat per serving.

Milk products with lower-fat contents are required to be nutritionally equivalent to full-fat milk and provide at least the same amount of fat-soluble vitamins A and D as full-fat milk. These two vitamins are lost when milk fat is removed or reduced and are replaced later in the process.

### Dietary Impact

Nutrition experts believe that the new milk labeling will not only help consumers differentiate between reduced-fat milk and low-fat milk, it might also encourage them to switch from the former to the latter. Two percent milk has almost twice the amount of total fat as 1 percent milk.

## NUTRITION INFORMATION ON FRESH FOODS

In 1991, in accordance with the NLEA, the FDA established guidelines for voluntary nutrition labeling on fresh fruits, vegetables, and fish. The program will remain voluntary only if at least 60 percent of retailers continue to participate in the program. According to the FDA, a 1996 survey (the latest available data) showed that more than 70 percent of U.S. food retailers participated in the voluntary point-of-purchase nutrition information program.

As of August 2003 nutrition labeling is available for the 20 most frequently eaten raw fruits, vegetables, and fish. Grocers can convey nutrition information through stickers, posters, brochures, leaflets, or any other method, as long as the information is readily available to consumers. Although participation is voluntary, the FDA regulates the information offered. The information must include serving size; calories per serving; amount of protein; total carbohydrate, total fat, and sodium; and percent of the Reference Daily Intakes for iron, calcium, and vitamins A and C per serving.

The Food Safety and Inspection Service (FSIS) of the USDA has established a similar voluntary program for raw meat and poultry. The program includes major cuts of raw, single-ingredient meat and poultry products. As with raw fruits, vegetables, and fish, nutrition information may be displayed on posters, brochures, and other point-of-purchase materials, as long as they are located near the food. The information may also be included on the package label. The information must include serving size based on raw or cooked weight; calories per serving; calories from total fat per serving; amount per serving (by weight and by Percent Daily Values) for total fat, saturated fat, cholesterol, sodium, total carbohydrate, and dietary fiber; amount by weight of sugars and protein; and Percent Daily Values per serving for vitamins A and C, calcium, and iron.

## NUTRITION LABELING EXEMPTIONS

Under the NLEA some foods are exempt from nutrition labeling. These include:

- Food served for immediate consumption, such as that served in hospital cafeterias and airplanes, and that sold by food-service vendors—for example, mall cookie counters, sidewalk vendors, and vending machines.

- Ready-to-eat food that is not for immediate consumption, but is prepared primarily on-site—for example, bakery, deli, and candy store items.

- Food shipped in bulk, as long as it is not for sale in that form to consumers.

- Medical foods, such as those used to address the nutritional needs of patients with certain diseases.

- Plain coffee and tea, some spices, and other foods that contain no significant amounts of any nutrients.

## SHOPPERS READ FOOD LABELS

It is the position of the American Dietetic Association that nutrition label education is an effective way of helping consumers to make food choices. The Food Marketing Institute (FMI), in *Trends in the United States: Consumer Attitudes & the Supermarket, 2003* (Washington, D.C., 2003), found that nearly half of shoppers (46 percent) believe they are primarily responsible for making sure that the food they buy is nutritious. Among the factors they look at in deciding to purchase a food item for the first time, health claims were third most important, after price and brand name.

## CHAPTER 7
# FOOD SAFETY

## FOODBORNE ILLNESSES

In the United States, where food is often sold pre-packaged and has government seals of inspection, consumers expect food to be safe. Outbreaks of foodborne illness do occur, however, and have caused public concern about the safety of food. Today, the public realizes that any kind of food can be tainted with bacteria at any point, from the processing plant to the consumer's kitchen.

In 1993 three children and one adult died, and many more got sick, from contaminated hamburgers in the Pacific Northwest. In 1998 a juice maker agreed to what is believed to be the biggest settlement involving food poisoning from ingestion of fresh food. The families of five children who suffered severely from drinking fresh-squeezed apple juice may have received as much as $15 million. A total of 70 people became ill from this food-poisoning outbreak, including an infant who died.

The U.S. Department of Agriculture (USDA) reports, citing the Centers for Disease Control and Prevention (CDC), that foodborne pathogens cause an estimated 76 million illnesses each year, resulting in 325,000 hospitalizations and 5,200 deaths (*Economics of Foodborne Disease: Food and Pathogens,* Economic Research Service, USDA, July 17, 2001).

## FOODBORNE PATHOGENS

According to the CDC an estimated 250 pathogens are associated with foodborne illnesses (harmful bacteria, viruses, chemicals, and parasites). Bacterial pathogens are the most commonly identified cause of foodborne illnesses. Chemical pathogens are usually natural toxins in food and in such metals as copper and cadmium. Viruses, such as hepatitis A, are transmitted by infected food handlers or through contact with sewage. Parasites can also grow in host animals. For example, *Trichinella* is found in raw or undercooked pork.

In 2000 the CDC reported 26,021 cases of foodborne illness outbreaks in the United States. (See Table 7.1.) Of the cases in which the cause of the illness was identified, 51 percent were viral in origin and 46 percent were attributed to bacteria. Nearly half (46 percent) of all cases of foodborne illnesses in 2000 were attributed to unknown causes.

### Bacterial Pathogens

According to the CDC, ailments resulting from bacterial pathogens can cause serious complications beyond the immediate food-poisoning crisis. Arthritis, organ failures, stillbirths, and other complications may follow an episode of food poisoning. (See Table 7.2.)

The Economic Research Service (ERS) of the USDA reported that, in 1999, five foodborne bacterial pathogens (*Campylobacter, Salmonella, Escherichia coli* O157:H7, *E. coli* non-O157 STEC, and *Listeria monocytogenes*) were responsible for more than 31,000 hospitalizations

**TABLE 7.1**

**Total number of foodborne disease outbreaks by cause, 2000**

| Cause | Number of outbreaks | Number of cases |
|---|---|---|
| Bacterial | 223 | 6,506 |
| Chemical | 37 | 185 |
| Parasitic | 6 | 169 |
| Viral | 176 | 7,208 |
| Multiple causes | 3 | 22 |
| Total confirmed causes | 445 | 14,090 |
| Total unknown causes | 969 | 11,931 |
| Total 2000 | 1,414 | 26,021 |

SOURCE: "The Total Number of Foodborne Disease Outbreaks by Etiology," in *2000 Summary Statistics,* Centers for Disease Control and Prevention, Foodborne Outbreak Response and Surveillance Unit, Atlanta, GA, April 14, 2003 [Online] http://www.cdc.gov/foodborneoutbreaks/us_outb/fbo2000/summary00.htm [accessed August 1, 2003]

TABLE 7.2

**Some foodborne pathogens that can cause serious illnesses**

| Foodborne pathogen | Serious illnesses that can result | Foods in which pathogens have been found |
|---|---|---|
| **Bacteria** | | |
| Campylobacter | Arthritis, blood poisoning, Guillain-Barre syndrome (paralysis), chronic diarrhea, meningitis, and inflammation of the heart, gallbladder, colon, and pancreas | Poultry, raw milk, and meat |
| E. coli O157:H7 | HUS,[a] which is associated with kidney failure and neurologic disorders; and other illnesses | Meat, especially ground beef; raw milk; and produce |
| Listeria | Meningitis, blood poisoning, stillbirths, and other disorders | Soft cheese, other dairy products, meat, poultry, seafood, fruits, and vegetables |
| Salmonella | Reactive arthritis, blood poisoning, Reiter's disease (inflammation of joints, eye membranes, and urinary tract) and inflammation of the pancreas, spleen, colon, gallbladder, thyroid, and heart | Poultry, meat, eggs, dairy products, seafood, fruits, and vegetables |
| Shigella | Reiter's disease, HUS, pneumonia, blood poisoning, neurologic disorders, and inflammation of the spleen | Salads, milk and dairy products, and produce |
| Vibrio vulnificus | Blood poisoning | Seafood |
| Yersinia enterocolitica | Reiter's disease, pnemonia, and inflammation of vertebrae, lymphatic glands, liver, and spleen | Pork and dairy products |
| **Parasites** | | |
| Toxoplasma gondii | Central nervous system disorders | Meat, primarily pork |
| Trichinella spiralis | Heart and neurologic disorders | Pork |

[a]Hemolytic-uremic syndrome.

SOURCE: "Some Foodborne Pathogens That Can Cause Serious Illnesses" in *Food Safety: Information on Foodborne Illnesses,* U.S. General Accounting Office, Washington, DC, 1996

and 1,229 deaths. (See Table 7.3.) The STEC abbreviation stands for Shiga toxin–producing *E. coli.*

The federal government is working to reduce the number of illnesses related to foodborne pathogens. In addition to providing American consumers and retailers with information on safe food-handling practices, it has targeted food safety as one of the key objectives of Healthy People 2010, an initiative designed to promote health and prevent disease in the United States (Department of Health and Human Services, November 2000, available online at http://healthypeople.gov/ [accessed October 20, 2003]). Some of the specific goals of the initiative include:

- Cutting by 50 percent the number and rates of infection caused by foodborne pathogens, especially *Campylobacter, E. coli* O157:H7, *L. monocytogenes,* and *Salmonella.* Progress in this area is measured against the baseline rate. (The baseline rate is the rate of infections attributed to these pathogens in 1997. For example, there were 13.7 cases of *Salmonella*-related illnesses per 100,000 persons in 1997; the goal is to reduce this figure to 6.8 cases per 100,000 by the end of 2010.)

- Increasing the percentage of the population who apply food-safety practices.

- Lowering the risk of human exposure to pesticides in food.

*CAMPYLOBACTER JEJUNI.* The CDC reported that *Campylobacter jejuni* is the major cause of bacterial diarrheal illnesses in the United States ("Foodborne Diseases," National Institute of Allergy and Infectious Diseases, Bethesda, MD). The bacterium can infect anyone of any age, but typically is found in young children and young adults. The CDC estimates that more than 10,000 cases of the infection are reported in the United States each year.

*Campylobacter* infection is caused mainly by raw poultry and beef, unpasteurized milk, polluted water, and pets. The illness lasts 2–10 days. While some infected persons have no symptoms at all, others experience diarrhea, fever, headache, and chills. In persons with compromised immune systems, *Campylobacter* sometimes spreads to the bloodstream and causes a life-threatening infection (campylobacteriosis). Between 200 and 730 victims die from campylobacteriosis annually. (See Table 7.4.)

Tracking foodborne pathogens is one of the major functions of the CDC's Foodborne Diseases Active Surveillance Network (FoodNet). FoodNet conducts surveillance of nine foodborne pathogens and one syndrome in

TABLE 7.3

## Estimated annual cost due to selected foodborne bacterial pathogens, 2000[1]

| Pathogen | Estimated annual foodborne bacterial illnesses[2] | | | Costs[3,4] |
| | Cases | Hospitalizations | Deaths | |
|---|---|---|---|---|
| | Number | | | Billion 2000 dollars |
| *Campylobacter* spp | 1,963,141 | 10,539 | 99 | 1.2 |
| *Salmonella*[5] | 1,341,873 | 15,608 | 553 | 2.4 |
| *E. coli* O157 | 62,458 | 1,843 | 52 | 0.7 |
| *E. coli*, non-O157 STEC | 31,229 | 921 | 26 | 0.3 |
| *Listeria monocytogenes* | 2,493 | 2,298 | 499 | 2.3 |
| Total | 3,401,194 | 31,209 | 1,229 | 6.9 |

[1] These estimates of foodborne illness costs are not directly comparable to earlier Economic Research Service (ERS) estimates of the costs of foodborne disease, which were based on earlier data and methodologies for valuing costs.

[2] Data from the Centers for Disease Control and Prevention, *Food-Related Illness and Death in the United States*.

[3] The total estimated costs include specific chronic complications in the case of *Campylobacter* (Guillian-Barré syndrome), *E. coli* O157 (hemolytic uremic syndrome), and *Listeria monocytogenes* (congenital and newborn infections resulting in chronic disability or impairment). Estimated costs for *Listeria monocytogenes* exclude less serious cases that do not require hospitalization.

[4] ERS currently measures the productivity losses due to nonfatal foodborne illnesses by the value of forgone or lost wages, regardless of whether the lost wages involved a few days missed from work or a permanent disability that prevented an individual from returning to work. Using the value of lost wages for cases resulting in disability probably understates an individual's willingness to pay to avoid disability because it does not account for the value placed on avoiding pain and suffering. The willingness-to-pay measure derived from labor market studies that ERS uses to value a premature death is not an appropriate measure of willingness to pay to avoid disability, because it measures the higher wages paid to workers to accept a higher risk of premature death, not disability. Methods have been suggested to adjust willingness to pay to reduce the risk of premature death downward to estimate willingness to pay to avoid disability, such as the approach based on measuring "Quality Adjusted Life Years" (QALYs). As yet, there is no consensus among economists about how to use these methods to value willingness to pay to avoid the disability, pain, and suffering associated with foodborne illnesses. ERS's conservative estimates of the annual costs due to foodborne illnesses (particularly the chronic conditions associated with *Campylobacter*) would be substantially increased if willingness to pay to avoid disability, pain, and suffering were also taken into account.

[5] For ERS estimates for *Salmonella* released in 2003, see the related chapter in the Economics of Foodborne Illness briefing room, and the ERS *Foodborne Illness Cost Calculator*.

SOURCE: "Estimated annual costs due to selected foodborne pathogens, 2000," in *Economics of Foodborne Disease: Feature*, U.S. Department of Agriculture, Economic Research Service, Washington, DC, May 12, 2003 [Online] http://www.ers.usda.gov/briefing/FoodborneDisease/features.htm [accessed August 1, 2003]

TABLE 7.4

## Seven pathogens found in food and nonfood sources

| Pathogen, acute illness, and complication | Estimated total annual | | Estimated share foodborne |
| | Cases | Deaths | |
| | Number | | Percent |
|---|---|---|---|
| **Bacteria:** | | | |
| *Campylobacter jejuni* or *coli*– | | | |
| Campylobacteriosis | 2,000,000–10,000,000 | 200–730 | 55–70 |
| Guillain–Barré Syndrome | 532–3,830 | 10–76 | 55–70 |
| Subtotal | N/A | 210–806 | N/A |
| *Clostridium perfringens*– | | | |
| *C. perfringens* intoxications | 10,000 | 100 | 100 |
| *Escherichia coli* O157:H7– | | | |
| *E. coli* O157:H7 disease | 20,000–40,000 | 50–100 | 80 |
| Hemolytic uremic syndrome[1] | 1,000–2,000 | 29–58 | 80 |
| Subtotal | N/A | 79–158 | N/A |
| *Listeria monocytogenes*[2]– | | | |
| Listeriosis | 1,092–1,860 | 270–510 | 85–95 |
| Complications | 26–43 | 0 | 85–95 |
| Subtotal | N/A | 270–510 | N/A |
| *Salmonella* (non-typhoid)– | | | |
| Salmonellosis | 800,000–4,000,000 | 1,000–2,000 | 87–96 |
| *Staphylococcus aureus*- | | | |
| *S. aureus* intoxications | 8,900,000 | 2,670 | 17 |
| **Parasite:** | | | |
| *Toxoplasma gondii*[3]– | | | |
| Toxoplasmosis | 520 | 80 | 50 |
| Complications | 3,120 | 0 | 50 |
| Subtotal | N/A[4] | 80 | N/A |
| **Total** | **11,700,000–23,000,000** | **4,400–6,300** | **N/A** |

Notes: N/A = Not applicable. Subtotal and totals may not add due to rounding. Totals are rounded down to reflect the uncertainty of the estimates. Nonfood sources include drinking or swimming in contaminated water and contact with infected people or anima

[1] Kidney failure.

[2] Includes only hospitalized patients because of data limitations.

[3] Includes only toxoplasmosis cases related to fetuses and newborn children who may become blind or mentally retarded. Does not include all other cases of toxoplasmosis. Another high-risk group for this parasite is the immunocompromised, such as patients with AIDS.

[4] Of the 4,000 infections from this parasite each year, 520 develop acute illness and later die prematurely or develop some degree of chronic complication because of the illness, and 2,680 do not have noticeable acute illness at birth but develop complications by age 17. Therefore, a total of 3,200 develop either acute illness, chronic complication, or both.

SOURCE: Jean C. Buzby and Tanya Roberts, "Guillain-Barré Syndrome Increases Foodborne Disease Costs," in *FoodReview*, vol. 20, issue 3, September-December 1997

nine locations throughout the United States: California, Colorado, Connecticut, Georgia, Maryland, Minnesota, New York, Oregon, and Tennessee. These locations represent 37.6 million people, or 13.8 percent of the U.S. population in 2003, according to the CDC. Preliminary data from FoodNet indicated that, in 2002, there were 5,006 confirmed (laboratory-diagnosed) cases of *Campylobacter* in the nine surveyed locations. California had the highest rate of infection, with 31.67 cases per 100,000 persons, while Tennessee had the lowest, with 6.37 cases per 100,000. (See Table 7.5.) The overall rate for the nine surveyed sites was 13.37 cases per 100,000, compared with the Healthy People goal of 12.3, indicating that progress is being made toward the objective.

***CAMPYLOBACTER*-ASSOCIATED GUILLAIN-BARRÉ SYNDROME (GBS).** In the United States, Guillain-Barré Syndrome (GBS), characterized by nerve damage that may develop into paralysis, is currently the leading cause of paralysis from a disease.

Medical studies worldwide have found that 20–40 percent of GBS patients had been afflicted with *Campylobacter* infection 1–3 weeks before exhibiting GBS symptoms. *Campylobacter,* the leading bacterial cause of foodborne illnesses in the United States, has significantly increased the instances and, therefore, the financial costs of these ailments. Almost all afflicted individuals need hospitalization, and some suffer relapses. About 20 percent of

TABLE 7.5

**Incidence of cases of infection with nine pathogens and of one syndrome under surveillance in the Foodborne Diseases Active Surveillance Network, by site, compared with national health objectives for 2010, 2002**

(Cases per 100,000 persons.)

| Syndrome | California | Colorado | Connecticut | Georgia | Maryland | Minnesota | New York | Oregon | Tennessee | Overall | Objective |
|---|---|---|---|---|---|---|---|---|---|---|---|
| *Campylobacter* | 31. 67 | 13.99 | 15.79 | 7.58 | 6.72 | 18.95 | 12.97 | 16.01 | 6.37 | 13.37 | 12.30 |
| *Escherichia coli* O157 | 0.99 | 2.12 | 1.37 | 0.67 | 0.48 | 3.62 | 1.69 | 5.13 | 0.70 | 1.73 | 1.00 |
| *Listeria* | 0.37 | 0.12 | 0.47 | 0.18 | 0.43 | 0.10 | 0.45 | 0.26 | 0.11 | 0.27 | 0.25 |
| *Salmonella* | 15.85 | 13.46 | 13.28 | 21.43 | 17.13 | 11.87 | 16.22 | 9.53 | 19.61 | 16.10 | 6.80 |
| *Shigella* | 11.45 | 5.53 | 3.04 | 19.06 | 21.53 | 4.46 | 1.60 | 2.71 | 5.07 | 10.34 | NA[1] |
| *Vibrio* | 0.37 | 0.12 | 0.32 | 0.32 | 0.35 | 0.10 | 0.12 | 0.43 | 0.25 | 0.27 | NA |
| *Yersinia* | 0.50 | 0.12 | 0.47 | 0.51 | 0.26 | 0.38 | 0.63 | 0.49 | 0.60 | 0.44 | NA |
| *Cryptosporidium* | 0.99 | 0.88 | 0.55 | 1.43 | 0.52 | 4.10 | 1.75 | 1.15 | 0.46 | 1.42 | NA |
| *Cyclospora* | 0.05 | NR[2] | 0.20 | 0.27 | 0.05 | NR | 0.33 | NR | 0.04 | 0.11 | NA |
| HUS[3] | 1.01 | 2.62 | 1.79 | 0.84 | NR | 2.42 | 0.49 | 8.96 | NR | 1.78 | NA |
| Population in surveillance (millions)[4] | 3.20 | 2.46 | 3.43 | 8.38 | 5.38 | 4.97 | 3.32 | 3.47 | 2.84 | — | — |

[1] Not applicable.

[2] None reported.

[3] Hemolytic uremic syndrome. Incidence per 100,000 children aged < 5 years.

[4] Population for some sites is entire state, for other sites, selected counties. For some sites, the catchment area for *Cryptosporidium* and *Cyclospora* is larger than for bacterial pathogens.

SOURCE: "TABLE. Incidence of cases of infection with nine pathogens and of one syndrome under surveillance in the Foodborne Diseases Active Surveillance Network, by site, compared with national health objectives for 2010—United States, 2002," in *Morbidity and Mortality Weekly Report,* vol. 52, no. 15, April 18, 2003

GBS patients become significantly disabled, and 2 percent die. (See Table 7.4.)

***ESCHERICHIA COLI (E. COLI)* O157:H7.** *E. coli* O157:H7 food poisoning occurs when meat comes in contact with animal feces carrying the bacterium, usually at the slaughterhouse or at the packing plant. People have billions of the *E. coli* bacteria in their intestines, and many strains are harmless. However, the CDC estimates that between 20,000 and 40,000 Americans are infected with *E. coli* O157:H7 disease each year. About 50–100 die. (See Table 7.4.)

*E. coli* infection tends to strike the very young or very old and those with weak or immature immune systems. Most cases are mild to moderate, occurring 2–5 days after eating contaminated food. Diarrhea can last 6–8 days, and bloody diarrhea occurs in about half these cases.

Less than 5 percent (1,000–2,000) of cases lead to hemolytic uremic syndrome (HUS), a disease characterized by red blood cell destruction, kidney failure, seizures, and strokes. Most cases occur among children under 5 years old, although the frail elderly also may be at risk. Death results in about 29–58 cases annually. (See Table 7.4.) The CDC reports that, as of 2000, *E. coli* O157:H7 infection was the leading cause of acute kidney failure in children.

While raw or undercooked ground beef is the most likely source of *E. coli* O157:H7 contamination, the bacterium has also been traced to unpasteurized apple cider, unpasteurized milk, water, some fresh produce, turkey roll,

and mayonnaise. The infection can spread from person to person.

In 1997 the USDA recalled 25 million pounds of beef believed contaminated with this type of *E. coli*. This was the largest meat recall in U.S. history, and, as a result, the Nebraska plant where the beef had been processed was shut down.

According to researchers at the ERS, foodborne illness–related recalls of meat and poultry products rose dramatically between 1990 and 2000 (Michael Ollinger and Nicole Ballinger, "Weighing Incentives for Food Safety in Meat and Poultry," *Amber Waves,* vol. 1, no. 2, April 2003). They estimated that the number of Class I recalls (the more dangerous type, that involve meat and poultry that could, if improperly handled and cooked, cause illness or death) averaged about 24 per year and led to the recall of about 1.5 million pounds of meat each year between 1993 and 1996. (See Figure 7.1). In stark contrast, between 1997 and 2000, the number of Class I recalls averaged 41 per year and affected 24 million pounds of meat annually. The authors believe that the contrast between these time periods likely is due to changes in food-safety regulation. They point to more stringent Food Safety and Inspection Service (FSIS) regulations, which led to a zero-tolerance policy regarding *L. monocytogenes* in 1989. In 1994 the FSIS applied the same standards to O157:H7-infected ground beef. They also attribute the difference between the two time periods to the increasing improvement in methods used by the CDC to identify foodborne illnesses.

FIGURE 7.1

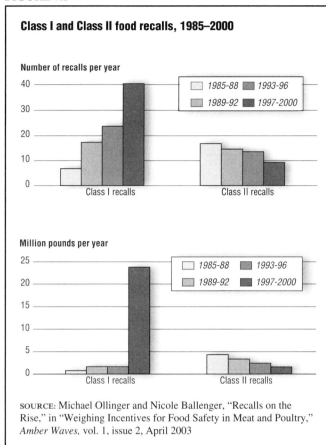

**Class I and Class II food recalls, 1985–2000**

Number of recalls per year

*1985-88* *1993-96*
*1989-92* *1997-2000*

Million pounds per year

*1985-88* *1993-96*
*1989-92* *1997-2000*

SOURCE: Michael Ollinger and Nicole Ballenger, "Recalls on the Rise," in "Weighing Incentives for Food Safety in Meat and Poultry," *Amber Waves,* vol. 1, issue 2, April 2003

In 1999, according to data from the ERS, *E. coli* O157:H7 infection caused 1,843 hospitalizations and 52 deaths. (See Table 7.3.) Of the $6.9 billion in costs for five foodborne bacterial infections (*Campylobacter, E. coli* O157:H7, *E. coli* non-O157 STEC, *Salmonella,* and *L. monocytogenes*) *E. coli* O157:H7 accounted for $0.7 billion of that total. Preliminary FoodNet data indicate that the incidence of infection from *E. coli* O157:H7 in the nine sites surveyed in 2002 was the highest in Oregon, with 5.13 cases per 100,000 population. (See Table 7.5.) Tennessee reported the lowest rate, with 0.70 cases per 100,000. The overall rate for the nine surveyed sites was 1.73—nearly two times higher than the goal of 1.0 cases per 100,000 population set by Healthy People 2010.

*LISTERIA* MONOCYTOGENES. About 1,092–1,860 cases of listeriosis occur each year, with 270–510 victims dying. (See Table 7.4.) Soft and semi-soft cheese, processed meats, undercooked chicken, and delicatessen salads are the usual sources of contamination. Unlike other bacteria, *Listeria* thrives in cold temperatures and can grow under refrigeration.

Listeriosis may be mild or severe. The symptoms of milder cases are sudden fever, headache, and other characteristics resembling influenza. The infection may last 3–4 weeks. A pregnant woman afflicted with listeriosis may pass the infection to her fetus, resulting in stillbirth or mental retardation in the baby. *Listeria* can travel from the gastrointestinal tract to the brain, causing meningitis. Blood poisoning may also occur. (See Table 7.2.)

Preliminary data from the FoodNet survey indicated that there were 101 reported cases of *Listeria*-associated illnesses in 2002. Connecticut, with a rate of 0.47 cases per 100,000 population, ranked highest among the sites surveyed in 2002. (See Table 7.5.) Minnesota ranked lowest, with 0.10 cases per 100,000 population. The overall rate for the nine sites surveyed was 0.27—very close to the objective of 0.25 cases per 100,000 set by Healthy People 2010.

*SALMONELLA.* According to the CDC, 40,000 cases of *Salmonella* infection are reported in the United States each year. However, the CDC believes that as many as 800,000 to 4 million people may be mildly infected without the disease being reported. (See Table 7.4.)

Only a handful of the more than 2,000 types of *Salmonella* cause food poisoning. As many as 1,000–2,000 of those infected die. (See Table 7.4.) The illness begins 6–72 hours after infection. The symptoms include severe diarrhea, nausea, vomiting, and fever, lasting 1–2 days.

Raw or undercooked chicken, beef, and eggs are the foods most likely to be contaminated with *Salmonella,* but it has also been found in unpasteurized milk, cheese, chocolate, fruits, and vegetables. People who have come in contact with infected stools can spread the infection. Most people know to take precautions with raw chicken, but recently the organism has flourished because it can now be transmitted from hens to the yolks of intact eggs.

According to the ERS, of five selected foodborne bacterial pathogens (*Campylobacter, Salmonella, E. coli* O157:H7, *E. coli* non-O157 STEC, and *L. monocytogenes*), *Salmonella* infections accounted for the highest number of hospitalizations (15,608), the highest number of deaths (553), and the second-highest number of cases (1,341,873) in 2000. (See Table 7.3.) The infection also accounted for $2.4 billion of the $6.9 billion in costs attributed to the five selected foodborne bacterial pathogens studied by the ERS.

The FoodNet Survey of *Salmonella* outbreaks in nine sites in 2002 indicated that the overall rate of infections (16.10 cases per 100,000 persons) among the nine sites surveyed is nearly three times higher than the Healthy People 2010 objective of 6.80 cases per 100,000. (See Table 7.5.) In fact, among the pathogens *Campylobacter, E. coli* O157:H7, *Listeria,* and *Salmonella,* the rate of outbreaks of *Salmonella* was the highest above its Healthy People 2010 goal.

**"MAD COW DISEASE."** In 1996 Europeans were frightened by a small outbreak of brain disease in Great Britain that resembled Creutzfeldt-Jakob disease (CJD). CJD, a very rare degenerative condition, usually affects people over 65, causing dementia and muscular contractions. The new variant CJD, a fatal illness, has been linked to bovine spongiform encephalopathy (BSE), more commonly known as "mad cow disease."

BSE first plagued cows in Great Britain in 1986, causing animals to develop spongy areas in their brains, to stagger, behave strangely, and to die by the thousands. It was believed that the disease was caused by infected, ground-up animal parts used as animal feed. Consumers were warned to stay away from beef, and 1.7 million cattle were destroyed in an effort to eliminate the disease. Mad cow disease has been confirmed among native-born cattle in Belgium, France, Switzerland, Germany, and Spain.

As of July 10, 2003, the FDA and USDA reported that BSE has never been found in the United States ("Bovine Spongiform Encephalopathy (BSE)," available online at http://www.usda.gov/news/releases/2003/05/bg0166.htm [accessed October 20, 2003]). The FDA and state regulatory agencies have undertaken a number of measures to prevent BSE in the United States, including increased inspections of renderers, animal feed manufacturers, and feed mills. Since 1990 the USDA has tested more than 48,000 cattle for BSE. The USDA also inspects all cattle slated for slaughter and tests ground beef for contaminants.

## COMPUTER TRACKING OF FOODBORNE ILLNESSES

In May 1998 the federal government introduced a new computer tracking system to expedite the identification of foodborne illnesses throughout the United States. The PulseNet computer network links the CDC, the FDA, the USDA, four laboratories, and state health departments.

When an outbreak of a foodborne illness occurs, the agencies identify the pathogen quickly, using the genetic code of the bacteria (DNA) in the tainted food and in afflicted individuals. The bacterial DNA code is then sent to agencies throughout the 50 states to determine if a similar illness has occurred in another site. Protective safeguards, such as a product recall, can then be initiated immediately.

## COSTS OF FOODBORNE ILLNESSES

Economists use two methods to estimate the financial costs of foodborne illnesses. The labor market approach estimates the statistical value of a life by using records that show consumers' willingness to pay to reduce the risks of death and poor health. This is based on labor market data indicating how much increased salary employers must offer workers to take a job with some injury risk. This method values the cost of a premature death at $5 million.

The human capital approach estimates the value of lost productivity (loss of income from death or disability). Lost productivity is calculated using a combination of lost income estimates and willingness-to-pay estimates. On this basis, the statistical value of a life tends to range from $15,000 to $1.9 million, depending on age. Jean C. Buzby and Tanya Roberts, in "Guillain-Barré Syndrome Increases Foodborne Disease Costs" (*FoodReview,* vol. 20, no. 3, September–December 1997), based the estimated costs of foodborne illnesses on the human capital approach. In 1996 dollars, the cost of a premature death, depending on age, was between $15,000 and $2,037,000.

The authors noted that both methods undervalued the true costs of foodborne illnesses to society because they mainly included medical costs and lost productivity. Total costs would be higher if the expenses resulting from complications, such as arthritis or meningitis, were added. The costs would also increase if societal costs, such as pain and suffering, travel to obtain medical care, and lost leisure time, were included.

CDC investigators gathered data in 1999, using reports from various years, in an attempt to estimate the average annual incidence of foodborne diseases in the United States (Paul S. Mead et al., "Food-Related Illness and Death in the United States," *Emerging Infectious Diseases,* September–October 1999). The data show that known pathogens cause 14.1 million foodborne illnesses annually, resulting in 60,000 hospitalizations and 1,800 deaths. Unknown agents cause 62 million illnesses, 263,000 hospitalizations, and 3,400 deaths; these are cases where inflammation of stomach and intestinal membranes (acute gastroenteritis) causes the hospitalizations and deaths, but the active agent remains undetermined. With all of our knowledge today about bacterial and viral agents, in 65 percent of food-related deaths every year the cause remains undetermined.

## FOOD-SAFETY PRECAUTIONS

There are a number of precautions consumers should take to minimize the chances of foodborne illness. The following includes general rules for food handling, storage, and consumption:

- When shopping, do not buy anything you will not use before the use-by or sell-by date.

- Refrigerate or freeze perishables, ready-to-eat foods, and leftovers as soon as possible. Freeze fresh meat and fish immediately if you will not use them within a few days.

## FIGURE 7.2

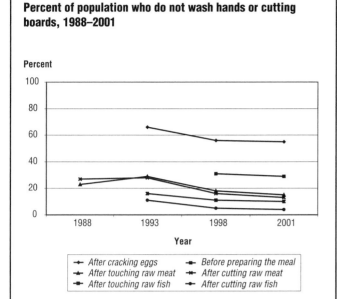

**Percent of population who do not wash hands or cutting boards, 1988–2001**

SOURCE: Sara Fein, Alan Levy, and Amy Lando, "Chart 1: FDA/FSIS Food Safety Survey. Cross-Contamination Measures: Percent of U.S. Population Who do Not Wash Hands or Cutting Boards," in *Food Safety Survey: Summary of Major Trends in Food Handling Practices and Consumption of Potentially Risky Foods,* U.S. Food and Drug Administration, Center for Food Safety and Applied Nutrition, Consumer Studies Branch, College Park, MD, August 27, 2002 [Online] http://www.cfsan.fda.gov/~dms/fssruvey.html [accessed September 2, 2003]

## FIGURE 7.3

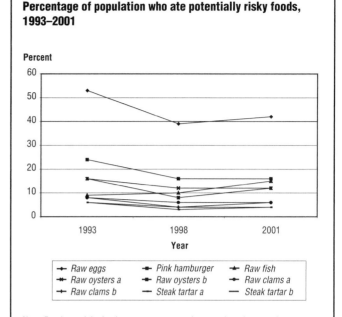

**Percentage of population who ate potentially risky foods, 1993–2001**

Note: For three of the foods, raw oysters, raw clams, and steak tartar, there are two numbers reported for 1998. This is because the wordings of these questions changed between 1993 and 2001 and were asked both ways in 1998. "A" after the food name is the 1993–1998 comparison; "b" is the 1998–2001 comparison.

SOURCE: Sara Fein, Alan Levy, and Amy Lando, "Chart 2: FDA/FSIS Food Safety Survey. Eating Potentially Risky Foods: Percent of US Population Who Ate Each Food," in *Food Safety Survey: Summary of Major Trends in Food Handling Practices and Consumption of Potentially Risky Foods,* U.S. Food and Drug Administration, Center for Food Safety and Applied Nutrition, Consumer Studies Branch, College Park, MD, August 27, 2002 [Online] http://www.cfsan.fda.gov/~dms/fssurvey.html [accessed September 2, 2003]

• Thaw frozen foods in the refrigerator or microwave, not on the kitchen counter. When marinating food, keep it in the refrigerator.

• Wash hands with hot soapy water before and after food preparation. Also, wash hands after using the bathroom, changing diapers, and handling pets.

• When preparing raw meats, keep knives and cutting boards separate from other ingredients and wash them thoroughly with hot water and soap. If possible, use separate cutting boards for fresh produce and for raw meats and fish. Never brush a marinade that has been in contact with raw meat on cooked meat. Wash counter tops with hot soapy water.

• Buy only clean, uncracked eggs, keep them refrigerated, and avoid eating raw or undercooked eggs. Make mayonnaise and caesar salad dressings with egg substitutes or pasteurized eggs. Do not eat raw cake batter or cookie dough.

• Wash all fruits and vegetables before eating, including those that will be peeled.

• Do not eat hamburgers that are pink in the center or steaks that are not thoroughly cooked.

Data from the FDA's Center for Food Safety and Applied Nutrition suggest that American consumers are making an effort to employ food-safety practices. The *FDA/FSIS Food Safety Survey* collected information on cross-contamination of foods and consumption of potentially risky foods in the years 1988, 1993, 1998, and 2001 ("Food Safety Survey: Summary of Major Trends in Food Handling Practices and Consumption of Potentially Risky Foods," Center for Food Safety and Applied Nutrition, FDA, August 27, 2002). Consumers were asked if they cleaned their hands and cutting boards after handling raw fish, meat, and chicken, and whether they ate raw or undercooked foods from animals, including pink hamburgers, steak tartare, raw fish, and eggs.

Researchers used two different criteria for asking consumers about food consumption in 1998: half the respondents were asked the questions with exactly the same wording that was used in 1993; the other half were asked about consumption within a more stringently defined time period. In 2001 all participants were asked about food consumption using the more precise time period. By employing these methods, researchers were able to obtain two estimates for 1998 data—one to compare with 1993 data, the other to compare with 2001 data.

FIGURE 7.4

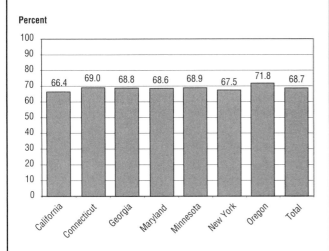

**Percentage of population who wash cutting boards with soap or bleach and water after cutting raw meat or poultry in general, FoodNet sites, 1998–99**

SOURCE: "Graph 1: Percent by State (N=12755) Wash Cutting Board w/Soap or Bleach and Water After Cutting Raw Meat or Poultry in General," in "1998–1999 Population Survey Atlas of Exposures," *CDC's Emerging Infections Program: Foodborne Diseases Active Surveillance Network (FoodNet),* Centers for Disease Control and Prevention, Atlanta, GA, 1999 [Online] http://www.cdc.gov/foodnet/surveys/pop/question/Qbwash.htm [accessed September 2, 2003]

FIGURE 7.5

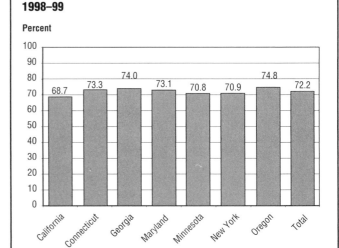

**Percent of population who wash their hands with soap and water after touching chicken in general, FoodNet sites, 1998–99**

SOURCE: "Graph 1: Percent of State (N=12755) Wash Hands w/Soap and Water After Touching Chicken in General," in "1998–1999 Population Survey Atlas of Exposures," *CDC's Emerging Infections Program: Foodborne Diseases Active Surveillance Network (FoodNet),* Centers for Disease Control and Prevention, Atlanta, GA, 1999 [Online] http://www.cdc.gov/foodnet/surveys/pop/question/Qbwash.htm [accessed September 2, 2003]

The survey found that, between 1993 and 1998, there was considerable improvement on every measure of cross-contamination and on four of the six measures of eating potentially dangerous foods. For the time period between 1998 and 2001 the survey found that most of the measures of cross-contamination of foods showed slight improvement. (See Figure 7.2.) Findings on the consumption of potentially harmful foods, however, showed no change for some measures since the 1998 survey, but others showed an increase. (See Figure 7.3.) Researchers reported that, while consumption of pink meats such as hamburger and steak tartar remained stable, consumption of raw clams, oysters, and fish had increased.

Findings from the CDC's *Population Survey Atlas of Exposures* tend to corroborate the results of the FDA's *FDA/FSIS Food Safety Survey.* The FoodNet sites comprised 29 million persons, or 11 percent of the United States population, in 1998–99. Consumers surveyed in these sites indicated that they practiced food-safety measures such as washing hands and/or cutting boards after handling raw meat or poultry. Sixty-nine percent of consumers surveyed said they washed their cutting boards with soap or bleach and water after cutting raw meat or poultry. (See Figure 7.4.) Seventy-two percent of consumers reported that they washed their hands with soap and water after touching chicken. (See Figure 7.5.) Eighty-six percent of consumers

reported that they washed lettuce before eating it at home. (See Figure 7.6.)

The CDC survey found that consumers' food-safety practices needed improvement in other areas, however. In the 2000 survey only three percent of consumers surveyed at FoodNet sites reported that they used a thermometer to check the internal temperature of a hamburger patty before eating the food. (See Figure 7.7.)

Despite findings by the FDA that there has been an increase during the last few years (2000–2002) in the proportion of foodborne illnesses linked to some fresh fruits and vegetables ("FDA Survey of Domestic Fresh Produce, FY 2000/2001 Field Assignment," FDA, January 2003) consumers appeared willing to consume potentially harmful foods. The 2000 CDC survey found that 16.6 percent of individuals at the eight surveyed sites had eaten uncooked parsley in the month preceding the survey, and 13.7 percent had eaten uncooked cilantro. (See Table 7.6.)

The FDA has also found evidence that links listeriosis outbreaks to consumption of some ready-to-eat foods such as deli and luncheon meats and hot dogs ("HHS and USDA Release Listeria Risk Assessment and Listeria Action Plan," *HHS News,* FDA, January 18, 2001). Nonetheless, the CDC survey found that consumers were not averse to eating some of these potentially harmful foods, as well as other products such as seafood. At the eight sites surveyed in 2000, 59.2 percent of consumers ate deli meats, 47.9

FIGURE 7.6

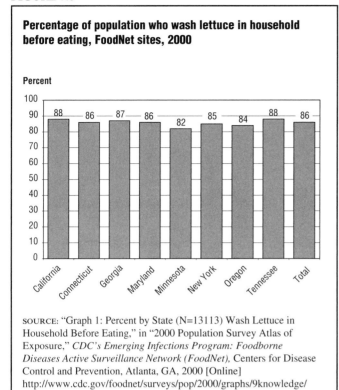

**Percentage of population who wash lettuce in household before eating, FoodNet sites, 2000**

SOURCE: "Graph 1: Percent by State (N=13113) Wash Lettuce in Household Before Eating," in "2000 Population Survey Atlas of Exposure," *CDC's Emerging Infections Program: Foodborne Diseases Active Surveillance Network (FoodNet),* Centers for Disease Control and Prevention, Atlanta, GA, 2000 [Online] http://www.cdc.gov/foodnet/surveys/pop/2000/graphs/9knowledge/3wash_lettuce/graph.htm [accessed September 2, 2003]

FIGURE 7.7

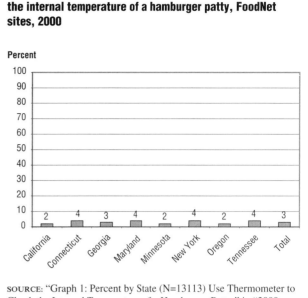

**Percentage of population who use a thermometer to check the internal temperature of a hamburger patty, FoodNet sites, 2000**

SOURCE: "Graph 1: Percent by State (N=13113) Use Thermometer to Check the Internal Temperature of a Hamburger Patty," in "2000 Population Survey Atlas of Exposures," *CDC's Emerging Infections Program: Foodborne Diseases Active Surveillance Network (FoodNet),* Centers for Disease Control and Prevention, Atlanta, GA, 2000 [Online] http://www.cdc.gov/foodnet/surveys/pop/2000/graphs/9knowledge/4thermometer/graph.htm [accessed September 2, 2003]

percent consumed fresh fish, and 13.6 percent had eaten cold smoked salmon, lox, and other smoked fish during the month before the survey. (See Table 7.7.)

## REGULATING FOOD SAFETY

Food safety is a growing problem, especially because the pool of people at risk grows as the population ages and the number of people with illnesses or conditions that suppress the immune system (AIDS, organ-transplant patients, etc.) increases. An aging population also means greater concern about the chronic effects of both microbial and chemical contaminants (pesticides). These may have long-term effects that only become apparent with longer life spans.

As noted earlier, multiple agencies are involved in food-safety regulation. The USDA inspects meat, poultry, and egg products. The FDA has regulatory responsibility for the rest of the food products, while the Environmental Protection Agency (EPA) establishes the levels of pesticide residues that can be tolerated by humans.

In 1994 the USDA established a requirement for labels with handling instructions on raw or partially cooked meat and poultry. The labels were designed to reduce the risk of foodborne illness attributable to unsafe handling, preparation, and storage.

Also in 1994 FDA Commissioner David Kessler turned to the National Aeronautics and Space Administration

(NASA) to copy NASA's program for ensuring safe food. NASA knew it would be disastrous to have an astronaut in outer space with food poisoning. The agency developed the Hazard Analysis and Critical Control Points (HACCP) program to prevent food poisoning before it could occur. Instead of looking for bacteria in finished products, manufacturing plants would have to identify the points where infection is most likely to occur ("Critical Control Points"—CCP) and design a plan to prevent contamination, keeping careful records to document their efforts.

For example, poultry producers would have to certify that feces are not rubbed into the bird's skin as it is defeathered, that the chill tank is not a "fecal soup," and that the birds are chilled quickly enough to prevent the growth of bacteria. The HACCP program has been adapted and applied to meat and fish processing.

As a consequence of the September 11, 2001, terrorist attacks on the United States, there is increased concern about the vulnerability of the food supply to acts of bioterrorism. The Public Health Security and Bioterrorism Preparedness and Response Act of 2002 allows the FDA to take additional measures to protect the U.S. food supply. In January 2003 the FDA proposed the measures to ensure a safe national food supply ("FDA Actions on New Bioterrorism Legislation," *Protecting the Food Supply,* FDA, January 2003). Food producers, processors, and packers

**TABLE 7.6**

**Herbs eaten in the past month, FoodNet sites, 2000**

| State | Uncooked parsley | Uncooked cilantro |
|---|---|---|
| California (n = 1,566) | | |
| Number | 406 | 572 |
| Percent | 25.9 | 36.5 |
| Connecticut (n = 1,587) | | |
| Number | 358 | 172 |
| Percent | 22.6 | 10.8 |
| Georgia (n = 1,514) | | |
| Number | 155 | 135 |
| Percent | 10.2 | 8.9 |
| Maryland (n = 1,574) | | |
| Number | 291 | 139 |
| Percent | 18.5 | 8.8 |
| Minnesota (n = 1,785) | | |
| Number | 221 | 159 |
| Percent | 12.4 | 8.9 |
| New York (n = 1,683) | | |
| Number | 311 | 107 |
| Percent | 18.5 | 6.4 |
| Oregon (n = 1,726) | | |
| Number | 267 | 355 |
| Percent | 15.5 | 20.6 |
| Tennessee (n = 1,678) | | |
| Number | 166 | 154 |
| Percent | 9.9 | 9.2 |
| Total (n = 13,113) | | |
| Number | 2,175 | 1,793 |
| Percent | 16.6 | 13.7 |

SOURCE: "Herbs eaten in the past month by site," in *2000 Population Survey Atlas of Exposures,* Centers for Disease Control and Prevention, Atlanta, GA, 2000 [Online] http://www.cdc.gov/foodnet/surveys/pop/2000/tables/table8.htm [accessed September 3, 2003]

must register with the FDA. Importers must notify FDA of each shipment of food into the U.S. New record-keeping rules have been added. And the FDA is authorized to hold food if "the agency has credible evidence or information that the food presents a threat of serious adverse health consequences or death to humans and animals."

## Meat Regulations

Before the present system, the USDA used inspection based on human senses—so-called organoleptic inspection—to test for food safety. Inspectors judged the safety of the meat by what they could see, feel, and smell. While organoleptic inspection could identify grossly visible lesions or diseases, it could not identify microbial pathogens, the cause of today's principal health risks. In poultry inspections, for example, the inspector had approximately two seconds to visually examine the inside and outside surfaces of each bird and feel the eviscerated (removed) internal organs.

In July 1996 the government instituted new regulations for meat inspections. Bacterial levels for salmonella were regulated. Processors were required to test all of their products for *E. coli* O157:H7. Critical points of contamination were required to be identified in processing. And all plants were required to have written plans to prevent contamination.

## Seafood Regulations

The FDA also developed a NASA-like HACCP program for the seafood industry, which took effect in early 1996. Seafood contaminants include the deadly *Vibrio vulnificus,* which kills half those it infects, as well as other bacteria, viruses, natural toxins, parasites, and chemicals.

## Food Additive Regulations

Whole foods, as opposed to functional foods (foods that contain a substance or substances that, manufacturers claim, perform a function in the body), are generally not required to undergo premarket review or approval by the FDA, but they are subject to postmarket surveillance for adulteration. The FDA, however, can regulate additives if they could potentially cause harm. Food manufacturers are responsible for proving that additives are safe before their products go to market. Manufacturers of food and color additives must demonstrate a reasonable certainty that their products are harmless. Furthermore, if any food additive is found to induce cancer in animals or people, its use will be prohibited.

EXEMPTIONS. Two categories of substances are exempt from food additive regulations. Prior-sanctioned substances are substances that were approved by the FDA or the USDA before 1958. "Generally recognized as safe" (GRAS) substances are substances that "experts qualified by scientific training and experience" have generally recognized as safe when used as intended in food. For example, salt, pepper, vinegar, vegetable oil, spices, and natural flavors, as well as some preservatives and sweeteners, are legally considered GRAS.

## NEW FOOD TECHNOLOGIES

Food technology is changing rapidly. Scientists continue to research ways to increase crop yields; produce more nutritious foods; grow plants that naturally resist disease, pests, and adverse weather, as well as tolerate chemical herbicides; and get rid of bacteria responsible for foodborne illnesses.

## Biotechnology

The shelves of most American supermarkets are lined with foods that have been genetically altered to improve the product's taste, shelf life, or resistance to insects and other pests while growing. Tomatoes, potatoes, squash, corn, and soybeans have been genetically altered through the emerging science of biotechnology. So have ingredients in everything from ketchup and cola to hamburger buns and cake mixes.

TABLE 7.7

**Meat, poultry, and seafood eaten in the past month, FoodNet sites, 2000**

| State | Deli meats | Uncooked or unheated salami | Jellied meats | Hot dogs | Ate any hot dogs and cooked hot dog before eating it | Fresh fish | Raw fresh fish | Oysters | Raw oysters | Cold smoked salmon, lox, lox spread, or other smoked fish |
|---|---|---|---|---|---|---|---|---|---|---|
| California (n = 1,566) | | | | | | | | | | |
| Number | 873 | 255 | 63 | 622 | 588 | 1,004 | 262 | 169 | 90 | 393 |
| Percent | 55.7 | 16.3 | 4.0 | 39.7 | 37.5 | 64.1 | 16.7 | 10.8 | 5.7 | 25.1 |
| Connecticut (n = 1,587) | | | | | | | | | | |
| Number | 1,125 | 229 | 35 | 831 | 799 | 884 | 86 | 74 | 41 | 196 |
| Percent | 70.9 | 14.4 | 2.2 | 52.4 | 50.3 | 55.7 | 5.4 | 4.7 | 2.6 | 12.4 |
| Georgia (n = 1,514) | | | | | | | | | | |
| Number | 794 | 111 | 37 | 851 | 827 | 681 | 49 | 121 | 46 | 126 |
| Percent | 52.4 | 7.3 | 2.4 | 56.2 | 54.6 | 45.0 | 3.2 | 8.0 | 3.0 | 8.3 |
| Maryland (n = 1,574) | | | | | | | | | | |
| Number | 1,090 | 151 | 29 | 844 | 817 | 800 | 55 | 140 | 55 | 211 |
| Percent | 69.3 | 9.6 | 1.8 | 53.6 | 51.9 | 50.8 | 3.5 | 8.9 | 3.5 | 13.4 |
| Minnesota (n = 1,785) | | | | | | | | | | |
| Number | 963 | 278 | 48 | 855 | 818 | 679 | 34 | 57 | 19 | 221 |
| Percent | 53.9 | 15.6 | 2.7 | 47.9 | 45.8 | 38.0 | 1.9 | 3.2 | 1.1 | 12.4 |
| New York (n = 1,683) | | | | | | | | | | |
| Number | 1,169 | 188 | 22 | 931 | 896 | 750 | 54 | 46 | 14 | 137 |
| Percent | 69.5 | 11.2 | 1.3 | 55.3 | 53.2 | 44.6 | 3.2 | 2.7 | 0.8 | 8.1 |
| Oregon (n = 1,726) | | | | | | | | | | |
| Number | 878 | 176 | 41 | 734 | 694 | 799 | 77 | 137 | 26 | 341 |
| Percent | 50.9 | 10.2 | 2.4 | 42.5 | 40.2 | 46.3 | 4.5 | 7.9 | 1.5 | 19.8 |
| Tennessee (n = 1,678) | | | | | | | | | | |
| Number | 874 | 116 | 34 | 866 | 815 | 682 | 47 | 78 | 41 | 156 |
| Percent | 52.1 | 6.9 | 2.0 | 51.7 | 48.6 | 40.6 | 2.8 | 4.6 | 2.4 | 9.3 |
| Total (n = 13,113) | | | | | | | | | | |
| Number | 7,766 | 1,504 | 309 | 6,534 | 6,524 | 6,279 | 664 | 822 | 322 | 1,781 |
| Percent | 59.2 | 11.5 | 2.4 | 49.8 | 49.8 | 47.9 | 5.1 | 6.3 | 2.5 | 13.6 |

SOURCE: "Meat, poultry, and seafood eaten in the past month by site," in *2000 Population Survey Atlas of Exposures,* Centers for Disease Control and Prevention, Atlanta, GA, 2000 [Online] http://ww.cdc.gov/foodnet/surveys/pop/2000/tables/table4.htm [accessed September 2, 2003]

Biotechnology enables scientists to modify DNA, the genetic material in living cells. Using recombinant DNA methods, scientists identify a desirable gene or several genes in a plant, make copies of those genes, and introduce the gene copies into the genetic code of another plant. The process is called genetic engineering. Usually, the genes are crossed to other crops, allowing rapid development of new varieties.

In 1990 the FDA approved the commercial use of a recombinant DNA–produced enzyme called chymosin (rennet), issuing the first regulation for use of such genetically engineered product. Rennet, used to help milk clot in making cheese, comes from the lining of calves' stomachs. Scientists copied the gene that produces rennet and reproduced it inside a bacterium. Today, about 50 percent of the rennet used in cheese-making is produced by this technique.

In 1992 the FDA announced that food and food ingredients produced by biotechnology are regulated under the Federal Food, Drug, and Cosmetic Act of 1938 (52 Stat 1040.) The FDA proposed mandatory rules in January 2001 that would tighten the scrutiny of bioengineered foods. The rules required that manufacturers of plant-derived, bioengineered foods and animal feeds notify the FDA at least 120 days before the products are marketed.

As part of the notification, the manufacturers have to provide information showing that the foods are as safe as their conventional counterparts. Manufacturers have completed voluntary consultations on roughly 50 bioengineered foods using scientific guidelines published by the FDA in 1992. The new rules make voluntary consultations mandatory and require manufacturers to submit safety and nutritional information to the FDA.

In 1994, for the first time, the FDA approved a whole food derived from a plant modified by biotechnology. The FDA found the fresh tomato Flavr Savr as safe as tomatoes produced by conventional methods. Grocers began selling the Flavr Savr tomato in 1994. The Flavr Savr took longer to ripen, could remain on the vine longer, and was expected to be of better quality than other tomatoes available in winter.

Experiments are now under way to develop tomatoes that have enhanced levels of lycopene, a plant chemical that gives them their red color. Researchers say lycopene also may offer health benefits because of its apparent antioxidant properties. Antioxidants are thought to neutralize harmful molecules in the human body called "free radicals." These substances, which result from cell metabolism and other causes, may contribute to cancer and cardiovascular disease.

Many genetic modifications have been designed to improve production. About half the soybeans and about 25 percent of the corn grown in the United States has been bioengineered, according to the USDA. Most of these crop varieties have been designed either to tolerate herbicides better or to resist insects without the need for extensive pesticide spraying. An estimated two-thirds of the processed foods in U.S. supermarkets contain genetically engineered corn, soybeans, or other crops.

Genetically engineered foods that have already been approved, that are awaiting approval, or are being developed include:

- Higher-protein rice.
- Potatoes with higher starch content, which will help reduce the oil absorbed during frying.
- Strawberries with increased ellagic acid, a natural cancer-fighting agent.
- Bananas resistant to fungus.
- Peanuts with improved protein balance.
- Other fruits and vegetables to contain vitamins C and E to protect against heart disease and cancer.

A federally funded study by the National Research Council released in 2000 concluded that there is no evidence to suggest that bioengineered food is unsafe.

OPPOSITION. The debate over genetically engineered plants began almost as soon as scientists altered plant genes in the early 1980s. Opposition to bioengineered foods has been especially strong in Europe and Japan.

Many consumer and environmental groups believe that genetic engineering is a radical new technology, not an extension of traditional plant breeding. Some of the adverse results that they think are at least theoretically possible with new biotechnology include:

- An increase in levels of naturally occurring toxins and allergens (substances that produce an allergic reaction) or the activation of dormant toxins or allergens.

- A change in the absorption or metabolism of important nutrients.
- A reduction in the effectiveness of some antibiotics through the use of antibiotic-resistant genes.
- Harmful environmental consequences, including negative effects on wildlife and ecosystems.
- A decrease in the quality and nutritional adequacy of animal feed or an increase in the toxins in animal feed.

In September 2000 a consumer group reported that a bioengineered variety of corn not approved for human consumption had been found in taco shells. The corn, dubbed StarLink, was modified to contain a gene from the bacterium *Bacillus thuringiensis* that expressed a protein—Cry9C—toxic to certain insects that endanger the profits of corn growers.

Although StarLink's developer, Aventis, was required to ensure that the bioengineered corn did not go into food, some became mingled with corn destined for human consumption. The presence of an unapproved pesticide in food means that the food is adulterated under the Federal Food, Drug, and Cosmetic Act, enforced by the FDA.

Upon learning of allegations that the taco shells contained StarLink corn, the FDA began a thorough investigation. Kraft Foods, producer of the taco shells, initiated its own investigation and voluntarily recalled millions of taco shells when an independent laboratory found that the shells contained the Cry9C gene. The FDA subsequently confirmed the presence of StarLink in the taco shells.

LABELING. FDA policy dictates that foods derived from biotechnology need not be specially labeled. The FDA will, however, require labeling of genetically engineered food products if the new product differs significantly from its traditional counterpart. For example, labeling would be required if a genetically engineered tomato no longer contained vitamin C. The FDA will also require labeling if a gene from a commonly allergenic food is introduced into a food that was not previously considered allergenic or if the food contains a known toxic substance.

Consumer and environmental groups want the FDA to require premarket testing, a mandatory premarket notification system, and labeling. Some groups that object to genetically engineered foods for moral, ethical, religious, or scientific reasons have threatened legal action against the FDA policy. Critics of the FDA policy insist all genetically engineered foods should be labeled so that consumers can avoid them if they choose. For example, identifying the presence of animal genes in plants may be important for individuals whose diets are restricted for religious reasons. The FDA asserts that in the few cases in which an animal gene might be inserted into a plant, the characteristics of the plant food would not change in a manner relevant to religious beliefs.

Most critics are concerned that the proposed regulations will be inadequate to warn consumers who suffer from allergies when an allergenic protein has been transferred. A study conducted at the University of Nebraska involved feeding subjects modified soybeans injected with a gene from a Brazil nut. Those with an allergy to the nut had an adverse reaction, while those with no allergy were not affected.

Supporters of the FDA policy counter that across-the-board labeling would be expensive and impractical. The components of processed food would be difficult to track, and analytic tests would not always reveal if a food had been genetically engineered. In addition, labels imply a level of risk that is scientifically unsupported and might alarm consumers and jeopardize their acceptance of this technology. Consumer acceptance is key to realizing the potential of new biotechnology.

## Will Consumers Pay for Genetically Modified Food?

Data from a study by researchers at the ERS suggest that consumers tend to shy away from purchasing or eating genetically altered foods (Abebayehu Tegene et al., "The Effects of Information on Consumer Demand for Biotech Foods: Evidence from Experimental Auctions," March 2003, available online at http://www.ers.usda.gov/publications/tb1903/tb1903.pdf [accessed October 20, 2003]). The researchers designed and performed an experimental auction to gauge the willingness of consumers to buy genetically altered tortilla chips, russet potatoes, and vegetable oil. Labels for these products were of two types: one with a notation that the food had been genetically altered, one without such mention. Consumers also were provided with three sources of information about the products: one source with a pro-biotechnology bias, one with an anti-biotechnology bias, and one from an independent third party.

The study showed that participants, on average, paid 14 percent less for genetically modified food, regardless of the slant of the information they received. The study also showed that, nevertheless, the information and its source influenced the buyers. Those receiving anti-biotechnology information paid on average 35–38 percent less. Those who, in addition to negative information, were also given information from independent sources, paid 15–22 percent less for genetically modified foods.

The authors also suggested that the use of the term "genetically modified" instead of "bioengineered" or "biotech" may have influenced the outcome of the auctions. They pointed out that the FDA and USDA prefer the terms "bioengineered" and "biotech" to describe foods produced with the aid of biotechnology.

## Novel Macroingredients

Novel macroingredients are typically large quantities of digestible, partially digestible, or non-digestible substances, sometimes 10 percent above the weight of the overall food product. In comparison, food additives are used in amounts below 1 percent by weight. Food producers are developing macroingredients in response to research about the relationship of diet and disease. Their goal is to modify traditional foods so that consumers who want to adhere to diets lower in fat and sugar can achieve this without having to change their eating habits. Olestra is the first macroadditive approved by the FDA.

The government is uncertain how to test the safety of novel macroingredients because there is no precedent for evaluating the effects of these products. Conventional methods of animal testing may be inadequate because these ingredients may be chemically more complex than traditional foods and may comprise a greater proportion of the human diet. The usual method for testing toxicity of food additives—giving laboratory animals more than 100 times the likely human intake of the substance—is impractical. Scientists would have to feed laboratory animals quantities they could not physically tolerate. Human testing may be the only way to assess the safety of novel macroingredients. The FDA has not developed a policy or regulations for human clinical trials or determined whether they should be required for novel macroingredients.

OLESTRA. In 1996 the FDA approved olestra, a fat substitute developed by Procter & Gamble, for use in salty and spicy snacks. Although olestra, or sucrose polyester, has properties similar to natural fat, it provides no calories or fat because it is indigestible.

Olestra was approved despite several problems. It absorbs fat-soluble vitamins, such as vitamins A, D, E, and K, from foods eaten at the same time as olestra. It also reduces the absorption of carotenoids—nutrients found in carrots, sweet potatoes, green leafy vegetables, and some animal tissues. Although research on the effects of carotenoids is not conclusive, some studies have shown that they help protect against cancer.

Studies also found that olestra caused severe intestinal cramps, more frequent bowel movements, and diarrhea in some people. The FDA claims these gastrointestinal effects do not have medical consequences and, in response to these problems, has required that all foods with olestra be labeled with a warning about nutrient loss and possible intestinal distress. Critics, however, charge that Procter & Gamble plans to use olestra in other food items (see Table 7.8), which would lead to an increase in olestra consumption.

Marion Nestle, in "The Selling of Olestra" (*Public Health Reports,* vol. 113, no. 6, November/December

TABLE 7.8

**Some potential uses of olestra, according to the Procter & Gamble Company**

| Snack foods | Restaurant foods |
|---|---|
| Potato chips[1] | French fries |
| Corn chips[1] | Fried chicken |
| Cheese puffs[1] | Fried fish |
| Crackers[1] | Onion rings |
| Doughnuts | |
| Pastries and pies | **Table spreads** |
| Cakes and cookies | Margarines[2] |
| Ice cream[2] | Cheeses[2] |

**Home use**
Fried chicken
Grilled meats and vegetables
Sauteed meats and vegetables
Baked desserts and snacks

[1] Use of olestra in savory (salty and spicy) snacks was approved by the FDA on January 24, 1996
[2] Not included in P&G's 1987 petition to the FDA, which excluded uses in table spreads and ice cream

SOURCE: Marion Nestle, "Table 7.5: Some Potential Uses of Olestra, According to the Procter & Gamble Company," in "The Selling of Olestra," *Public Health Reports*, vol. 113, no. 6, November/December 1998 used with the permission of Oxford University Press

1998), noted that while olestra snacks may be fat free, they are not calorie free. In fact, they reduce by one-half the calories of natural fat products. Nestle believes that just as artificial sweeteners have not lowered overall sugar intake, olestra would probably not reduce the total fat intake.

In March 2001 *Discover Magazine* reported that olestra sales had tumbled from $400,000 in 1998 to $200,000 in 2000 as a result of factors such as the unattractive wording on the label.

On August 1, 2003, the FDA announced that it will no longer require the warning statement on products containing olestra ("FDA Changes Labeling Requirement for Olestra," *FDA Talk Paper*, August 1, 2003).

Studies submitted by Procter & Gamble and the Center for Science in the Public Interest led the FDA to conclude that gastrointestinal upsets from consumption of products containing olestra typically are not severe enough to warrant the warning label. However, the FDA still requires that manufacturers add vitamins A, D, E, and K to products containing olestra. The vitamins will be listed on the label with the indicator "dietarily insignificant."

**Functional Foods**

Gingko biloba, St. John's Wort, echinacea, and phosphatidyl serine are just a few dietary supplements found in functional foods—foods that contain a substance or substances that, manufacturers claim, perform a useful function in the body. For example, calcium-fortified orange juice is a functional food that "strengthens the bone." Other functional foods have been touted as capable of increasing energy, preventing depression, boosting the immune system, and increasing mental acuity. Functional foods are one of the fastest-growing sectors of the food industry, showing annual retail sales of $10 billion. Several large food companies, such as Kellogg and Pillsbury, have produced functional foods in response to the growing demands for them.

In "Functional Foods" (*Nutrition Action Health Letter*, Center for Science in the Public Interest, Washington, D.C., April 1999) Beth Brophy and David Schardt pointed out that it was not until 1993 that the FDA allowed "health claims" on food labels. Prior to this, labels could not claim that foods were capable of preventing a disease. Any reference to a disease meant that the particular food was considered an "unapproved" or illegal drug.

Starting in 1993 Congress told the FDA it could allow a food label to state, for example, that "a diet low in saturated fat and cholesterol can reduce the risk of heart disease," but only if it has the FDA's approval and only if the food isn't unhealthy. Nonetheless, the FDA strictly regulates health claims on food labels and as of September 2003 had approved only 14 such claims.

In 1994 dietary supplement companies found a loophole in FDA regulations. With the enactment of the Dietary Supplement Health and Education Act (DSHEA; PL 103-417) Congress indicated that there may be a link between dietary supplements and disease prevention, and manufacturers were allowed to claim that a certain supplement can affect the structure or function of the body. For example, the supplement label may claim that it "promotes a healthy heart." Without mention of a disease, such a claim does not require FDA approval.

Large food companies that prepare functional foods are using the same structure and function claims. Some have gone so far as to call their products dietary supplements. In December 1998 McNeil Consumers Healthcare, the U.S. distributor of a Finnish margarine called Benecol, announced that it would sell its product as a dietary supplement.

In May 1999 the FDA approved the sale of Benecol, while announcing that it does not endorse Benecol or its claims. The FDA had simply reviewed the testing done by McNeil and told the company it would not violate FDA labeling regulations if the product label states Benecol contains an ingredient that "helps promote healthy cholesterol levels."

Brophy and Schardt are concerned that, unlike food additives or drugs, ingredients in functional foods are not required to undergo premarket evaluations to determine if they might cause serious conditions, such as cancer or liver toxicity. Some individuals have been known to develop severe allergies to dietary supplements, the health-claim

TABLE 7.9

**Estimated annual quantities and percentage of consumption for irradiated food, as of January 2000**

| Food product | Amount irradiated (millions of pounds) | Percentage of annual consumption |
|---|---|---|
| Spices and dry or dehydrated aromatic vegetable substances | 95.0 | 9.5 |
| Fruits and vegetables | 1.5 | 0.002 |
| Fresh and frozen uncooked poultry | 0.5 | 0.002 |
| **Total** | **97.0** | |

Notes: Refrigerated and frozen uncooked beef, pork, lamb, and goat have been approved for irradiation; however, as of January 2000, these products were not available commercially.

SOURCE: "Estimated Annual Quantities and Percentage of Consumption for Irradiated Food in the United States, as of January 2000" in *Food Irradiation: Available Research Indicates that Benefits Outweigh Risks,* U.S. General Accounting Office, Washington, DC, 2000

FIGURE 7.8

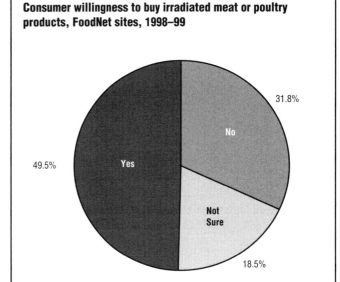

**Consumer willingness to buy irradiated meat or poultry products, FoodNet sites, 1998–99**

SOURCE: Paul D. Frenzen et. al., "Figure 3. Only half of adult consumers in the FoodNet sites were willing to buy irradiated meat or poultry products in 1998–99," in *Issues in Food Safety Economics,* Agriculture Information Bulletin No. 757, U.S. Department of Agriculture, Economic Research Service, Washington, DC, August 2000

components of functional foods. Still others have suffered adverse reactions from mixtures of medicine and dietary supplements.

## Irradiation

The term irradiation refers to the exposure of food to radiation in order to eliminate bacteria. In 1963 irradiation was first approved by the FDA for wheat and wheat flour. Since then the FDA has approved irradiation for spices and seasonings, enzymes, fruits, vegetables, grain products, and poultry. In December 1997 the FDA concluded that irradiation is safe for raw meat. However, since the USDA regulates the processing and labeling of red meat, irradiation was not authorized until the FSIS implemented regulations on December 23, 1999 (64 FR 72150). Additional regulations were issued by the FSIS in February 2000.

According to FDA scientists, irradiation eliminates or decreases bacterial pathogens, insects, and parasites. It diminishes spoilage and, in some fruits and vegetables, prevents sprouting and delays the ripening process. They claim the process is safe and does not remove nutrients from the food or make it radioactive. It also does not noticeably change food taste, texture, or appearance.

According to the USDA, as of May 2003, there are 37 countries that have approved the use of irradiation on more than 40 food products ("USDA Releases Specifications for the Purchase of Irradiated Ground Beef in the National School Lunch Program," *USDA News Release,* May 29, 2003). Some of these countries—including Canada, France, China, Japan, Italy, Russia, and Mexico—have been using food irradiation since the 1960s. American astronauts have eaten irradiated foods since 1972, and such professional organizations as the American Medical Association and the American Dietetic Association have endorsed irradiation. However, not everyone approves of exposing food to radiant energy. Opponents are concerned that irradiation facilities could threaten worker safety and public health. Some believe that irradiation may result in carcinogenic food.

As of early 2000 the majority of irradiated foods consumed in the U.S. were in the category of spices or other dried vegetable substances, accounting for 95 million of the 97 million pounds of irradiated food product. (See Table 7.9.)

Despite government sanction and the willingness of food manufacturers to use irradiation to combat foodborne pathogens, irradiated products account for a very small portion of the estimated 51.4 billion pounds (boneless equivalent weight) of meat and poultry consumed in the United States. According to the USDA (Paul D. Frenzen et al., "Consumer Acceptance of Irradiated Meat & Poultry Products," *Issues in Food Safety Economics,* August 2000) the perception by meat and poultry manufacturers that consumers are unwilling to buy irradiated meat was borne out by the results of a FoodNet survey. The survey showed that only 50 percent of adult consumers were willing to buy irradiated products such as ground beef and chicken. (See Figure 7.8.) Additional findings showed that only about 25 percent of adult consumers were willing to pay the more expensive prices charged for irradiated ground beef and chicken. (See Table 7.10.) Table 7.11 provides a list of the reasons adult consumers gave for their reluctance to buy irradiated meat products.

TABLE 7.10

**Consumer willingness to pay more for irradiated ground beef and chicken, FoodNet sites, 1998–99**

| Response | Ground beef | Chicken |
|---|---|---|
| | *Percent* | |
| Willing to buy irradiated meat or poultry: | | |
| Would pay more | 22.7 | 24.5 |
| Wouldn't pay more | 7.0 | 7.2 |
| Not sure about paying more | 17.5 | 16.5 |
| Not willing to buy or unsure about buying irradiated meat or poultry | 52.8[1] | 51.9[2] |
| **Total** | 100.00 | 100.0 |

[1] Includes 2.3 percent of respondents who were willing to buy irradiated meat or poultry but did not buy ground beef.
[2] Includes 1.4 percent of respondents who were willing to buy irradiated meat or poultry but did not buy chicken.
Note: Totals may not sum to 100.0 percent due to rounding.

SOURCE: Paul D. Frenzen et al., "Table 1. Consumer willingness to pay more for irradiated ground beef and chicken, FoodNet sites, 1998–99," in *Issues in Food Safety Economics,* Agriculture Information Bulletin No. 757, U.S. Department of Agriculture, Economic Research Service, Washington, DC, August 2000

TABLE 7.11

**Most important reason why adults would not buy irradiated meat or poultry, FoodNet sites, 1998–99**

| Most important reason | Percent |
|---|---|
| Insufficient information about risks and/or benefits | 35.0 |
| Concerned about safety of eating irradiated food | 22.7 |
| Irradiation doesn't make food safer | 4.2 |
| Doesn't eat meat or poultry | 4.0 |
| Concerned about environmental impact of irradiation | 3.9 |
| Doesn't need irradiation to make food safe | 3.5 |
| Doesn't like trying new foods/products | 3.3 |
| Price of irradiated food | 2.5 |
| Taste/appearance of irradiated food | 1.4 |
| Other, unspecified reasons | 10.2 |
| Doesn't know/not sure | 7.9 |
| Refused to answer | 1.4 |
| **Total** | 100.0 |

Note: Includes only those respondents (31.8 percent of total) who would not buy irradiated meat or poultry.

SOURCE: Paul D. Frenzen et al., "Table 2. Most important reason why adults would not buy irradiated meat or poultry, FoodNet sites, 1998–99," in *Issues in Food Safety Economics,* Agriculture Information Bulletin 757, U.S. Department of Agriculture, Economic Research Service, Washington, DC, August 2000

FIGURE 7.9

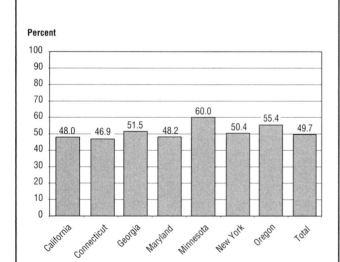

**Percentage of population who would purchase irradiated meat or poultry if available, selected states, 1998–99**

SOURCE: "Graph 1: Percent by State (N=12755) Would Purchase Irradiated Meat or Poultry if Available," in "1998–1999 Population Survey Atlas of Exposures," *CDC's Emerging Infections Program: Foodborne Diseases Active Surveillance Network (FoodNet),* Centers for Disease Control and Prevention, Atlanta, GA, 1999 [Online] http://www.cdc.gov/foodnet/surveys/pop/question/Q40.htm [accessed August 28, 2003]

These findings are borne out by the CDC's *Population Survey Atlas of Exposures.* According to the survey, only half the respondents surveyed in seven locations in 1998–99 said they were willing to buy irradiated meat or poultry if these products were available. (See Figure 7.9.)

Willingness to buy irradiated meat and poultry was highest in Minnesota (60 percent) and lowest in Connecticut (47 percent).

## PESTICIDES

### Regulatory Monitoring

Three federal agencies share responsibility for regulating pesticides. The FDA is charged with enforcing pesticide residue tolerances and ensuring that environmental contaminants in food and animal feed are within safe levels. (Residue tolerance refers to the maximum amount of a pesticide residue that is permitted in or on a food.) The EPA is responsible for registering the use of pesticides after ensuring that their use will not cause an unreasonable risk. The EPA also establishes the legal maximum level of pesticide residues allowed in each specific food. In addition the EPA obtains information on industrial chemical effects that present unreasonable risks to people and the environment, and controls their production, distribution, and disposal. The third agency, the USDA, is responsible for regulating pesticides in meat, poultry, and egg products.

FDA DOMESTIC MONITORING. In *Food and Drug Administration Pesticide Program—Residue Monitoring 2001* (Washington, D.C., 2001) the FDA analyzed 2,101 food samples from 41 states (no samples were collected from Alabama, Connecticut, Hawaii, Maine, Mississippi, Nevada, South Dakota, Tennessee, or Vermont) and Puerto Rico. Three-fifths of samples (60.2 percent) had no detectable pesticide residues and only 1.1 percent had violative residues. The FDA defines a violative residue as "a residue

FIGURE 7.10

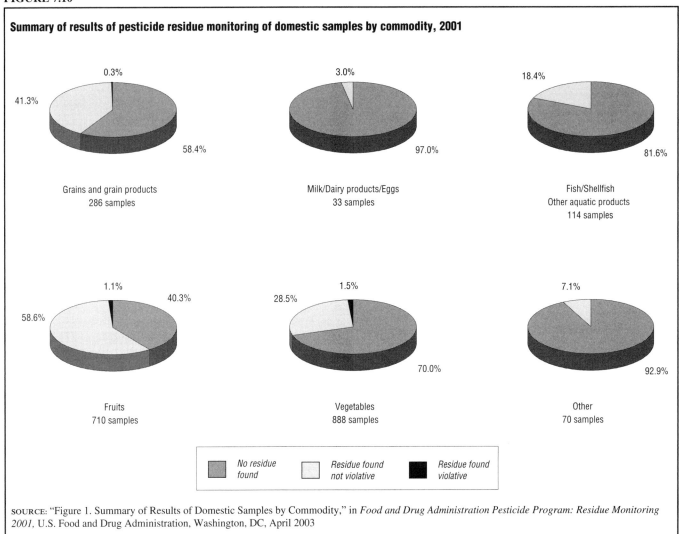

**Summary of results of pesticide residue monitoring of domestic samples by commodity, 2001**

SOURCE: "Figure 1. Summary of Results of Domestic Samples by Commodity," in *Food and Drug Administration Pesticide Program: Residue Monitoring 2001*, U.S. Food and Drug Administration, Washington, DC, April 2003

that exceeds a tolerance or a residue at a level of regulatory significance for which no tolerance has been established in the sampled food." Figure 7.10 shows the proportions of the domestic samples by commodity group with no residues found, non-violative residues found, and violative residues found.

The FDA's Total Diet Study, conducted in 2001, is different from regulatory monitoring in that it determined pesticide residues in 1,030 food items prepared for consumption. As Table 7.12 indicates, the pesticide residues shown were found in more than 2 percent of samples. The five most frequently occurring residues have been the same for several years. All, however, are below regulatory limits.

**FDA IMPORT MONITORING.** In 2001 the FDA also analyzed food samples from 99 countries. Mexico was the source of the largest number of samples, reflecting the volume and diversity of commodities imported from that country. Of the 4,374 samples analyzed, 72 percent had no

pesticide residues detected, and 4.8 percent had violative residues. (See Figure 7.11.)

**Problems with Monitoring Pesticides in Imports**

The United States has no jurisdiction over food producers in other countries. Consequently, federal agencies must rely on the foreign countries' food-safety systems and/or U.S. inspection at the port of entry. The U.S. General Accounting Office (GAO) has repeatedly reported to Congress that this is a flawed food-safety system, but nothing has been done to correct it.

While the USDA has the power to require that an exporting country's meat-inspection system meet American standards before that country can ship products to the United States, the FDA has no such power. The FDA must rely on exporting countries to comply voluntarily with U.S. food standards. In addition, produce importers retain possession of their shipments during investigation of suspected unsafe food and can distribute them for sale while the FDA conducts pesticide residue testing. Consequently,

## TABLE 7.12

**Frequency of occurrence of pesticide residues found in total diet study foods, 2001[1]**

| Pesticide[2] | Total number of findings | Occurrence, % | Range, ppm |
|---|---|---|---|
| DDT | 234 | 23 | 0.0001–0.031 |
| chlorpyrifos-methyl | 201 | 20 | 0.0001–0.537 |
| endosulfan | 185 | 18 | 0.0001–0.266 |
| malathion | 164 | 16 | 0.0007–0.080 |
| dieldrin | 152 | 15 | 0.0001–0.020 |
| chlorpropham | 73 | 7 | 0.0006–1.029 |
| chlorpyrifos | 71 | 7 | 0.0001–0.058 |
| permethrin | 60 | 6 | 0.0004–1.856 |
| carbaryl[3] | 55 | 5 | 0.0004–1.459 |
| iprodione | 39 | 4 | 0.0003–3.541 |
| dicloran | 36 | 3 | 0.0002–0.197 |
| heptachlor | 35 | 3 | 0.0001–0.0005 |
| lindane | 28 | 3 | 0.0001–0.002 |
| hexachlorobenzene | 28 | 3 | 0.0001–0.002 |
| thiabendazole[4] | 27 | 3 | 0.015–0.524 |
| methamidophos | 25 | 2 | 0.001–0.243 |
| acephate | 24 | 2 | 0.002–0.505 |
| methoxychlor | 24 | 2 | 0.0002–0.020 |
| quintozene | 22 | 2 | 0.0001–0.0043 |

[1] Based on 4 market baskets analyzed in 2001 consisting of 1030 total items. Only those found in > 2% of the samples are shown.

[2] Isomers, metabolites, and related compounds are included with the "parent" pesticide from which they arise.

[3] Reflects overall incidence; however, only 93–95 selected foods per market basket (*i.e.,* 377 items total) were analyzed for N-methylcaramates.

[4] Reflects overall incidence; however, only 67 selected foods per market basket (*i.e.,* 268 items total) were analyzed for the benzimidazole fungicides thiabendazole and benomyl.

SOURCE: "Table 6. Frequency of Occurrence of Pesticide Residues Found in Total Diet Study Foods in 2001," *Food and Drug Administration Pesticide Program: Residue Monitoring 2001*, U.S. Food and Drug Administration, Washington, DC, April 2003

perishable fruits and vegetables may be sold and consumed before the results of testing are available.

### Children Are Vulnerable to Pesticides

Children are at greater risk of harm from pesticides than are adults. Relative to their size, they eat more than adults do, and their bodies are still developing.

The FDA's Total Diet Study included analysis of pesticide residues found in about 20 different types of baby food. (See Table 7.13.) The pesticide residue found most often in these foods was carbaryl, with 16 total findings and a 21 percent occurrence rate.

According to *America's Children and the Environment: Measures of Contaminants, Body Burdens, and Illnesses* (EPA, Washington, D.C., February 2003) children are exposed to organophosphate pesticides through ingesting foods such as corn, fruits, vegetables, and nuts. Figure 7.12 shows the percentage of fruits, vegetables, and grains with detectable residues of these pesticides for the years 1994–2001. This percentage declined from 1997 to 1998, and again from 1999 to 2001.

### Regulation Affecting Cancer-Causing Pesticide Residues

In 1996 Congress passed legislation changing the rules governing cancer-causing ingredients in foods. The Delaney Clause, passed in 1958, banned any cancer-causing residues in processed foods. The new provisions (part of the Food Protection Act; PL 104-170) would allow pesticide residues only if there was a "reasonable certainty" that they would cause no harm. ("Reasonable certainty" has been defined as a lifetime risk of developing cancer of no more than one in 1 million.) Special attention would be required to ensure that no harm would result to infants and children from cumulative effects. The legislation applies equally to raw and processed foods. One of the reasons for the change was that scientists were now able to detect residues in amounts far lower than they once could.

### ORGANIC FOODS

The word "organic," as it pertains to food, usually means that the food has been grown without synthetic pesticides and/or fertilizers. In 1990 the Organic Foods Production Act (PL 101-624) mandated that the USDA develop national standards and a certification program for organically grown agricultural products. In December 1997 the USDA proposed a national standard for the production, handling, and processing of organically grown agricultural products.

Essentially, the new organic standard offers a national definition for the term "organic." It details the methods, practices, and substances that can be used in producing and handling organic crops and livestock, as well as processed products. It established clear organic labeling criteria and specifically prohibited the use of genetic engineering methods, ionizing radiation, and sewage sludge for fertilization.

All agricultural products labeled organic must originate from farms or handling operations certified by a state or private agency accredited by the USDA. Farms and handling operations that sell less than $5,000 worth per year of organic agricultural products are exempt from certification. The new organic labeling rules came into effect in October 2002.

Because organic farming is labor-intensive and done on a relatively small scale (accounting for only 1.2 percent of U.S. food sales) organic products cost more than other foods, sometimes as high as 50 percent more. Nonetheless, organic farming has become a $4 billion business, increasing about 20 percent annually since 1990. The industry is supported by people who want healthy food free of chemicals.

It is important to remember that the label "certified organic" is not a nutrition claim. Organic foods do not contain more or different nutrients than regular food.

FIGURE 7.11

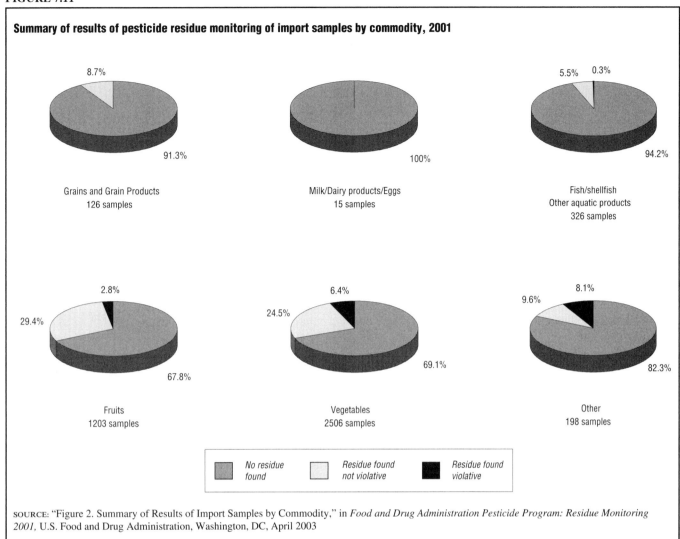

**Summary of results of pesticide residue monitoring of import samples by commodity, 2001**

SOURCE: "Figure 2. Summary of Results of Import Samples by Commodity," in *Food and Drug Administration Pesticide Program: Residue Monitoring 2001*, U.S. Food and Drug Administration, Washington, DC, April 2003

Furthermore, while organic foods are produced without the use of artificial chemicals, the possibility remains that they were exposed to disease-carrying bacteria or to residual chemicals in the environment. A "certified organic" label is not a guarantee of safety. Still, organic products should have been exposed to far fewer chemicals and other high-technology treatments than non-organic foods. For many people this difference alone justifies the purchase of organic food.

According to the National Organic Program of the USDA, as of October 21, 2002, all producers and handlers of any product carrying the word "organic" on its label, or displaying the USDA Organic Seal (see Figure 7.13), must be certified by a USDA-accredited agent.

## DIETARY SUPPLEMENTS

### Definition of Dietary Supplements

For many years the FDA regulated dietary supplements as food, considering them to consist of essential nutrients, such as proteins, vitamins, and minerals. In 1990 the Nutrition Labeling and Education Act (PL 101-535) included "herbs, or similar nutritional substances" under the category of dietary supplements. In 1994, as a result of vigorous lobbying by the dietary supplement industry, Congress indicated that there might be a link between dietary supplements and disease prevention. Under the DSHEA, Congress added items such as ginseng, fish oils, psyllium (a seed used as a mild laxative), enzymes, and mixtures of any of these ingredients to the definition of dietary supplements.

Unlike prescription and over-the-counter drugs, dietary supplements are not required to undergo evaluations for safety or effectiveness before they are sent to market. The DSHEA allows dietary supplement manufacturers to make almost any claim for their products, as long as they print the disclaimer on the label that the products "have not been evaluated by the Food and Drug Administration." After the passage of the DSHEA, dietary supplement sales climbed from $8 billion in 1994 to $12 billion in 1997.

TABLE 7.13

**Frequency of occurrence of pesticide residues found in selected baby foods, 2001[1]**

| Pesticide[2] | Total number of findings | Occurrence, % | Range, ppm |
|---|---|---|---|
| carbaryl[3] | 16 | 21 | 0.002–0.035 |
| endosulfan | 10 | 13 | 0.0001–0.0035 |
| chlorpyrifos-methyl | 8 | 10 | 0.001–0.176 |
| malathion | 8 | 10 | 0.008–0.046 |
| chlorpyrifos | 7 | 9 | 0.0002–0.002 |
| iprodione | 7 | 9 | 0.0002–0.084 |
| permethrin | 7 | 9 | 0.0005–0.018 |
| ethylenethiourea[4] | 7 | 9 | 0.003–0.012 |
| thiabendazole[5] | 5 | 6 | 0.010–0.043 |
| benomyl[5] | 3 | 4 | 0.039–0.064 |
| dicloran | 2 | 3 | 0.0008–0.002 |
| dimethoate | 2 | 3 | 0.001–0.003 |
| DDT | 1 | 1 | 0.0006 |
| esfenvalerate | 1 | 1 | 0.007 |
| methoxychlor | 1 | 1 | 0.0005 |
| dieldrin | 1 | 1 | 0.0001 |
| phosmet | 1 | 1 | 0.011 |

[1] Based on 4 collections consisting of 78 total items.
[2] Isomers, metabolites, and related compounds are included with the "parent" pesticide from which they arise.
[3] Reflects overall incidence; however, only 12–14 selected foods per collection (i.e., 53 items total) were analyzed for N-methylcarbamates.
[4] Reflects overall incidence; however, only 11–12 selected foods per collection (i.e., 47 items total) were analyzed for ethylenethiourea.
[5] Reflects overall incidence; however, only 13–14 selected foods per collection (i.e., 54 items total) were analyzed for the benzimidazole fungicides (thiabendazole and benomyl).

SOURCE: "Table 7. Frequency of Occurrence of Pesticide Residues Found in Selected Baby Foods in 2001," in *Food and Drug Administration Pesticide Program: Residue Monitoring 2001*, U.S. Food and Drug Administration, Washington, DC, April 2003

FIGURE 7.12

**Percentage of fruits, vegetables, and grains with detectable residues of organophosphate pesticides, 1994–2001**

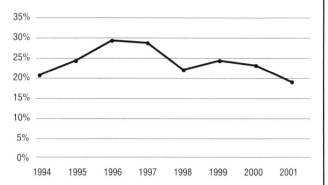

SOURCE: "Percentage of fruits, vegetables, and grains with detectable residues of organophosphate pesticides," in *America's Children and the Environment: Measures of Contaminants, Body Burdens, and Illnesses, Second Edition*, EPA 240-R-03-001, U.S. Environmental Protection Agency, Office of Children's Health Protection, National Center for Environmental Economics, Washington, DC, February 2003

As a result of a 1999 ruling by the U.S. Court of Appeals for the D.C. Circuit in the case of *Pearson v. Shalala* (64 3d 650, D.C. Cir. 1999) the FDA can permit dietary supplement manufacturers to make qualified health claims on the labels of their products. These are claims that do not meet the criteria known as "significant scientific agreement," but do have a preponderance of scientific evidence in their favor. The FDA allows these qualified claims in the belief that not including them would be misleading to consumers ("Labeling of Dietary Supplements," available online at http://www.cfsan.fda.gov/~dms/ds-labl.html [accessed October 20, 2003]).

**New FDA Regulation for Dietary Supplements**

Effective March 23, 1999, the FDA required that dietary supplement labels include a Supplement Facts panel, patterned after the Nutrition Facts panel on food items. According to the FDA, labels must identify dietary supplements as such. Products with botanical ingredients must identify the part of the plant used. Supplements labeled "high potency" and "antioxidant" must also meet FDA criteria. (See Figure 7.14.)

On March 23, 2003, the FDA proposed a new regulation regarding the packaging and labeling of dietary supplements ("FDA Proposes Labeling and Manufacturing Standards for All Dietary Supplements," *FDA News*, March 7, 2003). The proposed regulation requires that there be no contaminating substances in the supplements, and that the labels present accurate information.

**Some Dietary Supplements Are Dangerous**

In 1998 the *New England Journal of Medicine* reported a number of adverse effects among individuals using dietary supplements. Robert S. DiPaola et al., in "Clinical and Biologic Activity of an Estrogenic Herbal Combination (PC-SPES) in Prostate Cancer" (Vol. 339, No. 12, September 17, 1998), found that PC-SPES, an unregulated combination of eight herbs, produced unexpected effects similar to that of estrogen.

Richard J. Ko, of the California Department of Health Services, in "Adulterants in Asian Patent Medicines" (*New England Journal of Medicine*, Vol. 339, No. 12, September 17, 1998), reported that toxic levels of metals such as lead, arsenic, and mercury have been found in Asian patent medicines collected from California retail herbal stores. Chemicals such as ephedrine were also common components not declared on the supplement label.

Many cases of immediate adverse reactions to dietary supplements have also been reported. Kava has been known to cause drowsiness, and echinacea has brought on allergic reactions. According to the FDA, since 1993, the herbal stimulant Ma-huang, or Chinese ephedra, has caused at least 30 deaths and more than 800 cases of adverse

## FIGURE 7.13

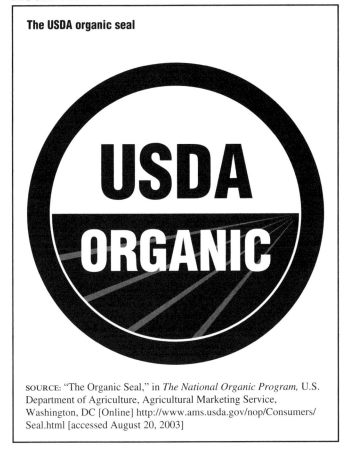

The USDA organic seal

SOURCE: "The Organic Seal," in *The National Organic Program,* U.S. Department of Agriculture, Agricultural Marketing Service, Washington, DC [Online] http://www.ams.usda.gov/nop/Consumers/Seal.html [accessed August 20, 2003]

## FIGURE 7.14

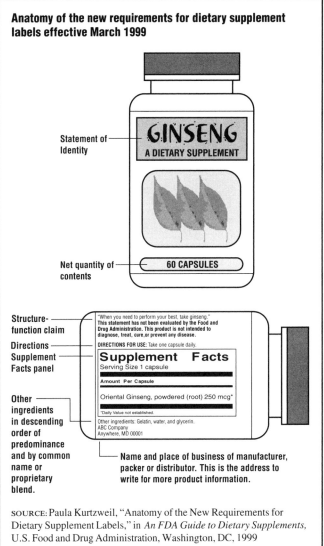

Anatomy of the new requirements for dietary supplement labels effective March 1999

SOURCE: Paula Kurtzweil, "Anatomy of the New Requirements for Dietary Supplement Labels," in *An FDA Guide to Dietary Supplements,* U.S. Food and Drug Administration, Washington, DC, 1999

side-effects, including strokes, heart attacks, seizures, and high blood pressure. Ephedra, an amphetamine-like compound, exerts powerful stimulant effects on the nervous system and heart. So-called herbal fen-phen products contain ephedra as their main ingredient. Table 7.14 shows dietary supplements that have been associated with illnesses and injuries.

In 2002–03 the FDA issued safety alerts to people in health professions about a number of dietary supplements ("2002 Safety Alerts for Drugs, Biologics, Medical Devices, and Dietary Supplements," available online at http://www.fda.gov/medwatch/SAFETY/2002/safety02.htm [accessed October 20, 2003]):

• Dietary supplements containing kava—there is a possibility of liver damage.

• Milk-based powdered infant formulas—should not be given to newborns because there is a risk of *Enterobacter sakazakii* infection.

• Nettle capsules made by Nature's Way Products Inc.—the company is recalling the product because of potentially damaging levels of lead.

• PC/SPES and SPES dietary and herbal supplements in capsule form—they contain undeclared prescription drugs and should only be used under direction of a physician.

• Dietary supplements containing ephedra—evidence suggests that there are health risks.

## PUBLIC OPINION

### Food-Safety Information and Concerns

Nutrition and product safety are important to food shoppers. In the 2003 Food Marketing Institute (FMI) survey *Trends in the United States: Consumer Attitudes & the Supermarket, 2003* (Washington, D.C., 2003) 79 percent of consumers expressed confidence that the food in their supermarket was safe.

Consumers believed that food-safety problems could occur at various points in the food distribution chain, from the farm to the home. Shoppers thought that food processors (35 percent) and restaurants (15 percent) were the most likely sources of food-safety problems. (See Figure 7.15.) Third most likely was the home, according to 10 percent of shoppers. Only 6 percent of respondents felt

TABLE 7.14

**Supplements associated with illnesses and injuries, 1998**

| Name | Possible health hazards |
|---|---|
| **Herbal Ingredients** | |
| *Chaparral*<br>(a traditional American Indian medicine) | liver disease, possibly irreversible |
| *Comfrey* | obstruction of blood flow to liver, possibly leading to death |
| *Slimming/dieter's teas* | nausea, diarrhea, vomiting, stomach cramps, chronic constipation, fainting, possibly death |
| *Ephedra*<br>(also known as Ma huang, Chinese Ephedra and epitonin) | ranges from high blood pressure, irregular heartbeat, nerve damage, injury, insomnia, tremors, and headaches to seizures, heart attack, stroke, and death |
| *Germander* | liver disease, possibly leading to death |
| *Lobelia*<br>(also known as Indian tobacco) | range from breathing problems at low doses to sweating, rapid heartbeat, low blood pressure, and possibly coma and death at higher doses |
| *Magnolia-Stephania preparation* | kidney disease, possibly leading to permanent kidney failure |
| *Willow bark* | Reye syndrome, a potentially fatal disease associated with aspirin intake in children with chickenpox or flu symptoms; allergic reaction in adults. (Willow bark is marketed as an aspirin-free product, although it actually contains an ingredient that converts to the same active ingredient in aspirin.) |
| *Wormwood* | neurological symptoms, characterized by numbness of legs and arms, loss of intellect, delirium, and paralysis |
| **Vitamins and Essential Minerals** | |
| *Vitamin A*<br>in doses of 25,000 or more International Units a day | birth defects, bone abnormalities, and severe liver disease |
| *Vitamin B₆*<br>in doses above 100 milligrams a day | balance difficulties, nerve injury causing changes in touch sensation |
| *Niacin*<br>in slow-released doses of 500 mg or more a day or immediate-release doses of 750 mg or more a day | range from stomach pain, vomiting, bloating, nausea, cramping, and diarrhea to liver disease, muscle disease, eye damage, and heart injury |
| *Selenium*<br>in doses of about 800 micrograms to 1,000 mcg a day | tissue damage |
| **Other Supplements** | |
| *Germanium*<br>(a nonessential mineral) | kidney damage, possibly death |
| *L-tryptophan*<br>(an amino acid) | eosinophilia myalgia syndrome, a potentially fatal blood disorder that can cause high fever, muscle and joint pain, weakness, skin rash, and swelling of the arms and legs |

SOURCE: "An FDA Guide to Dietary Supplements," in *FDA Consumer*, U.S. Food and Drug Administration, Washington, DC, 1998

FIGURE 7.15

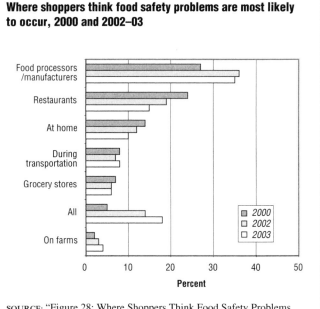

**Where shoppers think food safety problems are most likely to occur, 2000 and 2002–03**

SOURCE: "Figure 28: Where Shoppers Think Food Safety Problems Are Most Likely to Occur," in *Trends in the United States: Consumer Attitudes & the Supermarket, 2003,* Food Marketing Institute (FMI), Washington, DC, 2003

FIGURE 7.16

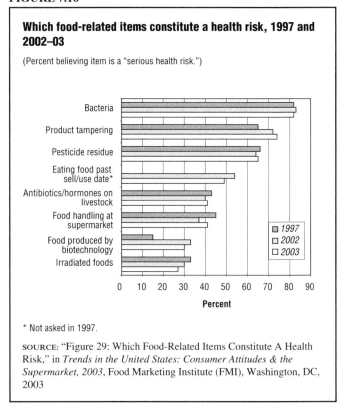

**Which food-related items constitute a health risk, 1997 and 2002–03**

(Percent believing item is a "serious health risk.")

* Not asked in 1997.

SOURCE: "Figure 29: Which Food-Related Items Constitute A Health Risk," in *Trends in the United States: Consumer Attitudes & the Supermarket, 2003*, Food Marketing Institute (FMI), Washington, DC, 2003

that grocery stores were likely to experience food-safety problems.

## Shoppers Aware of Foodborne Illness Risk

While shoppers recognized the dangers of mishandling food, there was a significant decrease in those who reported that it was very or fairly common for people to become ill because of the way food was handled or prepared in their homes. In 2003, 20 percent thought this was very or fairly common, compared with 41 percent in 1999.

Survey respondents felt that the most common sources of food poisoning were bacteria (82 percent), product tampering (74 percent), and pesticide residue (65 percent). (See Figure 7.16.)

Shoppers were aware of proper food handling to keep food safe. They mentioned a number of things they did in their own kitchens. Many of these food-handling practices were publicized in the Fight Bac! campaign, sponsored by the Partnership for Food Safety Education, a national organization dedicated to informing consumers about the importance of food safety. The action most frequently mentioned was washing hands and surfaces, followed by washing vegetables and cleaning food, keeping the food preparation area insect-free, cooking properly, and refrigerating foods promptly.

**Attitudes Toward Biotechnology**

Consumers were more willing to buy biotechnology-modified products if it meant resistance to insect damage and fewer required pesticide applications. Over half (57 percent) of respondents were very or somewhat likely to buy these types of products, though this was down from 77 percent in 1996.

# CHAPTER 8
# PERCEPTION AND REALITY IN AMERICAN DIETS

Most Americans have received information about the health benefits of lowering cholesterol intake, cutting back on fat, and eating more fruits and vegetables—but has this led people to change their eating habits? While many are aware of the importance of a healthful diet, they are often confused by conflicting messages from health providers and food companies. Others, while they might know what a healthful diet is, put convenience and taste ahead of healthful eating.

According to the Behavioral Risk Factor Surveillance System (BRFSS) of the Centers for Disease Control and Prevention (CDC), only 22.6 percent of Americans ate fruits and vegetables 5 or more times a day in 2002. (See Table 8.1 and Figure 8.1.) More than one-third (36 percent) ate fruits and vegetables between 1 and 3 times per day. Considering that *Dietary Guidelines for Americans,* a joint publication of the U.S. Department of Health and Human Services and the U.S. Department of Agriculture (USDA), recommends 5–9 servings of fruits and vegetables daily, most Americans still have a way to go. Another indication that Americans have not improved their eating habits, despite greater knowledge of the nutritional benefits of a healthful diet, is the growing prevalence of overweight American adults and children.

## PERCEIVED INTAKE VERSUS ACTUAL CONSUMPTION

P. P. Basiotis, Mark Lino, and Julia Dinkins ("Consumption of Food Group Servings: People's Perception vs. Reality," *Nutrition Insights,* USDA, Washington, D.C., October 2000) compared the number of food-group servings that people thought they were consuming with the number of servings from records they kept over a two-week period. As Table 8.2 indicates, all gender and age groups perceived consuming fewer grain servings (2.5–3.2) daily than they actually ate (4.2–6.2 servings). Although their consumption of grains per day was above

what they believed, it was still below Food Guide Pyramid recommendations. For example, females ages 19–50 consumed 4.2–4.6 servings of grains per day, while the recommendation is 9 servings.

On average, each gender/age group perceived consuming more fruit servings daily than was actually the case. Males ages 19–50 believed they consumed 2.1–2.2 servings of fruit on a given day. Based on their food diaries, they actually consumed less than 1 serving per day. The recommendation for this group is 4 servings per day.

Adult females believed they consumed more vegetable servings per day than they actually consumed: 2.5–2.6 versus 1.7–2.2 actual servings. Adult males, on the other hand, believed they consumed slightly fewer vegetable servings per day than they actually

**TABLE 8.1**

### Average frequency of fruit and vegetable consumption per day, 2002

(Median percentage answering the question "What is your average frequency of fruit and vegetable consumption per day?")

| | Median % | Number of states[1] |
|---|---|---|
| Never or < 1 a day | 4.7 | 54 |
| 1 to < 3 times a day | 35.9 | 54 |
| 3 to < 5 times a day | 36.1 | 54 |
| 5+ times a day | 22.6 | 54 |

[1] Number of states includes District of Columbia, Puerto Rico, Virgin Islands, and Guam.

SOURCE: "What is your average frequency of fruit and vegetable consumption per day?" in *Behavioral Risk Factor Surveillance System Online Prevalence Data,* Centers for Disease Control and Prevention, National Center for Chronic Disease Prevention and Health Promotion, Division of Adult and Community Health, Atlanta, GA, August 20, 2003 [Online] http://apps.nccd.cdc.gov/brfss/display.asp?cat=NU&yr=2002&qkey=4340&state=US [accessed August 26, 2003]

FIGURE 8.1

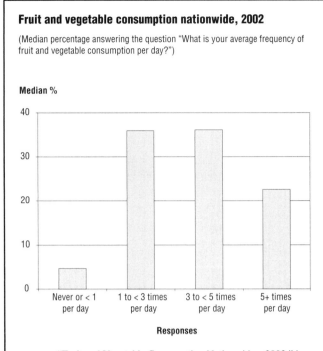

**Fruit and vegetable consumption nationwide, 2002**

(Median percentage answering the question "What is your average frequency of fruit and vegetable consumption per day?")

SOURCE: "Fruit and Vegetable Consumption Nationwide—2002," in *Behavioral Risk Factor Surveillance System Online Prevalence Data,* Centers for Disease Control and Prevention, National Center for Chronic Disease Prevention and Health Promotion, Division of Adult and Community Health, Atlanta, GA, August 20, 2003 [Online] http://apps.nccd.cdc.gov/brfss/display.asp?cat=NU&yr=2002 &qkey=4340&state=US [accessed August 26, 2003]

consumed. Both women and men consumed less than the daily recommendation of 3.5–5 servings for their gender/age group.

All gender/age groups believed their usual daily milk intake was far more than they actually consumed. They thought they consumed 2.1–3.2 servings or milk products per day, but their food diaries indicated they consumed 1–1.6 servings per day.

All gender/age groups perceived their typical servings of meat, poultry, fish, dry beans, eggs, and nuts as more than they actually consumed. They thought they ate 2.7–3.7 servings, but their food diaries indicated they consumed only 1.6–2.5 servings per day. Meat consumption was also below Pyramid recommendations.

Each gender/age group underestimated its average daily servings of fats, oils, and sweets, perceiving only 1.6–2.2 servings versus actually consuming 3.0–4.5 servings. The Food Guide Pyramid does not specify the number or size of servings, but recommends that people consume these foods sparingly.

The study concluded that people's perceptions of their food-group consumption were very different from their actual consumption.

## THE HEALTHY EATING INDEX

The Healthy Eating Index (HEI) was developed by the USDA's Center for Nutrition Policy and Promotion (CNPP) to measure and monitor the type and quantity of foods eaten and the extent that nutritional knowledge and diet-health awareness influence diet.

The HEI consists of 10 components, representing different aspects of a healthful diet:

- Components 1–5 measure the degree to which a person's diet conforms to the USDA's Food Guide Pyramid serving recommendations for the five major food groups: grains, vegetables, fruits, milk, and meat.

- Component 6 measures total fat consumption as a percentage of total food energy (calorie) intake.

- Component 7 measures saturated fat consumption as a percentage of total food energy intake.

- Component 8 measures total cholesterol intake.

- Component 9 measures total sodium intake.

- Component 10 measures variety in a person's diet.

The total HEI score is the sum of the 10 components, and the maximum score is 100. An HEI score over 80 indicates a "good" diet; a score between 51 and 80 indicates the diet "needs improvement"; and a score lower than 51 indicates a "poor" diet. The HEI reflects dietary intake in relation to the five major food groups of the Food Guide Pyramid. In developing the Index, the CNPP used the Pyramid's serving recommendations as shown in Table 8.3.

P. P. Basiotis et al., in *The Healthy Eating Index: 1999–2000* (CNPP, Washington, D.C., December 2002), concluded that although the diet quality of Americans has improved since 1989, it still does not meet the standards of a good, healthful diet. In fact, in 1999–2000 the diets of more people needed improvement than was the case in 1996, and the percentage of those whose diet quality was good dropped 18 percent from 1996. The authors found that 74 percent of the population in 1999–2000 had diets that needed improvement, an increase of 5 percent from 1996. (See Figure 8.2.) The percentage of those whose diet was considered good in 1996 (12.2 percent) dropped to just 10 percent in 1999–2000. However, the percentage of the population with a poor diet dropped 1.3 percent between 1996 and 1999–2000, from 17.3 percent to 16 percent.

Each component of the HEI has a maximum score of ten and a minimum score of zero. The lower the score, the less the compliance with recommended dietary intakes. Figure 8.3 shows that while the higher score (7.7) for cholesterol intake indicates that Americans are making an effort to follow health guidelines in this area, there is reason

TABLE 8.2

**Food group servings perceived, consumed, and recommended by gender/age group, 2000**

| | Grains | Fruits | Vegetables | Milk | Meat, etc. | Other (fats, oils, and sweets) |
|---|---|---|---|---|---|---|
| **Females 19-24** | | | | | | |
| Perceived | 3.2 | 2.6 | 2.6 | 3.2 | 3.5 | 2.2 |
| Consumed | 4.2 | 0.8 | 1.7 | 1.2 | 1.6 | 3.0 |
| Recommended | 9 | 3 | 4 | 2 | 2.4 | Use sparingly |
| **Females 25-50** | | | | | | |
| Perceived | 2.9 | 2.2 | 2.5 | 2.3 | 3.0 | 2.1 |
| Consumed | 4.6 | 0.8 | 2.0 | 1.0 | 1.7 | 3.2 |
| Recommended | 9 | 3 | 4 | 2 | 2.4 | Use sparingly |
| **Females 51 +** | | | | | | |
| Perceived | 2.5 | 2.4 | 2.6 | 2.1 | 2.7 | 1.6 |
| Consumed | 4.7 | 1.5 | 2.2 | 1.0 | 1.7 | 3.1 |
| Recommended | 7.4 | 2.5 | 3.5 | 3 | 2.2 | Use sparingly |
| **Males 19-24** | | | | | | |
| Perceived | 2.9 | 2.1 | 2.2 | 3.1 | 3.7 | 2.1 |
| Consumed | 5.5 | 0.6 | 2.3 | 1.6 | 2.3 | 4.1 |
| Recommended | 11 | 4 | 5 | 2 | 2.8 | Use sparingly |
| **Males 25-50** | | | | | | |
| Perceived | 2.9 | 2.2 | 2.4 | 2.2 | 3.4 | 2.1 |
| Consumed | 5.9 | 0.9 | 2.5 | 1.2 | 2.5 | 4.0 |
| Recommended | 11 | 4 | 5 | 2 | 2.8 | Use sparingly |
| **Males 51 +** | | | | | | |
| Perceived | 2.7 | 2.2 | 2.5 | 2.1 | 3.1 | 1.7 |
| Consumed | 6.2 | 1.3 | 2.7 | 1.1 | 2.4 | 4.5 |
| Recommended | 9.1 | 3.2 | 4.2 | 3 | 2.5 | Use sparingly |

*Recommended servings based on energy RDA for gender/age groups.

SOURCE: "Food group servings: Perceived, average daily consumed, and recommended* by gender/age group," in *Consumption of Food Group Servings: People's Perceptions vs. Reality,* Nutrition Insights 20, U.S. Department of Agriculture, Center for Nutrition Policy and Promotion, Washington, DC, 2000

for concern in other areas, such as fruit intake, which had the lowest score (3.8) of all the components in the HEI.

While Figure 8.4 confirms that Americans do not eat enough fruit (only 17 percent of individuals in the survey followed the dietary recommendations), it also demonstrates that more Americans are watching their cholesterol intake. More than two-thirds (69 percent) of individuals followed the dietary guidelines for cholesterol in 1999–2000.

## HEI Scores by Population Characteristics

For the *The Healthy Eating Index: 1999–2000,* the CNPP used data from the *National Health and Nutrition Examination Survey 1999–2000.* (Previous HEI reports were based on data from the USDA's *Continuing Survey of Food Intakes by Individuals.*) The CNPP looked at Americans' diet quality by selected demographics, including race/ethnicity, gender, and age. Table 8.4 shows the distribution of HEI scores overall and for individual components by selected demographics.

Children ages 2–3 had the highest overall HEI score of all the population subgroups (75.7). Females had a slightly higher score (64.5) than did males (63.2), and Mexican Americans had the highest score (64.5) of all the racial/ethnic groups. (See Table 8.4.)

The higher the level of educational attainment, the higher the HEI score. Individuals with education beyond high school had the highest HEI, 65.3. Those who had completed high school ranked second, with an HEI of 63.0, and those who did not have a high school diploma had the lowest score, 61.1.

HEI scores for individual components show that fruit consumption for both males (3.5) and females (4.1) was low. Females scored higher than males in following guidelines for cholesterol intake (8.3 versus 7.1) and sodium intake (7.0 versus 5.0). But females age 11 and older scored lower than males in the same age group for milk intake. This is especially important, given that calcium intake is necessary for healthy bones and teeth, and insufficient calcium intake has been linked to osteoporosis in females.

Table 8.5 shows that while some progress has been made in the overall HEI score since 1989, there was an even more positive change between 1996 and 2000. This is not the case for individual components of the index, however. HEI scores for vegetables, cholesterol, and sodium intake dropped between 1996 and 2000. Scores for milk, meat, and saturated fat were higher in 1999–2000 than they were in 1996, indicating some improvement within these individual areas.

TABLE 8.3

**Recommended number of servings per day for age/gender categories**

| Age/gender category | Kilocalories | Grains | Vegetables | Fruits | Milk | Meat |
|---|---|---|---|---|---|---|
| Children 1-3 | 1,300 | 6.0[a] | 3.0[a] | 2.0[a] | 2.0[a] | 2.0[a] |
| * | 1,600 | 6.0 | 3.0 | 2.0 | 2.0 | 2.0 |
| Children 4-6 | 1,800 | 7.0 | 3.3 | 2.3 | 2.0 | 2.1 |
| Females 51+ | 1,900 | 7.4 | 3.5 | 2.5 | 2.0 | 2.2 |
| Children 7-10 | 2,000 | 7.8 | 3.7 | 2.7 | 2.0 | 2.3 |
| Females 11-50 | 2,200 | 9.0 | 4.0 | 3.0 | 2.0 | 2.4 |
| Males 51+ | 2,300 | 9.1 | 4.2 | 3.2 | 2.0 | 2.5 |
| Males 11-14 | 2,500 | 9.9 | 4.5 | 3.5 | 3.0 | 2.6 |
| * | 2,800 | 11.0 | 5.0 | 4.0 | 2.0 | 2.8 |
| Males 19-50 | 2,900 | 11.0 | 5.0 | 4.0 | 2.0[b] | 2.8 |
| Males 15-18 | 3,000 | 11.0 | 5.0 | 4.0 | 2.0 | 2.8 |

[a] Portion sizes are reduced for children age 1-3.
[b] Is 3 servings for persons age 11 to 24.
* RDA levels included in the Food Guide Pyramid.

SOURCE: Jayachandran Variyam, James Blaylock, David Smallwood, and Peter Basiotis, "Table 2: Recommended number of servings per day for age/gender categories," in *USDA's Healthy Eating Index and Nutrition Information,* Technical Bulletin No. 1866, U.S. Department of Agriculture, Economic Research Service, Washington, DC, 1998

---

**FIGURE 8.2**

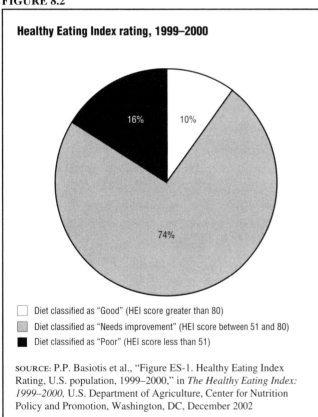

**Healthy Eating Index rating, 1999–2000**

□ Diet classified as "Good" (HEI score greater than 80)
▨ Diet classified as "Needs improvement" (HEI score between 51 and 80)
■ Diet classified as "Poor" (HEI score less than 51)

SOURCE: P.P. Basiotis et al., "Figure ES-1. Healthy Eating Index Rating, U.S. population, 1999–2000," in *The Healthy Eating Index: 1999–2000,* U.S. Department of Agriculture, Center for Nutrition Policy and Promotion, Washington, DC, December 2002

## The Effect of Nutrition Knowledge and Diet-Health Awareness

Jayachandran N. Variyam et al., in *USDA's Healthy Eating Index and Nutrition Information* (Economic Research Service, USDA, Washington, D.C., 1998), developed a model to measure how nutrition knowledge and diet-health awareness influence an individual's HEI.

**FIGURE 8.3**

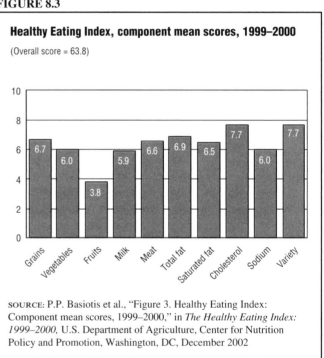

**Healthy Eating Index, component mean scores, 1999–2000**

(Overall score = 63.8)

SOURCE: P.P. Basiotis et al., "Figure 3. Healthy Eating Index: Component mean scores, 1999–2000," in *The Healthy Eating Index: 1999–2000,* U.S. Department of Agriculture, Center for Nutrition Policy and Promotion, Washington, DC, December 2002

Respondents were asked to identify, for example, which of two foods has a higher fiber content: fruit or meat, cornflakes or oatmeal, popcorn or pretzels. They also were asked to identify which foods contain more cholesterol: liver or T-bone steak, butter or margarine, skim or whole milk. Other questions probed knowledge of different kinds of fat, the types of foods that contain cholesterol, and the relationship between fat and cholesterol.

Respondents answered some questions more easily than they did others. More than 93 percent of individuals age 20 and older correctly identified whole milk as

FIGURE 8.4

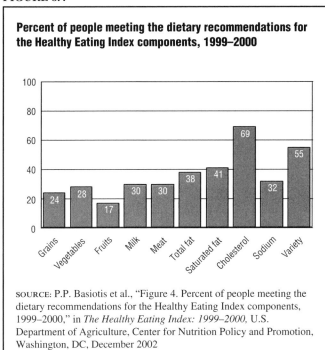

**Percent of people meeting the dietary recommendations for the Healthy Eating Index components, 1999–2000**

SOURCE: P.P. Basiotis et al., "Figure 4. Percent of people meeting the dietary recommendations for the Healthy Eating Index components, 1999–2000," in *The Healthy Eating Index: 1999–2000*, U.S. Department of Agriculture, Center for Nutrition Policy and Promotion, Washington, DC, December 2002

containing more saturated fat than skim milk. (See Table 8.6.) Nearly eight out of ten individuals (79 percent) knew that regular hamburger has more fat than ground round, but only 49 percent knew that porterhouse steak has more fat than round steak. Only 36 percent of respondents knew that cholesterol is contained in animal products such as meat and dairy products, but 86 percent knew that peanuts have more fat than popcorn. When respondents were asked what kind of fat, saturated or polyunsaturated, is more likely to be a liquid rather than a solid, only 27 percent knew the correct answer (polyunsaturated).

Table 8.7 lists the questions used to measure awareness of diet-health problems. Nearly all (95 percent) of individuals age 20 and older had heard of problems associated with being overweight, but only 66 percent were aware of health problems associated with insufficient intake of fiber.

## WHAT DO AMERICANS KNOW ABOUT NUTRITION?

Americans are generally aware of diet-disease relationships that have been widely publicized by the media and the government. But data in *Results from the USDA's 1994–96 Diet and Health Knowledge Survey* (Agricultural Research Service, USDA, Beltsville, MD, October 2000) suggest that many consumers need additional education in specific diet-disease areas, such as the possible link between dietary fats and higher blood cholesterol levels.

For example, although 95 percent of individuals age 20 and older were aware that being overweight can cause

health problems (see Table 8.7), only 23 percent knew that hypertension is one of the related problems. (See Table 8.8.) Nearly nine out of ten individuals in this age group (88 percent) knew that eating too much fat can lead to health problems (see Table 8.7), but only 26 percent knew of the link between fat consumption and obesity, and even fewer people—10.4 percent—knew of the relationship between fat consumption and the risk of hypertension. About two-thirds (66 percent) of individuals in the survey knew that there is a relationship between insufficient intake of fiber and potential health risks (see Table 8.7), but only 15 percent of them were aware that one of the potential health risks is cancer.

Consumers, however, often feel frustrated when they receive differing nutrition information. Forty percent of women and men age 20 and older "strongly agreed" with the survey statement "There are so many recommendations about healthy ways to eat, it's hard to know what to believe."

### Nutrition Awareness Does Not Necessarily Change Dietary Behavior

Nutrition scientists caution that just because a person is aware of certain diet-disease relationships, it does not necessarily mean he or she will put this knowledge into practice. For example, despite the growing awareness, especially among women, of the relationship between calcium and health, the USDA's 1994–96 *Continuing Surveys of Food Intakes by Individuals* found that calcium intake by female respondents age 20 and older fell below recommended levels. This group had a calcium intake that was only 75 percent of the Recommended Dietary Allowance (RDA), the same percentage that was reported in the 1989–91 survey.

Other factors also may counteract consumers' nutrition awareness. Many individuals misperceive their actual nutrient intakes. In addition, social and economic factors, such as the rising trend of away-from-home meals, may lead to less consumption of certain nutrients.

### SHOPPERS' CONCERN WITH NUTRITION

In the Food Marketing Institute's (FMI) annual survey of shopping behavior, *Trends in the United States: Consumer Attitudes & the Supermarket, 2003* (Washington, D.C., 2003), 1,001 individuals were asked about their concern with the nutritional content of what they eat. Among both genders, and in all age groups, types of households, and regions, there was a decrease in the number of people "very concerned" about nutritional content from 1996 to January 2002, when there was an increase from 46 percent to 50 percent. There also was an increase, from 50 percent to 53 percent, from January 2002 to January 2003. (See Table 8.9.) Vegetarians and those persons on

TABLE 8.4

**Healthy Eating Index, overall and component mean scores, by selected characteristics, 1999–2000**

| Characteristic | Overall | Grains | Vegetables | Fruits | Milk | Meat[1] | Total fat | Saturated fat | Cholesterol | Sodium | Variety |
|---|---|---|---|---|---|---|---|---|---|---|---|
| **Gender** | | | | | | | | | | | |
| Male | 63.2 | 6.9 | 5.9 | 3.5 | 6.3 | 7.2 | 6.9 | 6.5 | 7.1 | 5.0 | 8.0 |
| Female | 64.5 | 6.4 | 6.0 | 4.1 | 5.6 | 6.1 | 6.9 | 6.5 | 8.3 | 7.0 | 7.5 |
| **Age/gender** | | | | | | | | | | | |
| Children, 2-3[2] | 75.7 | 8.9 | 6.5 | 7.3 | 7.4 | 6.3 | 7.8 | 5.9 | 8.9 | 8.3 | 8.6 |
| Children, 4-6 | 66.9 | 7.4 | 5.0 | 4.9 | 7.2 | 4.9 | 7.1 | 5.7 | 9.1 | 7.8 | 7.8 |
| Children, 7-10 | 66.0 | 8.0 | 5.0 | 3.9 | 7.7 | 5.6 | 7.1 | 6.0 | 8.6 | 6.2 | 8.0 |
| Females, 11-14 | 61.4 | 6.5 | 5.0 | 3.6 | 5.3 | 5.3 | 7.0 | 6.0 | 8.8 | 7.0 | 7.0 |
| Females, 15-18 | 61.7 | 6.4 | 5.6 | 3.6 | 4.6 | 5.3 | 7.2 | 6.6 | 9.0 | 6.7 | 6.8 |
| Females, 19-50 | 63.2 | 6.1 | 6.2 | 3.3 | 5.5 | 6.5 | 6.9 | 6.6 | 8.1 | 6.5 | 7.5 |
| Females, 51+ | 66.6 | 6.4 | 6.4 | 5.3 | 5.3 | 6.2 | 6.8 | 6.7 | 8.1 | 7.7 | 7.7 |
| Males, 11-14 | 60.8 | 7.0 | 4.8 | 2.7 | 6.1 | 5.7 | 7.3 | 6.2 | 8.1 | 5.9 | 7.2 |
| Males, 15-18 | 59.9 | 7.0 | 5.1 | 2.5 | 6.1 | 6.8 | 7.2 | 6.3 | 7.0 | 4.4 | 7.5 |
| Males, 19-50 | 61.3 | 6.6 | 6.0 | 2.7 | 6.1 | 7.5 | 6.9 | 6.6 | 6.7 | 4.2 | 7.9 |
| Males, 51+ | 65.2 | 6.7 | 6.7 | 4.5 | 5.9 | 7.7 | 6.6 | 6.7 | 6.8 | 5.3 | 8.4 |
| **Race/ethnicity** | | | | | | | | | | | |
| Non-Hispanic White | 64.2 | 6.8 | 6.2 | 3.7 | 6.4 | 6.5 | 6.7 | 6.3 | 7.8 | 5.8 | 7.9 |
| Non-Hispanic Black | 61.1 | 6.2 | 5.2 | 3.7 | 4.5 | 7.0 | 7.0 | 6.9 | 7.4 | 6.3 | 7.0 |
| Mexican American | 64.5 | 6.5 | 5.6 | 4.1 | 5.5 | 6.7 | 7.3 | 6.8 | 7.3 | 6.8 | 7.8 |
| Other race[3] | 63.4 | 6.6 | 5.9 | 3.8 | 4.0 | 6.7 | 7.5 | 7.3 | 8.1 | 6.3 | 7.2 |
| Other Hispanic | 64.2 | 6.6 | 5.4 | 3.8 | 5.7 | 6.6 | 7.7 | 7.1 | 7.8 | 6.0 | 7.6 |
| **Place of birth** | | | | | | | | | | | |
| United States | 63.5 | 6.7 | 6.0 | 3.6 | 6.1 | 6.6 | 6.8 | 6.3 | 7.7 | 5.9 | 7.7 |
| Mexico | 66.0 | 6.4 | 5.4 | 4.5 | 5.2 | 7.1 | 7.8 | 7.6 | 7.1 | 7.0 | 8.0 |
| Other | 65.7 | 6.3 | 5.8 | 4.6 | 5.1 | 6.6 | 7.9 | 7.7 | 7.8 | 6.1 | 7.8 |
| **Education[4]** | | | | | | | | | | | |
| No high school diploma | 61.1 | 6.0 | 5.5 | 3.3 | 4.9 | 6.9 | 6.9 | 6.8 | 7.2 | 6.6 | 7.1 |
| High school diploma | 63.0 | 6.3 | 6.3 | 3.7 | 5.8 | 7.1 | 6.6 | 6.3 | 7.4 | 5.7 | 7.9 |
| More than high school diploma | 65.3 | 6.7 | 6.7 | 4.0 | 6.3 | 7.0 | 6.7 | 6.8 | 7.5 | 5.5 | 8.2 |
| **Income as percent of poverty** | | | | | | | | | | | |
| <100% | 61.7 | 6.2 | 5.4 | 3.5 | 5.3 | 6.4 | 7.1 | 6.5 | 7.5 | 6.8 | 7.0 |
| 100-184% | 62.6 | 6.6 | 5.6 | 3.4 | 5.7 | 6.3 | 7.0 | 6.5 | 8.0 | 6.3 | 7.2 |
| >184% | 65.0 | 6.8 | 6.3 | 4.0 | 6.3 | 6.7 | 6.8 | 6.5 | 7.7 | 5.7 | 8.2 |

[1] One serving of meat equals 2.5 ounces of lean meat.

[2] Portion sizes were reduced to two-thirds of adult servings except for milk for children age 2-3.

[3] Consists of Asian, Pacific Islander, American Indian, and Alaskan Native.

[4] Consists of people age 25 and over only.

Note: The overall HEI score ranges from 0 to 100. HEI component scores range from 0 to 10. For each subgroup, component scores may not exactly equal the overall score because of rounding.

SOURCE: P.P. Basiotis et al., "Table 3. Healthy Eating Index, overall and component mean scores, by selected characteristics, 1999–2000," in *The Healthy Eating Index: 1999–2000*, U.S. Department of Agriculture, Center for Nutrition Policy and Promotion, Washington, DC, December 2002

medically restricted diets accounted for the highest percentages among those very concerned, at 72 percent and 71 percent, respectively. Women (56 percent) were more likely to be concerned than men (46 percent). Among household types, those without children were more likely to express concern than households with children (57 percent versus 48 percent). Among age groups, persons ages 50–64 (63 percent) were more likely to be very concerned than persons in other age groups. People living in the South (55 percent) were the most likely to express concern than were persons living in other regions of the country. The higher the level of educational attainment, the more likely that individuals expressed concern. People with at least some college education (57 percent) ranked higher than did those with high school education or less (48 percent).

When asked about the food they eat at home and away from home, 68 percent of respondents said that their diets could be "somewhat" healthier or "a lot" healthier. (See Table 8.10.) In most categories, this represented a decrease from 2002 when 70 percent answered this question in the affirmative. Almost a quarter (22 percent) responded that their diets were "healthy enough."

In 2003 close to half (46 percent) of respondents felt that they, themselves, should be primarily responsible for ensuring that the food they buy is nutritious. Only 16 percent felt that this was the responsibility of food manufacturers and processors, a slight increase since 2000 and 2002 when 15 percent felt that food manufacturers and processors were responsible. (See Table 8.11.)

**TABLE 8.5**

### Trends in the Healthy Eating Index, overall and component mean scores, 1989, 1996, and 1999–2000

| | 1989 | 1996 | 1999–2000 |
|---|---|---|---|
| **Overall** | **61.5** | **63.8** | **68.3** |
| **Components** | | | |
| Grains | 6.1 | 6.7 | 6.7 |
| Vegetables | 5.9 | 6.3 | 6.0 |
| Fruits | 3.7 | 3.8 | 3.8 |
| Milk | 6.2 | 5.4 | 5.9 |
| Meat | 7.1 | 6.4 | 6.6 |
| Total fat | 6.3 | 6.9 | 6.9 |
| Saturated fat | 5.4 | 6.4 | 6.5 |
| Cholesterol | 7.5 | 7.9 | 7.7 |
| Sodium | 6.7 | 6.3 | 6.0 |
| Variety | 6.6 | 7.6 | 7.7 |

SOURCE: P.P. Basiotis et al., "Table 4. Trends in the Healthy Eating Index, overall and component mean scores," in *The Healthy Eating Index: 1999–2000,* U.S. Department of Agriculture, Center for Nutrition Policy and Promotion, Washington, DC, December 2002

**TABLE 8.7**

### Diet-health awareness, 1994–96

| Question | Yes | No |
|---|---|---|
| | *Percent* | |
| Are you aware of health problems related to: | | |
| Not eating enough calcium? | 82.0 | 18.0 |
| Being overweight? | 94.7 | 5.3 |
| Eating too much fat? | 88.0 | 12.0 |
| Eating too much cholesterol? | 89.8 | 10.2 |
| Not eating enough fiber? | 65.5 | 34.5 |
| Eating too much sugar? | 80.0 | 20.0 |
| Eating too much salt or sodium? | 88.5 | 11.5 |

SOURCE: Compiled by Information Plus from *Results from USDA's 1994–96 Diet and Health Survey, Table Set 19,* U.S. Department of Agriculture, Agricultural Research Service, Beltsville Human Nutrition Research Center, Food Surveys Research Group, Beltsville, MD, October 2000

## EATING OUT

The changing American scene—more women in the workforce, the increasing number of dual-earner households, smaller families (many consisting of empty-nester baby boomers)—is reflected in America's eating habits. Americans are eating out more often. In 1997 *Tableservice Restaurant Trends* (National Restaurant Association, Washington, D.C., 1997) reported that, for nearly 4 in 10 adults, restaurant meals were essential to the way they lived.

The National Restaurant Association, a trade association with more than 30,000 members representing more than 175,000 restaurants, is the leading source for research and information on the restaurant industry. In 1996 a nationwide survey by the association (*Meal Consumption Behavior,* Washington, D.C., 1996) found that the

**TABLE 8.6**

### Knowledge of nutrient content, 1994–96

| Question (correct answers are in bold) | Correct | Incorrect |
|---|---|---|
| | *Percent* | |
| Which kind of fat (saturated, **polyunsaturated**) is more likely to be a liquid than a solid? Or are they equally likely to be liquids? | 27.2 | 72.8 |
| If a food has no cholesterol, is it also low in saturated fat, high in saturated fat, or **could be either high or low in saturated fat?** | 53.3 | 46.7 |
| Is cholesterol found in vegetables and vegetable oils, **animal products like meat and dairy products,** or ALL foods containing fat or oil? | 35.9 | 64.1 |
| If a product is labeled as containing only vegetable oil is it low in saturated fat, high in saturated fat, or **could be either high or low in saturated fat?** | 46.1 | 53.9 |
| If a product is labeled "light" does that mean that compared to a similar product not labeled "light" it is lower in calories, lower in fat, **lower in calories and/or fat,** or something else? | 37.3 | 62.7 |
| Based on your knowledge, which has more fat? | | |
| **Regular hamburger** or ground round | 79.1 | 20.9 |
| Loin pork chops or **pork spare ribs** | 65.9 | 34.1 |
| **Hot dogs** or ham | 61.4 | 38.6 |
| **Peanuts** or popcorn | 86.1 | 13.9 |
| Yogurt or **sour cream** | 84.5 | 15.5 |
| **Porterhouse steak** or round steak | 48.7 | 51.3 |
| Based on your knowledge, which has more saturated fat? | | |
| Liver or **t-bone steak** | 61.9 | 38.1 |
| **Butter** or margarine | 74.2 | 25.8 |
| Egg white or **egg yolk** | 80.6 | 19.4 |
| Skim milk or **whole milk** | 93.4 | 6.6 |

SOURCE: Compiled by Information Plus from *Results from USDA's 1994–96 Diet and Health Knowledge Survey, Table Set 19,* U.S. Department of Agriculture, Agricultural Research Service, Beltsville Human Nutrition Research Center, Food Surveys Research Group, Beltsville, MD, October 2000

typical American (eight years old or older) ate an average of 4.1 commercially prepared (away-from-home) meals per week, up from 3.7 meals in 1981. Meanwhile, privately prepared (at-home) meals decreased from an average of 15.1 meals per week in 1981 to 14.4 meals in 1996.

USDA data on the share of food budgets confirm this. In 1960, 26 percent of total food expenditures were away from home; by 2001 that number had risen to 42 percent. (See Figure 8.5.) The percentage of the American food budget spent on food at home has been declining since 1970, while the share spent on food away from home has been increasing. Total expenditures on food away from home have risen from $39.6 million in 1970 to $414.9 million in 2002—an astonishing 948 percent increase. (See Table 8.12.) Figure 8.6 illustrates that eating and drinking establishments account for the largest portion of total food expenditures on food away from home. In 2002, in fact, eating and drinking places accounted for 73 percent of all spending on food away from home. (See Table 8.12.)

TABLE 8.8

**Health risk awareness, 1994–96**

| Health risk | Have heard of problem |
|---|---|
| | *Percent* |
| Not eating enough calcium and relationship to: | |
| Bone problems/osteoporosis | 74.4 |
| Dental problems | 14.2 |
| Being overweight and relationship to: | |
| Heart disease | 75.0 |
| Hypertension | 22.9 |
| Diabetes | 15.9 |
| Eating too much fat and relationship to: | |
| Heart disease | 68.5 |
| High blood cholesterol | 15.5 |
| Obesity | 25.9 |
| Hypertension | 10.4 |
| Eating too much cholesterol and relationship to: | |
| Heart disease | 76.5 |
| Hypertension | 11.4 |
| High blood cholesterol | 9.8 |
| Not eating enough fiber and relationship to: | |
| Bowel problems | 50.4 |
| Cancer | 15.2 |
| Eating too much sugar and relationship to: | |
| Dental problems | 12.8 |
| Diabetes | 50.7 |
| Obesity | 23.9 |
| Eating too much salt or sodium and relationship to: | |
| Heart disease | 27.5 |
| Hypertension | 57.7 |

SOURCE: Compiled by Information Plus from *Results from USDA's 1994–96 Diet and Health Survey, Table Set 19,* U.S. Department of Agriculture, Agricultural Research Service, Beltsville Human Nutrition Research Center, Food Surveys Research Group, Beltsville, MD, October 2000

## Eating-Out Trend May Lower Nutritional Quality of American Diets

TOTAL CALORIES. Biing-Hwan Lin et al., in "Away From Home Food Increasingly Important to Quality of American Diet" (*USDA Agricultural Information Bulletin* 749, Washington, D.C., 2000), reported that, over the past two decades, the proportion of total calories consumed in away-from-home meals increased. In 1977–78 food away from home (food consumed in fast-food places, restaurants, schools, and other public places) accounted for 18 percent of the total caloric intake. By 1995 eating out contributed to 34 percent of the total caloric intake.

In addition, the share of calories eaten at fast-food places (3 percent) and restaurants (3 percent) in 1977–78 rose to 12 percent and 8 percent, respectively, in 1995. (See Figure 8.7.) According to the USDA, consumers may not be as careful in monitoring their caloric consumption when eating out—they tend to consume more food or to eat higher-calorie food.

TOTAL FAT, SATURATED FAT, AND CHOLESTEROL. *Dietary Guidelines for Americans* recommends that total fat intake be limited to no more than 30 percent of total calories and to no more than 10 percent of calories from saturated fats. These percentages are the "benchmark densities" for the two substances. Since 1977 Americans have decreased the total fat density of food consumed both at home and away from home. However, while the total fat density for food eaten at home declined significantly between 1977–78 and 1995, from 41.1 percent to 31.5 percent, fat density for away-from-home food declined slightly during the same period, from 41.2 percent to 37.6 percent. (See Table 8.13.)

While all foods have dropped in fat content, only foods eaten at home in 1995 approached the 30 percent benchmark for dietary calories from fat. Foods eaten away from home remained at 32–40 percent fat content. (See Table 8.13.)

The National Research Council recommends a daily cholesterol intake of no more than 300 milligrams (mg), or about 166 mg per 1,000 calories, regardless of age, gender, or total caloric intake. As with saturated fat, the cholesterol content of Americans' diets was first measured in 1987–88. Since then, average cholesterol density has been lower than the 300-mg benchmark density, but restaurant food exceeds that density. (See Figure 8.8.)

SODIUM. The National Research Council recommends that daily sodium intake not exceed 2,400 mg, regardless of age or gender. Nonetheless, American sodium intakes remain above recommended levels. (See Figure 8.9.) While away-from-home foods generally contain more sodium than at-home foods, restaurant foods contain much more sodium than any other type of away-from-home food and are much higher than the benchmark sodium density of 1,175 mg per 1,000 calories. (See Figure 8.10.)

DIETARY FIBER. Although fiber densities for home and away-from-home foods have increased slightly since 1987, they have stayed far below the benchmark density of 10.5 grams per 1,000 calories. In 1995 foods consumed at home had a fiber density of 8.1 grams per 1,000 calories; those eaten away from home had a fiber density of 6.1 grams per 1,000 calories. (See Figure 8.11.) Health authorities are concerned that the rising frequency of eating out may offset the little progress made in increased fiber intake at home.

CALCIUM AND IRON. In 1995 away-from-home food had a calcium density of 343 mg per 1,000 calories—well below the benchmark density of 425 mg per 1,000 calories. (See Figure 8.12.)

Between 1977 and 1995 the iron density of at-home foods increased more rapidly than that of food consumed away from home. In 1995 three in five (61 percent) of all individuals satisfied their recommended iron intake, compared with two in five persons (42 percent) in 1977–78.

TABLE 8.9

## Shoppers' concern about nutritional content, 1996–2003

Would you say you are very concerned, somewhat concerned, not very concerned, or not at all concerned about the nutritional content of what you eat?

| | | Very concerned | | | | | | | | 2003 level of concern | | |
|---|---|---|---|---|---|---|---|---|---|---|---|---|
| | 2003 Base | 1996 % | 1997 % | 1998 % | 1999 % | 2000 % | 2002 % | 2003 % | Very % | Somewhat % | Not very/ not at all % |
| Total | | 58 | 52 | 50 | 49 | 46 | 50 | 53 | 53 | 39 | 7 |
| **Gender** | | | | | | | | | | | |
| Men | 252 | 49 | 41 | 42 | 41 | 40 | 42 | 46 | 46 | 43 | 11 |
| Women | 749 | 62 | 56 | 53 | 52 | 49 | 54 | 56 | 56 | 38 | 6 |
| Work 20+ hrs./wk. | 392 | 69 | 57 | 51 | 48 | 46 | 54 | 57 | 57 | 40 | 3 |
| Work 0-19 hrs./wk. | 357 | 65 | 54 | 56 | 56 | 52 | 54 | 54 | 54 | 37 | 8 |
| **Type of household** | | | | | | | | | | | |
| With children | 418 | 58 | 50 | 52 | 48 | 44 | 46 | 48 | 48 | 45 | 7 |
| Aged 0-6 | 203 | 57 | 51 | 52 | 51 | 44 | 44 | 45 | 45 | 47 | 8 |
| Aged 7-17 | 318 | 60 | 50 | 52 | 49 | 44 | 45 | 49 | 49 | 44 | 7 |
| No children | 573 | 58 | 53 | 49 | 49 | 48 | 52 | 57 | 57 | 35 | 8 |
| **Age** | | | | | | | | | | | |
| 15-24 | 81 | 47 | 36 | 40 | 33 | 32 | 27 | 36 | 36 | 48 | 15 |
| 25-39 | 311 | 54 | 48 | 44 | 48 | 45 | 44 | 44 | 44 | 51 | 5 |
| 40-49 | 208 | 60 | 55 | 59 | 51 | 50 | 54 | 56 | 56 | 37 | 7 |
| 50-64 | 257 | 66 | 63 | 54 | 52 | 49 | 55 | 63 | 63 | 33 | 4 |
| 65 and older | 97 | 64 | 47 | 52 | 52 | 49 | 59 | 57 | 57 | 27 | 13 |
| **Region** | | | | | | | | | | | |
| East | 190 | 59 | 54 | 51 | 49 | 47 | 48 | 53 | 53 | 41 | 6 |
| Midwest | 240 | 55 | 49 | 50 | 45 | 44 | 45 | 52 | 52 | 40 | 8 |
| South | 350 | 62 | 57 | 55 | 52 | 44 | 56 | 55 | 55 | 38 | 5 |
| West | 220 | 56 | 43 | 41 | 50 | 52 | 49 | 51 | 51 | 40 | 9 |
| **Education** | | | | | | | | | | | |
| High school or less | 403 | 57 | 47 | 47 | 46 | 40 | 49 | 48 | 48 | 41 | 9 |
| Some college/more | 583 | 59 | 55 | 53 | 51 | 52 | 51 | 57 | 57 | 38 | 5 |
| **Medically restricted diet** | | | | | | | | | | | |
| Yes | 148 | 73 | 64 | 65 | 64 | 58 | 67 | 71 | 71 | 25 | 4 |
| No | 853 | 55 | 49 | 47 | 45 | 43 | 47 | 50 | 50 | 42 | 8 |
| **Vegetarian** | | | | | | | | | | | |
| Yes | 51 | 78 | 74 | 58 | 63 | 57 | 74 | 72 | 72 | 24 | 4 |
| No | 950 | 57 | 50 | 50 | 47 | 45 | 49 | 52 | 52 | 40 | 7 |

Note: All data are for January of that year.

SOURCE: "Table 37. Shoppers' Concern About Nutritional Content, 1996–2003," in *Trends in the United States: Consumer Attitudes & the Supermarket, 2003,* Food Marketing Institute, Washington, DC, 2003

The USDA attributes this trend partly to the increased home consumption of iron-fortified breakfast cereals.

On the other hand, the increasing practice of eating out might have contributed to lower iron intake among some women—in 1995 only one in every three women ages 18–39 met her recommended iron intake. For these women, foods eaten away from home accounted for 6 mg of dietary iron per 1,000 calories, compared with 8.2 mg for at-home foods. The benchmark density was 8.4 mg per 1,000 calories.

### The Perception and Reality of Eating Out

The USDA points out that consumers seem to pay more attention to the nutritional properties of at-home foods than away-from-home foods. Although many people claim that nutritious foods are important to them, their eating-out practices do not support this claim.

The National Restaurant Association conducted a nationwide survey to find out if "concerns about health and nutrition influence the choice of restaurants and foods eaten away from home" (*Nutrition and Restaurants: A Consumer Perspective,* Washington, D.C., 1993). The survey asked how likely it was that the respondent would order specific foods. Most respondents (86 percent) indicated they would likely try fresh fruit at a restaurant if it were available. At least 80 percent claimed they would likely eat skinless poultry, Italian dishes, fruit salad, and broiled or baked fish or seafood. Also included in the top-ten food items most likely to be ordered were main-dish salads with vegetables and grains, Chinese dishes, steak or roast beef, and whole-grain muffins. The foods that the respondents thought they would be least likely to try included raw fish or shellfish, caffeine-free coffee, Greek dishes, and sugar substitutes.

TABLE 8.10

## Evaluation of diet, 1996–2003

Thinking of all the foods you eat at home and away from home, how would you describe your diet? Would you say that it could be a lot healthier, could be somewhat healthier, is healthy enough or is as healthy as it could possibly be?

| | | Could be somewhat or a lot healthier | | | | | | | | | 2003 | | |
|---|---|---|---|---|---|---|---|---|---|---|---|---|---|
| | 1996 Base | 1997 % | 1998 % | 1999 % | 2000 % | 2001 % | 2002 % | 2003 % | | A lot healthier % | Somewhat healthier % | Healthy enough % |
| Total | 1,001 | 73 | 73 | 70 | 68 | 68 | 70 | 68 | | 21 | 47 | 22 |
| **Gender** | | | | | | | | | | | | |
| Men | 252 | 74 | 69 | 72 | 69 | 69 | 69 | 67 | | 21 | 46 | 23 |
| Women | 749 | 73 | 74 | 68 | 68 | 67 | 71 | 68 | | 21 | 48 | 22 |
| Work 20+ hrs./wk. | 392 | 75 | 76 | 74 | 74 | 76 | 77 | 70 | | 21 | 49 | 23 |
| Work 0-19 hrs./wk. | 357 | 71 | 71 | 62 | 62 | 56 | 64 | 67 | | 21 | 46 | 21 |
| **Age** | | | | | | | | | | | | |
| 15-24 | 81 | 71 | 75 | 79 | 76 | 69 | 77 | 73 | | 23 | 50 | 18 |
| 25-39 | 311 | 78 | 80 | 74 | 72 | 77 | 75 | 74 | | 25 | 49 | 22 |
| 40-49 | 208 | 79 | 77 | 74 | 73 | 73 | 75 | 70 | | 21 | 49 | 21 |
| 50-64 | 257 | 75 | 65 | 66 | 68 | 69 | 71 | 67 | | 20 | 47 | 23 |
| 65 and older | 97 | 44 | 55 | 51 | 53 | 43 | 56 | 55 | | 15 | 40 | 22 |
| **Income** | | | | | | | | | | | | |
| $15,000 or less | 102 | 68 | 72 | 60 | 62 | 61 | 60 | 67 | | 25 | 42 | 17 |
| $15,001-$25,000 | 140 | 75 | 73 | 68 | 73 | 78 | 77 | 75 | | 32 | 43 | 15 |
| $25,001-$35,000 | 131 | 73 | 71 | 77 | 67 | 69 | 75 | 68 | | 21 | 47 | 20 |
| $35,001-$50,000 | 162 | 78 | 77 | 74 | 71 | 73 | 76 | 79 | | 24 | 55 | 13 |
| $50,001-$75,000 | 165 | 73 | 77 | 75 | 71 | 71 | 71 | 69 | | 19 | 50 | 27 |
| $75,001 or more | 163 | 73 | 68 | 63 | 69 | 66 | 69 | 62 | | 13 | 48 | 32 |
| **Type of household** | | | | | | | | | | | | |
| With children | 418 | 78 | 78 | 76 | 74 | 74 | 77 | 74 | | 24 | 51 | 20 |
| Aged 0-6 | 203 | 76 | 79 | 75 | 72 | 74 | 79 | 74 | | 25 | 49 | 21 |
| Aged 7-17 | 318 | 79 | 77 | 77 | 74 | 75 | 77 | 74 | | 24 | 50 | 20 |
| No children | 573 | 69 | 68 | 65 | 65 | 64 | 66 | 63 | | 19 | 44 | 25 |

Note: All data are for January of that year.

SOURCE: "Table 42. Evaluation of Diet, 1996–2003," in *Trends in the United States: Consumer Attitudes & the Supermarket, 2003,* Food Marketing Institute, Washington, DC, 2003

The foods that consumers actually ordered during 1993 revealed a few discrepancies between what they said they would try and what they ordered. The most commonly ordered foods were hamburgers (87 percent) and steak or roast beef (84 percent). Fresh fruit (83 percent) was the number three item ordered, followed by broiled or baked fish or seafood, French fries, and Italian dishes, all at 78 percent. The National Restaurant Association concluded that "consumers generally overstated their likelihood of trying foods lower in fat and calories while understating their likelihood of ordering foods that are high in fat and calories."

**REASONS FOR THE DISCREPANCY.** The USDA offers two reasons for the discrepancy between consumer perception and reality when it comes to eating out:

- Consumers may have different attitudes about food consumed away from home than food eaten at home. They may think that it is not as important to consider the nutritional quality of away-from-home food, or they might be less willing to give up taste when eating out. Although Americans are eating out far more often than they used to, they may still feel that eating out represents a treat, an occasion when they don't have to concern themselves with nutrition. Americans may not realize that away-from-home foods have become an integral part of their diets.

- Traditional nutrition education has been geared toward the purchase and preparation of home foods—for example, the advice to cook without added fat. When it comes to foods eaten outside the home, nutritional properties may not be as apparent to consumers. For one thing, consumers may not prepare at home the foods they order when eating out. Additionally, consumers can't see the amount of fat used by restaurant cooks. Finally, restaurants often serve much larger portions of food than Americans would serve and consume at home.

TABLE 8.11

## Those on whom shoppers rely to ensure that the foods they buy are nutritious, 1996–2003

Who do you feel should be primarily responsible for ensuring that the food you buy in your grocery store is nutritious? Please listen to entire list before answering. Would you say government institutions or agencies, consumer groups/organizations, manufacturers/food processors, food stores, farmers or yourself as an individual?

(Base: 1,001 shoppers)

| | 1996[1] | 1996[2] | 1997[1] | 1998 | 1999 | 2000 | 2002 | 2003 |
|---|---|---|---|---|---|---|---|---|
| | | | | | *Percent* | | | |
| Yourself as an individual | 50 | 42 | 54 | 55 | 28 | 47 | 44 | 46 |
| Manufacturers/food processors | 29 | 22 | 22 | 26 | 7 | 15 | 15 | 16 |
| Government institutions/agencies | 19 | 14 | 32 | 23 | 5 | 15 | 13 | 14 |
| All/everybody | 18 | 7 | 6 | 7 | 57 | 8 | 9 | 11 |
| Food stores | 13 | 7 | 18 | 16 | 3 | 5 | 8 | 5 |
| Consumer groups/organizations | 9 | 6 | 14 | 8 | 2 | 5 | 5 | 3 |
| Not sure | * | * | 1 | 1 | 1 | 3 | 2 | 2 |
| Farmers | 6 | 1 | 9 | 8 | 1 | 2 | 3 | 1 |
| Other (volunteered) | * | 1 | 1 | * | 1 | * | * | 1 |

* = Less than 0.5 percent.
Notes: All data are for January of that year. 1996[1] and 1997[1] split sample. Multiple responses accepted. 1996[1] single response accepted. Through 1998 and in 2000 and after, "all/everybody" was volunteered, therefore 1999 comparison with data may not be valid. Modification to question wording in 2000.

SOURCE: "Table 44. Those on Whom Shoppers Rely to Ensure That the Foods They Buy Are Nutritious, 1996–2003," in *Trends in Consumer Attitudes & the Supermarket 2003*, Food Marketing Institute, Washington, DC, 2003

---

**FIGURE 8.5**

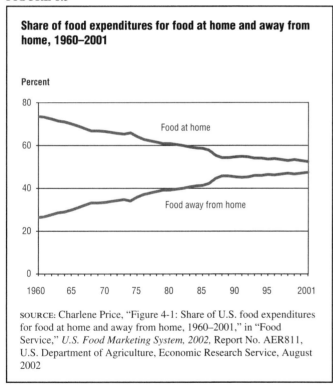

### Share of food expenditures for food at home and away from home, 1960–2001

SOURCE: Charlene Price, "Figure 4-1: Share of U.S. food expenditures for food at home and away from home, 1960–2001," in "Food Service," *U.S. Food Marketing System, 2002*, Report No. AER811, U.S. Department of Agriculture, Economic Research Service, August 2002

---

TABLE 8.12

## Total expenditures on food eaten away from home, 1970–2002[1]

| | Eating and drinking places[2] | Hotels and motels[2] | Retail stores, direct selling[3] | Recreational places[4] | Schools and colleges[5] | All other[6] | Total[7] |
|---|---|---|---|---|---|---|---|
| | | | | Million dollars | | | |
| 1970 | 22,617 | 1,894 | 3,325 | 721 | 4,475 | 6,551 | 39,583 |
| 1971 | 24,166 | 2,086 | 3,626 | 762 | 4,990 | 6,621 | 42,251 |
| 1972 | 27,167 | 2,390 | 3,811 | 832 | 5,370 | 7,017 | 46,587 |
| 1973 | 31,265 | 2,639 | 4,218 | 963 | 5,605 | 7,960 | 52,650 |
| 1974 | 34,029 | 2,864 | 4,520 | 1,167 | 6,287 | 9,178 | 58,045 |
| 1975 | 41,384 | 3,199 | 4,952 | 1,369 | 7,060 | 10,145 | 68,109 |
| 1976 | 47,536 | 3,769 | 5,341 | 1,511 | 7,854 | 10,822 | 76,833 |
| 1977 | 52,491 | 4,115 | 5,663 | 2,606 | 8,413 | 11,547 | 84,835 |
| 1978 | 60,042 | 4,863 | 6,323 | 2,810 | 9,034 | 13,012 | 96,084 |
| 1979 | 68,872 | 5,551 | 7,157 | 2,921 | 9,914 | 14,756 | 109,171 |
| 1980 | 75,883 | 5,906 | 8,158 | 3,040 | 11,115 | 16,194 | 120,296 |
| 1981 | 83,358 | 6,639 | 8,830 | 2,979 | 11,357 | 17,751 | 130,914 |
| 1982 | 90,390 | 6,888 | 9,256 | 2,887 | 11,692 | 18,663 | 139,776 |
| 1983 | 98,710 | 7,660 | 9,827 | 3,271 | 12,338 | 19,077 | 150,883 |
| 1984 | 105,836 | 8,409 | 10,315 | 3,489 | 12,950 | 20,047 | 161,046 |
| 1985 | 111,760 | 9,168 | 10,499 | 3,737 | 13,534 | 20,133 | 168,831 |
| 1986 | 121,699 | 9,665 | 11,116 | 4,059 | 14,401 | 20,755 | 181,695 |
| 1987 | 137,255 | 11,117 | 11,860 | 4,331 | 13,370 | 21,122 | 199,055 |
| 1988 | 151,138 | 11,905 | 12,973 | 4,669 | 13,934 | 22,542 | 217,160 |
| 1989 | 160,657 | 12,179 | 14,153 | 5,658 | 14,644 | 24,198 | 231,490 |
| 1990 | 172,024 | 12,508 | 15,764 | 6,798 | 15,598 | 25,773 | 248,465 |
| 1991 | 180,405 | 12,460 | 16,514 | 7,592 | 16,784 | 26,645 | 260,400 |
| 1992 | 182,327 | 13,204 | 13,586 | 8,602 | 17,755 | 27,946 | 263,420 |
| 1993 | 195,836 | 13,362 | 13,798 | 9,275 | 18,386 | 28,029 | 278,685 |
| 1994 | 205,768 | 13,880 | 14,203 | 9,791 | 19,361 | 28,208 | 291,211 |
| 1995 | 214,159 | 14,188 | 14,332 | 10,568 | 20,141 | 28,593 | 301,982 |
| 1996 | 221,834 | 14,510 | 14,466 | 11,360 | 20,941 | 28,985 | 312,095 |
| 1997 | 235,930 | 15,490 | 14,431 | 9,172 | 22,025 | 30,936 | 327,983 |
| 1998 | 249,310 | 15,835 | 15,231 | 10,019 | 23,233 | 31,944 | 345,573 |
| 1999 | 260,392 | 16,675 | 16,562 | 10,673 | 24,235 | 33,506 | 362,043 |
| 2000 | 280,742 | 17,479 | 16,821 | 11,351 | 24,848 | 34,501 | 385,743 |
| 2001 | 289,462 | 17,923 | 17,426 | 11,751 | 26,255 | 35,261 | 398,077 |
| 2002 | 304,606 | 17,912 | 18,274 | 11,843 | 26,978 | 35,344 | 414,957 |

[1] See *Developing an Integrated Information System for the Food Sector*, AER-575, U.S. Department of Agriculture, Economic Research Service, August 1987, for a description of USDA total food expenditures.

[2] Includes tips.

[3] Includes vending machine operators but not vending machines operated by organization.

[4] Motion picture theaters, bowling alleys, pool parlors, sports arenas, camps, amusement parks, golf and country clubs (includes concessions beginning in 1977).

[5] Includes school food subsidies.

[6] Military exchanges and clubs; railroad dining cars; airlines; food service in manufacturing plants, institutions, hospitals, boarding houses, fraternities and sororities, and civic and social organizations; and food supplied to military forces, civilian employees and child day care.

[7] Computed from unrounded data.

SOURCE: Adapted from "Table 3. Food away from home: Total expenditures," in *Briefing Room: Food CPI, Prices, and Expenditures: Food Away From Home,* U.S. Department of Agriculture, Economic Research Service, Washington, DC, June 2, 2003 [Online] http://www.ers.usda.gov/briefing/CPIFoodAnd Expenditures/Data/table3.htm [accessed August 26, 2003]

FIGURE 8.6

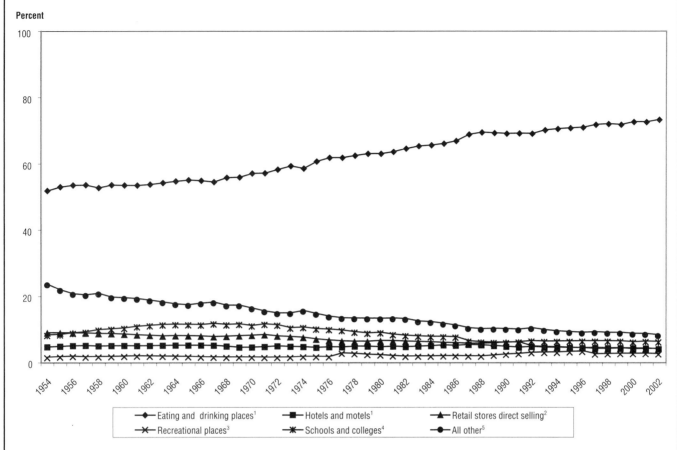

**Percentage of total expenditures on food away from home, 1954–2002**

Percent

*Legend:*
- ◆ Eating and drinking places[1]
- ■ Hotels and motels[1]
- ▲ Retail stores direct selling[2]
- ✕ Recreational places[3]
- ✱ Schools and colleges[4]
- ● All other[5]

[1] Includes tips.

[2] Includes vending machine operators but not vending machines operated by organization.

[3] Motion picture theaters, bowling alleys, pool parlors, sports arenas, camps, amusement parks, golf and country clubs (includes concessions beginning in 1977).

[4] Includes school food subsidies.

[5] Military exchanges and clubs; railroad dining cars; airlines; food service in manufacturing plants, institutions, hospitals, boarding houses, fraternities and sororities, and civic and social organizations; and food supplied to military forces, civilian employees and child day care.

SOURCE: Adapted from "Table 3. Food away from home: Total expenditures," in *Briefing Room: Food CPI, Prices, and Expenditures: Food Away From Home,* U.S. Department of Agriculture, Economic Research Service, Washington, DC, June 2, 2003 [Online] http://www.ers.usda.gov/briefing/CPIFoodAnd Expenditures/Data/table3.htm [accessed August 26, 2003]

FIGURE 8.7

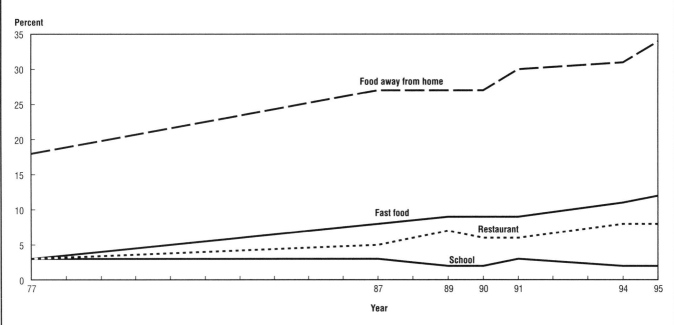

**Contributions of away-from-home sources to total calories, 1977–95**

SOURCE: Biing-Hwan Lin, Elizabeth Frazão, and Joanne Guthrie, "Figure 2: Contributions of away-from-home sources to total calories," in *Away-From-Home Foods Increasingly Important to Quality of American Diet,* Agricultural Information Bulletin #749, U.S. Department of Agriculture, Economic Research Service, and Food and Drug Administration, Washington, DC, January 1999

**TABLE 8.13**

## Fat and saturated fat intake levels and nutrient densities of foods at home and away from home, 1977–95

| Nutrient | 1977-78 | 1987-88 | 1989 | 1990 | 1991 | 1994 | 1995 |
|---|---|---|---|---|---|---|---|
| **Fat** | | | | *Grams* | | | |
| Average daily intake | 86.3 | 74.7 | 72.0 | 72.9 | 73.4 | 74.9 | 76.2 |
| | | | | *Percent of calories* | | | |
| Average intake | 41.1 | 37.0 | 35.3 | 35.4 | 35.1 | 33.6 | 33.6 |
| | | | | *Percent* | | | |
| People meeting recommendation[1] | 13 | 21 | 30 | 29 | 30 | 36 | 37 |
| | | | | *Percent of calories* | | | |
| Benchmark density[1] | 30.0 | 30.0 | 30.0 | 30.0 | 30.0 | 30.0 | 30.0 |
| Average fat density | 41.2 | 37.0 | 35.3 | 35.4 | 35.1 | 33.6 | 33.6 |
| Home foods | 41.1 | 36.3 | 34.4 | 34.5 | 33.8 | 31.9 | 31.5 |
| Away-from-home foods[2] | 41.2 | 38.7 | 37.8 | 38.1 | 38.2 | 37.4 | 37.6 |
| Restaurants | 46.2 | 41.3 | 40.7 | 40.7 | 41.2 | 40.0 | 40.1 |
| Fast-food places | 41.6 | 39.7 | 39.7 | 39.6 | 38.8 | 39.9 | 39.3 |
| Schools[3] | 40.1 | 38.0 | 37.7 | 36.1 | 36.8 | 36.1 | 35.7 |
| Other public places | 41.4 | 41.2 | 34.8 | 40.9 | 42.3 | 30.3 | 32.6 |
| Others | 38.6 | 36.4 | 33.9 | 33.1 | 34.2 | 34.1 | 34.9 |
| **Saturated fat** | | | | *Grams* | | | |
| Average daily intake | na | 27.7 | 25.7 | 26.0 | 26.0 | 25.6 | 26.2 |
| | | | | *Percent of calories* | | | |
| Average intake | na | 13.8 | 12.6 | 12.6 | 12.4 | 11.5 | 11.5 |
| | | | | *Percent* | | | |
| People meeting recommendation[1] | na | 17 | 29 | 29 | 31 | 40 | 39 |
| Nutrient density | | | | *Percent of calories* | | | |
| Benchmark density[1] | na | 10.0 | 10.0 | 10.0 | 10.0 | 10.0 | 10.0 |
| Average sat. fat density | na | 13.8 | 12.6 | 12.6 | 12.4 | 11.5 | 11.5 |
| Home foods | na | 13.5 | 12.3 | 12.2 | 12.1 | 11.1 | 10.9 |
| Away-from-home foods[2] | na | 14.7 | 13.5 | 13.8 | 13.3 | 12.4 | 12.8 |
| Restaurants | na | 15.5 | 14.3 | 13.5 | 14.0 | 12.3 | 12.5 |
| Fast-food places | na | 15.4 | 14.2 | 14.5 | 13.1 | 13.6 | 13.8 |
| Schools[3] | na | 13.9 | 15.4 | 16.1 | 15.4 | 14.4 | 14.2 |
| Other public places | na | 15.2 | 12.0 | 14.6 | 13.8 | 9.8 | 9.8 |
| Others | na | 13.7 | 12.0 | 11.8 | 12.0 | 11.1 | 12.1 |

na = not available.

[1] Recommendations are 30 percent or less of calories from fat and less than 10 percent of calories from saturated fat. These recommendations are the benchmark densities.

[2] Away from home presents the aggregate of fast foods, restaurants, schools, other public places, and others.

[3] Schools are classified as a separate category for children only; adults are included in "others."

SOURCE: Biing-Hwan Lin, Elizabeth Frazão, and Joanne Guthrie, "Table 6: Fat and saturated fat intake levels and nutrient densities of foods at home and away from home, 1977–95," in *Away-From-Home Foods Increasingly Important to Quality of American Diet,* Agricultural Information Bulletin #749, U.S. Department of Agriculture, Economic Research Service, and Food and Drug Administration, Washington, DC, January 1999

FIGURE 8.8

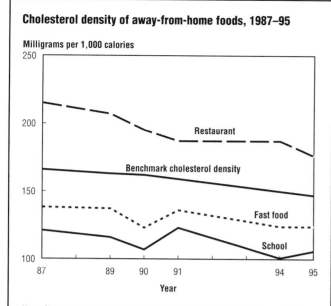

**Cholesterol density of away-from-home foods, 1987–95**

Milligrams per 1,000 calories

Note: Cholesterol intake was first measured in 1987. Healthful diets require the density to remain below the benchmark.

SOURCE: Biing-Hwan Lin, Elizabeth Frazão, and Joanne Guthrie, "Figure 8: Cholesterol density of away-from-home foods," in *Away-From-Home Foods Increasingly Important to Quality of American Diet,* Agricultural Information Bulletin #749, U.S. Department of Agriculture, Economic Research Service, and Food and Drug Administration, Washington, DC, January 1999

FIGURE 8.9

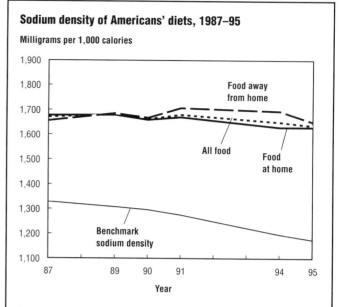

**Sodium density of Americans' diets, 1987–95**

Milligrams per 1,000 calories

Note: Sodium intake was first measured in 1987. Healthful diets require the density to remain below the benchmark.

SOURCE: Biing-Hwan Lin, Elizabeth Frazão, and Joanne Guthrie, "Figure 9: Sodium density of Americans' diets," in *Away-From-Home Foods Increasingly Important to Quality of American Diet,* Agricultural Information Bulletin #749, U.S. Department of Agriculture, Economic Research Service, and Food and Drug Administration, Washington, DC, January 1999

FIGURE 8.10

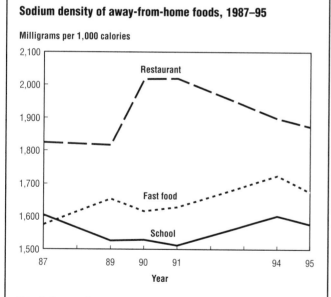

**Sodium density of away-from-home foods, 1987–95**

Milligrams per 1,000 calories

Note: Sodium was first measured in 1987. Healthful diets require the density to remain below the benchmark; the benchmark was 1,175 mg per 1,000 calories in 1995.

SOURCE: Biing-Hwan Lin, Elizabeth Frazão, and Joanne Guthrie, "Figure 10: Sodium density of away-from-home foods," in *Away-From-Home Foods Increasingly Important to Quality of American Diet,* Agricultural Information Bulletin #749, U.S. Department of Agriculture, Economic Research Service, and Food and Drug Administration, Washington, DC, January 1999

FIGURE 8.11

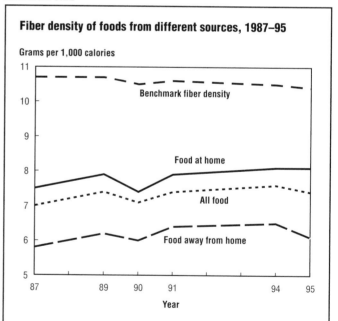

**Fiber density of foods from different sources, 1987–95**

Grams per 1,000 calories

Note: Dietary fiber was first measured in 1987. Healthful diets require the density to be above the benchmark.

SOURCE: Biing-Hwan Lin, Elizabeth Frazão, and Joanne Guthrie, "Figure 13: Fiber density of foods from different sources," in *Away-From-Home Foods Increasingly Important to Quality of American Diet,* Agricultural Information Bulletin #749, U.S. Department of Agriculture, Economic Research Service, and Food and Drug Administration, Washington, DC, January 1999

**FIGURE 8.12**

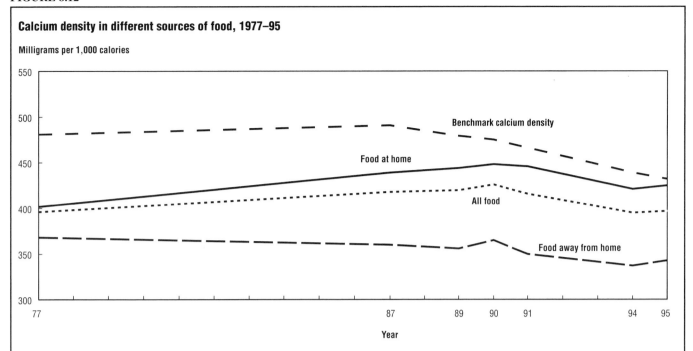

**Calcium density in different sources of food, 1977–95**

Milligrams per 1,000 calories

Note: Healthful diets require the density to be above the benchmark.

SOURCE: Biing-Hwan Lin, Elizabeth Frazão, and Joanne Guthrie, "Figure 11: Calcium density in different sources of food," in *Away-From-Home Foods Increasingly Important to Quality of American Diet,* Agricultural Information Bulletin #749, U.S. Department of Agriculture, Economic Research Service, and Food and Drug Administration, Washington, DC, January 1999

## CHAPTER 9
# WEIGHT, DIET, AND EXERCISE

Weight is a major issue for Americans. Some may look at the tall, slender models seen in every form of visual advertising and feel unnecessarily inadequate, but the Centers for Disease Control and Prevention (CDC) reports an upward trend in the prevalence of overweight and obesity among the American people. (See Figure 9.1.) Estimates by the CDC, based on data from the National Health Interview Surveys, show that obesity among U.S. adults has been steadily rising—from 13.5 percent of the adult population age 20 and over in 1960–62 to 30.8 percent of that population in 1999–2000.

## PREVALENCE OF OVERWEIGHT AND OBESITY

The National Center for Health Statistics (NCHS) of the CDC periodically surveys Americans to provide data and prevalence estimates for a variety of health measures. The center's National Health and Nutrition Examination Survey (NHANES) program collected weight and other health data in three surveys (1976–80, 1988–91, and 1991–94). Beginning in 1999 NHANES became a continuous annual survey. The survey used the body mass index (BMI) as a measure of weight relative to a person's height. The NHANES defined overweight as a BMI of 25 to 30 and obesity as a BMI of 30 or greater.

NHANES 1999–2000 found that 64.3 percent of U.S. adults age 20 and older were overweight. (See Figure 9.1 and Table 9.1.) The populations with the highest percentage of overweight members were black, non-Hispanic females (77.2 percent) and Mexican men (71.9 percent). The populations with the lowest percentage of overweight members were white, non-Hispanic females (58.1 percent) and black, non-Hispanic males (58.6 percent).

### Obesity Prevalence among Adults

Prevalence is the number of obese individuals in the population divided by the total number of individuals in the population. According to the CDC, the prevalence

of obesity in the adult population constitutes an "obesity epidemic."

**BY SEX.** As shown in Table 9.1 and Figure 9.1, obesity prevalence has risen steadily since 1960. Between 1991 and 2001 obesity prevalence among the adult population age 18 and older rose 74 percent, from 12 percent to 20.9 percent. (See Table 9.2.) In 2001 the prevalence of obesity in men (21 percent) and women (20.8) was about equal.

**FIGURE 9.1**

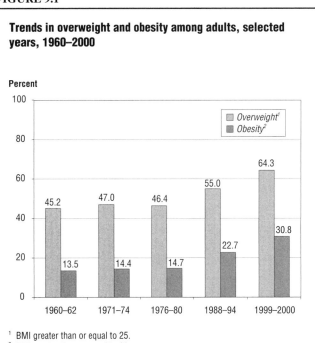

**Trends in overweight and obesity among adults, selected years, 1960–2000**

¹ BMI greater than or equal to 25.
² BMI greater than or equal to 30.

SOURCE: Adapted from "Table 70. Healthy weight, overweight, and obesity among persons 20 years of age and over, according to sex, age, race, and Hispanic origin: United States, 1960–62, 1971–74, 1976–80, 1988–94, and 1999–2000," in *Health, United States, 2002,* National Center for Health Statistics, Hyattsville, MD, 2002 [Online] http://www.cdc.gov/ nchs/data/hus/tables/2002/02hus070.pdf [accessed August 27, 2003]

TABLE 9.1

**Trends in overweight and obesity among adults aged 20–74 by sex and race/ethnicity, selected years, 1960–2000**

(Percent of population)

| | Overweight (BMI greater than or equal to 25) | | | | | Obesity (BMI greater than or equal to 30) | | | | |
|---|---|---|---|---|---|---|---|---|---|---|
| | 1960–62 | 1971–74 | 1976–80 | 1988–94 | 1999–2000 | 1960–62 | 1971–74 | 1976–80 | 1988–94 | 1999–2000 |
| Both sexes[1,2] | 45.2 | 47.0 | 46.4 | 55.0 | 64.3 | 13.5 | 14.4 | 14.7 | 22.7 | 30.8 |
| Male | 49.4 | 53.5 | 51.5 | 59.6 | 66.5 | 10.7 | 12.0 | 12.3 | 19.9 | 27.5 |
| Female | 41.2 | 41.0 | 41.6 | 50.5 | 62.0 | 16.1 | 16.7 | 16.8 | 25.5 | 34.0 |
| White male | 50.2 | 54.3 | 52.5 | 61.1 | X | 10.4 | 11.7 | 12.1 | 20.4 | X |
| White female | 38.9 | 39.1 | 39.4 | 49.0 | X | 14.7 | 15.4 | 15.3 | 24.0 | X |
| Black male | 43.9 | 49.3 | 48.5 | 56.7 | X | 14.1 | 16.0 | 15.0 | 20.9 | X |
| Black female | 58.8 | 58.2 | 60.0 | 65.9 | X | 26.6 | 28.7 | 29.8 | 37.0 | X |
| White, non-Hispanic male | X | X | 52.2 | 60.8 | 67.6 | X | X | 12.0 | 20.3 | 27.8 |
| White, non-Hispanic female | X | X | 38.9 | 47.1 | 58.1 | X | X | 15.2 | 23.1 | 30.9 |
| Black, non-Hispanic male | X | X | 48.4 | 57.0 | 58.6 | X | X | 14.9 | 21.1 | 28.5 |
| Black, non-Hispanic female | X | X | 59.4 | 66.2 | 77.2 | X | X | 29.5 | 37.2 | 50.3 |
| Mexican male | X | X | 57.0 | 64.0 | 71.9 | X | X | 14.6 | 20.7 | 29.6 |
| Mexican female | X | X | 57.4 | 66.2 | 69.5 | X | X | 23.8 | 33.6 | 38.1 |

X = Not available.

[1] Excludes pregnant women.

[2] Includes persons of all races and Hispanic origins, not just those shown separately.

SOURCE: Adapted from "Table 70. Healthy weight, overweight, and obesity among persons 20 years of age and over, according to sex, age, race, and Hispanic origin: United States, 1960–62, 1971–74, 1976–80, 1988–94, and 1999–2000," in *Health, United States, 2002,* National Center for Health Statistics, Hyattsville, MD, 2002 [Online] http://www.cdc.gov/nchs/data/hus/tables/2002/02hus070.pdf [accessed August 27, 2003]

**BY AGE AND RACE/ETHNICITY.** In 2001 the prevalence of obesity was highest for individuals ages 50–59 (26.1 percent) and lowest for those ages 18–29 (14.0 percent). (See Table 9.2.) Blacks had the highest prevalence of obesity (31.1 percent), followed closely by Hispanics (23.7 percent). Whites had the lowest prevalence (19.6 percent).

**BY EDUCATIONAL LEVEL AND SMOKING STATUS.** In 2001 the prevalence of obesity was lowest among those with or a college degree or above (15.7 percent) and highest among persons with less than a high school diploma (27.4 percent). (See Table 9.2.) Current smokers had the lowest prevalence of obesity (17.8 percent) and ex-smokers had the highest prevalence of obesity (23.9 percent). One-fifth (20.9 percent) of those who had never smoked were obese.

## Overweight and Obese Children

The CDC uses BMI-for-age growth charts, developed in 2000, to identify children who are overweight. Children who have BMI values at or above the 95th percentile of the sex-specific BMI growth charts are defined by the CDC as overweight. NHANES 1999–2000 found that approximately 15 percent of children and adolescents were overweight. (See Figure 9.2.) Note how the prevalence of overweight children and adolescents has grown since the 1963–65 survey, more than tripling for young children.

Using unpublished CDC data and a definition of obesity that corresponded to the CDC's definition of overweight, the American Obesity Association (AOA) reported that in 1999–2000, 16 percent of young boys (ages 6–11) and 14.5 percent of young girls were obese. Among adolescents ages 12–19, the obesity prevalence was reported as 15.5 percent for both boys and girls.

According to the National Institute of Diabetes and Digestive and Kidney Diseases (NIDDK), the part of the National Institutes of Health (NIH) chiefly responsible for obesity research, children become overweight for several reasons. Children whose parents or siblings are overweight are more likely to be overweight. Although heredity plays a role in overweight and obesity, shared family behaviors, such as eating habits and activity levels, also influence a child's weight.

Overweight children tend to eat foods high in fats and calories. An inactive lifestyle further contributes to overweight because children do not burn off the excess calories. Nielsen Media Research reported in 2000 that American children ages 2 to 17 spend an average of 19 hours and 40 minutes each week watching television. In addition, sitting in front of computers and playing video games has taken more time away from physical activities.

## Childhood Obesity and Type 2 Diabetes

Type 2 diabetes, also known as adult-onset diabetes, generally occurs in people over 40 and can be triggered by overweight. Today this disease is increasingly diagnosed in obese children, some younger than 10 years old. Type

TABLE 9.2

## Prevalence of adult obesity, by characteristics, 1991–2001

(In percent. BRFSS data by year.)

| Characteristics | 1991 | 1995 | 1998 | 1999 | 2000 | 2001 |
|---|---|---|---|---|---|---|
| Total | 12.0 | 15.3 | 17.9 | 18.9 | 19.8 | 20.9 |
| **Gender** | | | | | | |
| Men | 11.7 | 15.6 | 17.7 | 19.1 | 20.2 | 21.0 |
| Women | 12.2 | 15.0 | 18.1 | 18.6 | 19.4 | 20.8 |
| **Age groups** | | | | | | |
| 18–29 | 7.1 | 10.1 | 12.1 | 12.1 | 13.5 | 14.0 |
| 30–39 | 11.3 | 14.4 | 16.9 | 18.6 | 20.2 | 20.5 |
| 40–49 | 15.8 | 17.9 | 21.2 | 22.4 | 22.9 | 24.7 |
| 50–59 | 16.1 | 21.6 | 23.8 | 24.2 | 25.6 | 26.1 |
| 60–69 | 14.7 | 19.4 | 21.3 | 22.3 | 22.9 | 25.3 |
| >70 | 11.4 | 12.1 | 14.6 | 16.1 | 15.5 | 17.1 |
| **Race, ethnicity** | | | | | | |
| White, non Hispanic | 11.3 | 14.5 | 16.6 | 17.7 | 18.5 | 19.6 |
| Black, non Hispanic | 19.3 | 22.6 | 26.9 | 27.3 | 29.3 | 31.1 |
| Hispanic | 11.6 | 16.8 | 20.8 | 21.5 | 23.4 | 23.7 |
| Other | 7.3 | 9.6 | 11.9 | 12.4 | 12.0 | 15.7 |
| **Educational level** | | | | | | |
| Less than high school | 16.5 | 20.1 | 24.1 | 25.3 | 26.1 | 27.4 |
| High school degree | 13.3 | 16.7 | 19.4 | 20.6 | 21.7 | 23.2 |
| Some college | 10.7 | 15.1 | 17.8 | 18.1 | 19.5 | 21.0 |
| College or above | 8.0 | 11.0 | 13.1 | 14.3 | 15.2 | 15.7 |
| **Smoking status** | | | | | | |
| Never smoked | 12.0 | 15.2 | 17.9 | 19.0 | 19.9 | 20.9 |
| Ex-smoker | 14.0 | 17.9 | 20.9 | 21.5 | 22.7 | 23.9 |
| Current smoker | 9.9 | 12.3 | 14.8 | 15.7 | 16.3 | 17.8 |

SOURCE: "1991–2001 Prevalence of Obesity Among U.S. Adults, by Characteristics," Centers for Disease Control and Prevention, National Center for Health Statistics, Hyattsville, MD [Online] http://www.cdc.gov/nccdphp/dnpa/obesity/trend/prev_char.htm [accessed August 27, 2003]

2 diabetes is incurable and degenerative, causing kidney disease, blindness, frequent infection, and cardiovascular complications. In a study published in the journal *Pediatrics* (May 2002) Dr. William Dietz of the CDC reported "a disturbing increase" in the number of obesity-related childhood hospitalizations over the preceding 20 years, which included a near doubling of diabetes diagnoses and a fivefold increase in obesity-caused sleep apnea. Dietz noted that obese people can die from sleep apnea, because fat in the back of the throat, combined with large tonsils, blocks the airway.

## DETERMINING OVERWEIGHT AND OBESITY

In May 1998 the National Heart, Lung, and Blood Institute (NHLBI; also a part of the NIH) and the NIDDK released the first federal guidelines on the identification, evaluation, and treatment of overweight and obesity. The NHLBI and NIDDK reported that 97 million overweight Americans—55 percent of the population—are at increased risk for serious medical conditions, including higher rates of certain types of cancer.

Different methods are used for children and adults to find out if weight is appropriate for height. The federal standards for determining overweight or obesity in an adult are based on the body mass index, or BMI. The BMI uses a mathematical formula, incorporating a person's body weight and height to establish a value that determines his or her health risks. Scientists calculate the BMI by dividing a person's weight in kilograms by height in meters squared ($kg/m^2$). Figure 9.3 demonstrates adult BMI categories according to height and weight. The higher the BMI category, the greater the risk for health problems. Table 9.3 shows how to calculate BMI.

The new federal guidelines define overweight as a BMI of 25–29.9 and obesity as a BMI of 30 and above. This redefinition of overweight is based on research that relates BMI to risk of death and illness, and supports the *Dietary Guidelines for Americans.* The revised definition is consistent with the definition used by other countries and by the World Health Organization (WHO).

BMI numbers apply to both men and women. The new definition also means that many more Americans—about 29 million—previously considered at normal weight are now reclassified as overweight. In June 1998, a month after the new guidelines for overweight were released, the American Heart Association announced that obesity is now considered a major risk factor for a heart attack—not just a contributing risk, as previously described.

A person's waist circumference is associated with abdominal fat. A waist circumference of more than 40 inches

FIGURE 9.2

**Prevalence of overweight among children and adolescents, selected years, 1963–2000**

(Prevalence is the number of overweight individuals in the population divided by the total number of individuals in the population.)

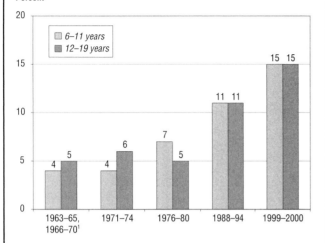

[1] Data for 1963-65 are for children 6-11 years of age; data for 1966-70 are for adolescents 12-17 years of age, not 12-19 years.

Note: Data excludes pregnant women starting with 1971-74. Pregnancy status not available for 1963-65 and 1966-70.

SOURCE: "Figure 1. Prevalence of overweight among children and adolescents ages 6–19 years," in *Prevalence of Overweight Among Children and Adolescents: United States 1999–2000,* Centers for Disease Control and Prevention, National Center for Health Statistics Hyattsville, MD [Online] http://www.cdc.gov/nchs/products/pubs/pubd/hestats/overwght99.htm [accessed August 26, 2003]

in men and more than 35 inches in women, along with a BMI of 25–34.9, means an increased risk of disease. The disease risks increase for obese and extremely obese individuals. (See Table 9.4.)

PLOTTING BMI IN YOUNG PEOPLE. For children and teens ages 2–20, BMI-for-age is plotted on gender-specific growth charts. Figure 9.4 is the growth chart for girls. (See Figure 9.4.) A girl with a BMI-for-age below the 5th percentile is considered underweight. A girl with a BMI-for-age greater than or equal to the 95th percentile is considered obese. (The growth chart for boys is available on-line at http://www.cdc.gov/nchs/data/nhanes/growthcharts/set2clinical/cj41l071.pdf.)

## CAUSES OF OVERWEIGHT AND OBESITY

The panel of NHLBI and NIDDK experts that developed the first federal obesity guidelines defines obesity as "a complex multifactorial chronic disease that develops from an interaction of genotype and the environment." The NIH believes that "increasing physiologic, biochemical and genetic evidence suggests that overweight is not a simple problem of will power as is sometimes implied,

but is a complex disorder of appetite regulation and energy metabolism." In 2002 the Internal Revenue Service designated obesity as a disease and, for the first time, allowed taxpayers to claim expenses associated with weight-loss programs as a medical deduction.

### Genetics

In 1994 scientists discovered a genetic mutation that may contribute to overweight. The mutation, first found in obese mice and then in humans, is thought to be responsible for at least some types of obesity. When mice with the defective gene, called "ob" for obese, were injected with leptin, a hormone normally secreted by fat cells, they underwent spectacular weight loss. Leptin caused even normal-weight mice to become thin. Initially, researchers hoped that the process would be the same in humans and that leptin was the missing key to weight control. Further research, however, found that, unlike the "ob" mice, who had no detectable levels of leptin, obese humans had leptin levels 20–30 times greater than normal-weight humans.

Scientists have speculated that the normal sequence of events is as follows: Fat cells produce leptin, which travels through the bloodstream to leptin receptors located in the hypothalamus, the portion of the brain that regulates unconscious body functions. If high levels of leptin are received, the receptor passes on a message of too much fat. The brain responds by reducing the appetite or increasing the rate at which fat is burned, or both.

Experts hypothesize that the problem in obese people may lie with leptin receptors that fail to send messages to the brain to stop eating. In addition, chronic high-fat diets may cause leptin insensitivity, creating a vicious cycle where the more the person eats, the less he or she is able to detect when the body is satisfied.

The NIDDK notes that there is growing evidence that obesity may have a genetic cause. The NIDDK cites a study of adults who were adopted as children. The study found that the subjects' adult weights were closer to the weights of their biological parents than to their adoptive parents' weights. However, the role of genetics in overweight and obesity remains controversial, and more research is needed to study the link between heredity and weight loss, gain, and maintenance.

### Environmental Factors

Researchers warn that no one knows what proportion of a population's obesity is actually caused by heredity. Leah Garnett, in "Is Obesity All in the Genes?" (*Harvard Health Letter,* vol. 21, no. 6, April 1996), observed, "Environmental factors are the weightiest determinants of who gets fat and who doesn't." The rate of obesity keeps rising, and yet the human gene pool has remained largely unchanged for several generations. Garnett believes that

FIGURE 9.3

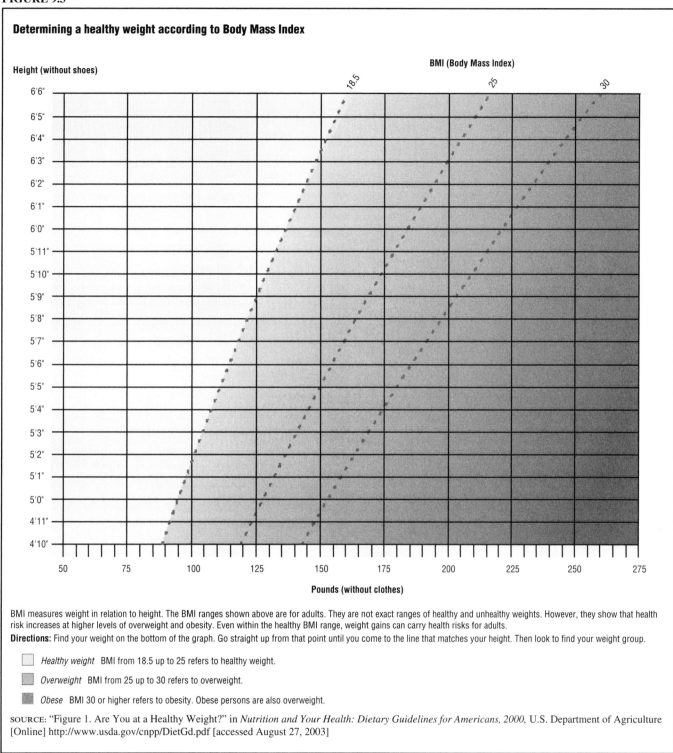

**Determining a healthy weight according to Body Mass Index**

BMI measures weight in relation to height. The BMI ranges shown above are for adults. They are not exact ranges of healthy and unhealthy weights. However, they show that health risk increases at higher levels of overweight and obesity. Even within the healthy BMI range, weight gains can carry health risks for adults.

**Directions:** Find your weight on the bottom of the graph. Go straight up from that point until you come to the line that matches your height. Then look to find your weight group.

*Healthy weight*  BMI from 18.5 up to 25 refers to healthy weight.

*Overweight*  BMI from 25 up to 30 refers to overweight.

*Obese*  BMI 30 or higher refers to obesity. Obese persons are also overweight.

SOURCE: "Figure 1. Are You at a Healthy Weight?" in *Nutrition and Your Health: Dietary Guidelines for Americans, 2000*, U.S. Department of Agriculture [Online] http://www.usda.gov/cnpp/DietGd.pdf [accessed August 27, 2003]

people with a genetic propensity for obesity live in an environment where excess is the norm. Because of this, they will probably gain more weight than people with a tendency toward leanness.

Many experts attribute the increasing proportions of overweight people to the environment in which they live. This environment includes many lifestyle behaviors that influence weight gain, such as eating habits and physical activity levels. Americans are eating out more, and restaurants not only serve bigger portions to attract more patrons, but also tend to serve foods higher in fat.

Modern technology has also affected our weight gain. Computers and televisions encourage a sedentary lifestyle. The remote control prevents the expenditure of energy, however minimal, of getting up to adjust a television or stereo dial. Social occasions typically revolve around eating, and sports events do not just involve the perennial hot dogs, but also high-calorie tailgate meals.

TABLE 9.3

**How to calculate Body Mass Index (BMI)**

$$BMI = \frac{\text{weight (in kilograms)}}{\text{height (in meters)}^2}$$

$$BMI = \frac{\text{weight (in pounds)} \times 705}{\text{height (in inches)}^2}$$

SOURCE: "Figure 9.1: How to Calculate BMI," Center for Nutrition Policy and Promotion, U.S. Department of Agriculture, Washington DC

## Physiological Factors

In 2002 researchers at the U.S. Department of Energy's Brookhaven National Laboratory conducted a brain-imaging study that seemed to show that obese people overeat simply because they find food more palatable than do non-obese people. In a June 20, 2002, Brookhaven news release, physician Gene-Jack Wang, lead author of the study, stated, "This enhanced activity in brain regions involved with sensory processing of food could make obese people more sensitive to the rewarding properties of food, and could be one of the reasons they overeat."

In "Study Finds Appetites Reduced by Hormone" (September 4, 2003), *New York Times* science writer Gina Kolata reported the results of a study published in *The New England Journal of Medicine* (September 4, 2003). The study showed that overweight people produced less of the hormone PYY (peptide YY 3-36), which is released by the intestine after a meal and signals fullness. Kolata commented, "Researchers have long noted that one reason people find it so hard to lose weight is that the body has many ways to thwart them."

## Psychological Factors

Psychological factors may also affect eating habits. Some people reach for food in response to stress. Others react to negative emotions, such as boredom, anger, or sadness, by overeating. Studies show that about 30 percent of people who are being treated for serious weight problems are binge eaters. During binge eating episodes, individuals consume large quantities of food, at the same time feeling they cannot control how much they are eating. Those who have severe binge eating problems are said to have a binge eating disorder.

## Other Causes

Certain drugs, such as steroids and anti-depressants, may cause weight gain. Some illnesses, including depression, and hormonal disorders such as hypothyroidism (loss of activity in the thyroid gland, often characterized by lower metabolism) and Cushing's syndrome (symptoms caused by overactivity of the adrenal glands' outer layers, or cortices), can predispose a person to overeat. About 1 percent of overweight cases result from these causes.

## CONSEQUENCES OF OBESITY

### Health Risks

According to a June 17, 1998, NIH news release, analysis of the NHANES III (1988–94) found that "As BMI levels rise, blood pressure and total cholesterol levels increase, and HDL or good cholesterol levels decrease. Men in the highest obesity category have more than twice the risk of hypertension [high blood pressure], high blood cholesterol, or both, compared to men with normal weight. Women in the highest obesity category have four times the risk of either or both of these health-risk factors."

High blood pressure is a major risk factor for heart disease and stroke. (See Table 9.5.) Very high levels of cholesterol and triglycerides (blood fats) can also lead to heart disease. Other diseases and health problems associated with obesity include hypertension; type 2 diabetes; gallbladder disease; osteoarthritis (deterioration of the joints); respiratory problems, including sleep apnea (interrupted breathing during sleep); and certain cancers.

Overweight men are more likely to develop cancer of the colon, rectum, and prostate. Overweight women, on the other hand, are at greater risk for developing cancer of the gallbladder, cervix, ovary, uterus, and breast.

### Psychological and Social Effects

Despite an increasing amount of research that shows obesity is a very complex medical problem, the obese in American society often suffer discrimination. People sometimes blame the obese for their condition, stereotyping them as lazy and undisciplined. Many think that if overweight people would watch what they eat and get some exercise, they could maintain a normal weight. The obese point out that they suffer job discrimination and are stigmatized by a society that places great importance on physical appearance, equating attractiveness with being slim.

## DIETING

Despite an abundance of diet books, many of which remain on the best-seller lists for months and sometimes years, there is no single satisfactory way to achieve long-term weight reduction. The American Dietetic Association reported in February 2002 that Americans spend $33 billion annually in the weight-loss industry. Some diets are not very effective; others might even be harmful.

An American Heart Association (AHA) analysis of hundreds of published studies on the safety and effectiveness of popular low-carbohydrate diets found that there is insufficient scientific evidence for or against the use of these diets ("Journal of the American Medical Association

**TABLE 9.4**

**Classification of overweight and obesity by Body Mass Index (BMI), waist circumference, and associated disease risk**

| | BMI (kg/m²) | Obesity class | Disease risk* relative to normal weight & waist circumference | |
| | | | Men: ≤ 102 cm (≤ 40 in)<br>Women: ≤ 88 cm (≤ 35 in) | Men: > 102 cm (> 40 in)<br>Women: > 88 cm (> 35 in) |
| --- | --- | --- | --- | --- |
| Underweight | <18.5 | | | |
| Normal | 18.5-24.9 | | | |
| Overweight | 25.0-29.9 | | Increased | High |
| Obesity | 30.0-34.9 | I | High | Very high |
| | 35.0-39.9 | II | Very high | Very high |
| Extreme Obesity | ≥40 | III | Extremely high | Extremely high |

*Disease risk for type 2 diabetes, hypertension and cardiovascular disease.

SOURCE: "Classification of Overweight and Obesity by BMI, Waist Circumference, and Associated Disease Risks," National Institutes of Health, National Heart, Lung and Blood Institute, Bethesda, MD [Online] http://www.nhlbi.nih.gov/health/public/heart/obesity/lose_wt/bmi_dis.htm [accessed August 26, 2003]

Study: Efficacy and Safety of Low-Carbohydrate Diets," April 8, 2003 [Online] http://www.americanheart.org/presenter.jhtml?identifier=3010801). According to Dr. Robert H. Eckel, chairman of the AHA's Nutrition, Physical Activity, and Metabolism Council, "In most of the studies contained in the analysis, weight loss occurred when study participants were on the diets for longer periods, and when they ate fewer calories." Experts, including the AHA, advise that to lose weight, one must expend more calories than are consumed.

## Who Is Dieting?

According to an ongoing survey by the Calorie Control Council, between 1986 and 2000 the percentage of American adults who were on a diet declined from 37 percent to 24 percent. (See Figure 9.5.) The council interpreted the low percentages to mean that "people continue to understand that traditional dieting (deprivation, short-term solutions) spell (sic) failure. Instead, it takes permanent lifestyle changes to take and keep weight off."

A March 11, 2003, survey by the Gallup Organization revealed that 15 percent of teens were on a diet to lose weight. (See Figure 9.6.) The CDC's ongoing survey Behavioral Risk Factor Surveillance System ("the world's largest telephone survey") queries respondents about behaviors that increase their risk for one or more of the leading causes of death. In 2000 nearly two-thirds (65.7 percent) of obese people and nearly half (45 percent) of overweight people were trying to lose weight. On the other hand, 13.5 percent of obese respondents and 20.1 percent of overweight respondents reported that they were trying neither to maintain nor lose weight. (See Table 9.6.)

DIET PLANS USED. According to the U.S. Department of Agriculture's Food Guide Pyramid, a "healthful" diet would include, among other things, 3–5 servings of vegetables and 2–4 servings of fruit a day. Table 9.6 shows

that more than a third of overweight (34.1 percent) and obese (35.7 percent) people reported eating fewer than 3 servings of fruit and vegetables each day. More than half (54.9 percent) of obese people who were trying to lose or maintain weight reported having received no professional weight-loss advice.

The Gallup Organization conducted consumer surveys in 2000 and 2002 for the Wheat Foods Council and the American Bakers Association (*Grains of Truth About Fad Diets & Obesity: Americans Realize Road to Good Health, Weight Loss a Long One,* Parker, CO, 2003). A low-fat diet was the most popular diet tried by those who were dieting; in 2002 more than half of respondents (60 percent) reported trying the low-fat diet. (See Figure 9.7.) Second in popularity was the Food Guide Pyramid diet (45 percent), followed by either a doctor-recommended diet (35 percent) or a high-protein, low-carbohydrate diet (35 percent).

Interestingly, although the majority (82 percent) of dieters agreed that "the Food Guide Pyramid [with a foundation of grains, fruits, and vegetables] is the basis of a sensible, healthful eating plan," more than a third (35 percent) of those same dieters indicated they had tried a high-protein, low-carbohydrate diet. More than half (56 percent) of respondents believed the high-protein, low-carbohydrate diet would help them lose weight; 61 percent believed such a diet was a safe way to lose weight; and 58 percent believed carbohydrates (found in grain foods) must be eliminated from the body for a person to lose weight. (See Figure 9.8.)

## Metabolism

One factor in the battle to lose weight and keep it off is metabolism. Rudolph L. Leibel et al., in "Changes in Energy Expenditure Resulting from Altered Body Weight" (*New England Journal of Medicine,* vol. 332, no. 10, March 9, 1995), found that the human body has a weight that it naturally gravitates to, whether fat or thin,

**FIGURE 9.4**

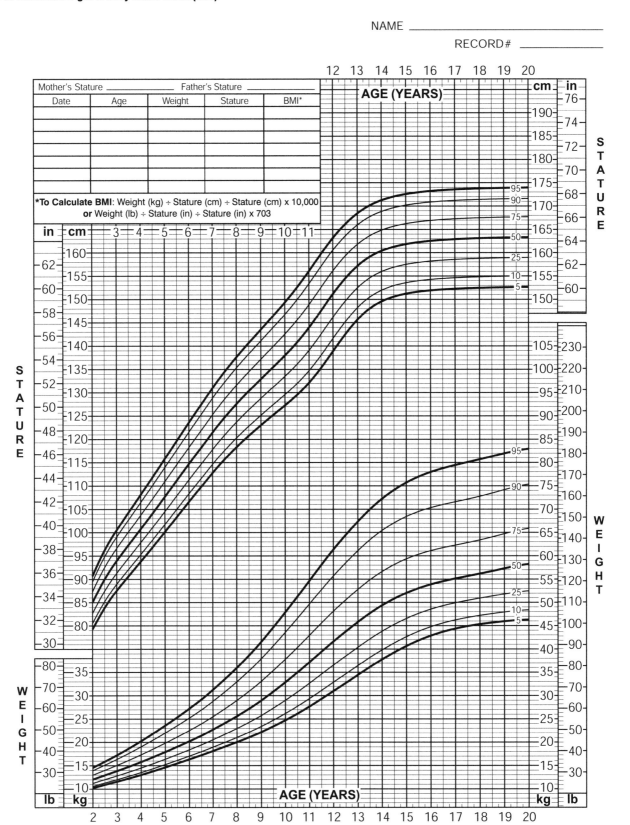

**How to calculate a girl's Body Mass Index (BMI)**

SOURCE: "2 to 20 years: Girls Stature-for-age and Weight-for-age percentiles," Centers for Disease Control and Prevention, National Center for Health Statistics, Hyattsville, MD [Online] http://www.cdc.gov/nchs/data/nhanes/growthcharts/set1clinical/cj41c022.pdf [accessed August 26, 2003]

TABLE 9.5

## Overweight and obesity risk factors

**Overweight and obesity are known risk factors for:**

• diabetes,
• heart disease,
• stroke,
• hypertension,
• gallbladder disease,
• osteoarthritis (degeneration of cartilage and bone of joints),
• sleep apnea and other breathing problems, and
• some forms of cancer (uterine, breast, colorectal, kidney, and gallbladder).

**Obesity is associated with:**

• high blood cholesterol,
• complications of pregnancy,
• menstrual irregularities,
• hirsutism (presence of excess body and facial hair),
• stress incontinence (urine leakage caused by weak pelvic-floor muscles),
• psychological disorders such as depression, and
• increased surgical risk.

SOURCE: *Statistics Related to Overweight and Obesity,* Publication 96-4158, National Institutes of Health, Weight Control Information Network, Bethesda, MD, 2000

---

**FIGURE 9.6**

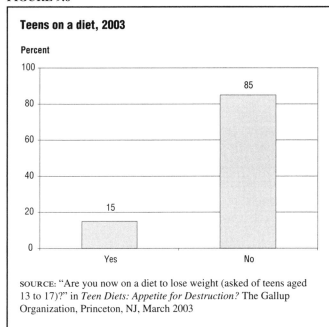

## Teens on a diet, 2003

SOURCE: "Are you now on a diet to lose weight (asked of teens aged 13 to 17)?" in *Teen Diets: Appetite for Destruction?* The Gallup Organization, Princeton, NJ, March 2003

---

and it works very hard to maintain that weight. The body adjusts itself to burn calories more slowly if weight is lost below that level and to burn them more quickly if weight is gained above that level.

For example, a 140-pound woman who has lost 10 pounds will burn about 10–15 percent fewer calories when she exercises than a woman who maintains that weight effortlessly. The same factors apply in the reverse scenario as well. If a woman has gained 10 pounds, her muscles during exercise will burn about 10–15 percent more calories to rid her body of the weight.

---

**FIGURE 9.5**

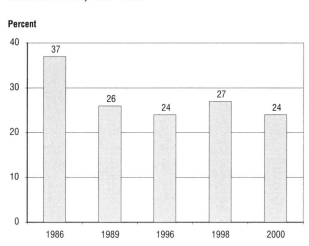

## Adults on a diet, 1986–2000

SOURCE: "Trends and Statistics: Adults on a Diet," *Calorie Control Council National Surveys,* Calorie Control Council, Atlanta, GA [Online] http://www.caloriecontrol.org/ dietfigs.html [accessed August 26, 2003]

---

**TABLE 9.6**

## Adults' weight-control practices by Body Mass Index, 2000

| Type of weight control practices | Body Mass Index | | | |
|---|---|---|---|---|
| | Total | Normal | Overweight | Obese |
| | *Percent* | | | |
| **Weight control practices** | | | | |
| Trying to lose weight | 38.5 | 20.7 | 45.0 | 65.7 |
| Trying to maintain weight | 35.9 | 43.6 | 34.9 | 20.8 |
| Neither | 25.6 | 35.7 | 20.1 | 13.5 |
| **Physical activity** | | | | |
| Inactive | 27.0 | 23.8 | 26.0 | 35.6 |
| Irregularly active | 28.2 | 27.8 | 28.7 | 28.1 |
| Regular not intense | 30.5 | 31.6 | 31.1 | 27.2 |
| Regular intense | 14.3 | 16.8 | 14.2 | 9.1 |
| **Fruit and vegetable intake, servings per day** | | | | |
| Less than 1 | 4.0 | 3.9 | 3.5 | 5.2 |
| 1 to less than 3 | 33.1 | 31.0 | 34.1 | 35.7 |
| 3 to less than 5 | 38.5 | 38.3 | 39.1 | 38.0 |
| 5 or more | 24.4 | 26.8 | 23.3 | 21.1 |
| **Professional advice on weight[1]** | | | | |
| Lose | 17.3 | 3.3 | 15.6 | 42.8 |
| Gain | 1.0 | 1.7 | 0.6 | 0.4 |
| Maintain | 2.7 | 3.2 | 2.8 | 1.9 |
| None | 79.0 | 91.8 | 81.0 | 54.9 |

[1] Questions were asked only to participants trying to lose or maintain weight; percentages are for persons who had a routine checkup in the previous 12 months.

SOURCE: "Obesity Trends: Percentage of United States Adults Who Use Specific Weight Control Practices by Body Mass Index," Centers for Disease Control and Prevention, National Center for Chronic Disease Prevention and Health Promotion, Atlanta, GA, 2002 [Online] http://www.cdc.gov/ nccdphp/dnpa/obesity/trend/prev_bmi.htm [accessed August 27, 2003]

---

This study challenged two myths about dieting. The first is that excessive dieting upsets the metabolism and makes it increasingly difficult to lose weight. Metabolism is controlled by the person's weight, not diet. The second

FIGURE 9.7

**Percentage of dieters who have tried various diets, 2000 and 2002**

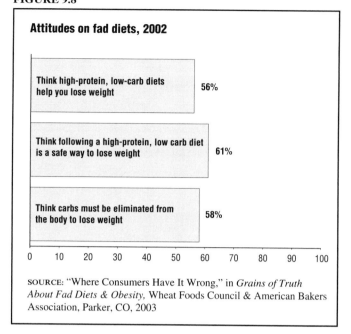

| | |
|---|---|
| Food Guide Pyramid diet | **45%** (41% in 2000) |
| Low-fat diet | **60%** (56% in 2000) |
| Doctor-recommended diet | **35%** (31% in 2000) |
| High-protein, low-carb diet | **35%** (30% in 2000) |
| Weight-loss organization diet | **27%** (25% in 2000) |
| Liquid diet/diet pills | **23%** (17% in 2000) |

☐ *2000* ■ *2002*

SOURCE: "Percentage of Dieters Who Have Tried a:" in *Grains of Truth About Fad Diets & Obesity,* Wheat Foods Council & American Bakers Association, Parker, CO, 2003

FIGURE 9.8

**Attitudes on fad diets, 2002**

| | |
|---|---|
| Think high-protein, low-carb diets help you lose weight | 56% |
| Think following a high-protein, low carb diet is a safe way to lose weight | 61% |
| Think carbs must be eliminated from the body to lose weight | 58% |

SOURCE: "Where Consumers Have It Wrong," in *Grains of Truth About Fad Diets & Obesity,* Wheat Foods Council & American Bakers Association, Parker, CO, 2003

myth is that obese people have slow metabolisms. The only people in the study who had sluggish metabolisms were those who were trying to maintain a body weight lower than their natural weight. Apparently, however, the body can be reset at a lower weight, as evidenced by those who are successful at weight loss. What that resetting process involves, however, is not yet understood.

## Weight Management versus Weight Loss

The National Academy of Sciences has studied weight-loss programs and concluded that program goals need to be changed from "weight loss" to "weight management." Individuals should aim to achieve the best weight possible for good health, not the lowest weight they think they should be. According to the federal guidelines to treat obesity, "The most successful strategies for weight loss include calorie reduction, increased physical activity, and behavior therapy designed to improve eating and physical activity habits" ("First Federal Obesity Clinical Guidelines Released," *NIH Press Release,* NIH, Washington, D.C., June 17, 1998).

## Characteristics of Successful Dieters

The National Weight Control Registry ([Online] http://www.lifespan.org/Services/Bmed/Wt_loss/NWCR/default.htm) has identified thousands of people who have lost weight and kept it off for long periods of time. The registry reveals a number of common characteristics among those who have succeeded in maintaining significant weight loss:

- Adherence to a low-calorie, low-fat diet.

- Participation in physical activities.

- Avoidance of diet fads, such as those that limit food intake to certain food groups.

## What to Eat?

A major problem with most weight-loss diets is that they are often unscientific and contradictory. Most diet plans are generally written by medical doctors with no formal nutrition training. In the 1970s carbohydrates were declared the cause of obesity, and high-fat, high-protein diets were promoted. Then fats were said to cause obesity, and high-fiber diets became the fad. Liquid diets were popular in the late 1980s. Then, when low fat, high-carbohydrate diets seemed to be the final answer, Americans were told that low-fat, high-carbohydrate foods such as pasta could make them fat. Finally, in the late 1990s, the high-fat, high protein, low-carbohydrate diet of the 1970s made a comeback.

Nutritionists warn against diets that limit the kinds of food a person can eat—diets, for example, that call for plenty of fats and very little or no carbohydrates. Such diets will likely throw off the body's metabolism. A metabolic disorder called ketosis occurs when, in the absence of carbohydrates, the body burns fats for energy. Compounds related to acetone, called ketones, accumulate in the blood and urine, causing symptoms including nausea, vomiting, bad breath, and lightheadedness. Left untreated, ketosis may lead to dehydration, confusion, or even death. The low-carbohydrate diets (notably the Atkins diet and Brownell's LEARN Program) are so popular that the NIH is conducting a one-year study to evaluate their safety and effectiveness.

## Fats Are Not Necessarily the Culprits in Obesity

It is believed that the return to a high-fat, high-protein, low carbohydrate diet is an indication of dieters' frustration that low-fat diets have not helped them lose weight. Some dieters think that if a product is labeled "fat-free" or "low-fat," it is all right to eat any quantity of it, regardless of the calories. Often, additional sugar is incorporated in the production of fat-free or low-fat food to make up for the loss of flavor due to the absence or low content of fat; this, in turn, increases the calorie count. Even if the lower-fat version may not have as many calories as the original product, people may consume more servings of it.

Experts agree that, in the long run, calories count in gaining or losing weight. An excess of calories means weight gain; reduction of calories means weight loss. They believe that the consumption of low-fat and fat-free foods loaded with extra sugars is responsible in part for the increasing weight gain among Americans.

## DIET DRUGS

In September 1997 the Food and Drug Administration (FDA) ordered the manufacturer of two diet drugs—fenfluramine, or Pondimin; and dexfenfluramine, commonly known as Redux—to take them off the market after they were linked to potentially fatal damage to the heart valves. Fenfluramine was often used in combination with phentermine, which increased the rate at which calories were burned; together the drugs were popularly called fen-phen. The FDA had approved the two drugs separately, and doctors could prescribe them in combination with each other.

In the mid-1990s some people considered fenfluramine and dexfenfluramine miracle appetite depressant pills to combat obesity. Researchers at the University of Rochester Medical School in New York who tested fen-phen reported that dieters who took the drugs lost an average of 16 percent of their body weight in 34 weeks, more than three times as much as the control group not taking the diet pills.

In 1996 doctors wrote 18 million prescriptions for Pondimin and Redux, usually in combination with phentermine. Weight-loss clinics mushroomed across the country, many doing business based on these "miracle pills." An estimated 2 million to 4 million people used the drugs. After the drugs were taken off the market, thousands of lawsuits were filed against the manufacturer. Under the terms of a settlement finalized in January 2002, American Home Products Corporation (now Wyeth, the distributor of Pondimin and Redux) agreed to compensate victims who claimed to have suffered heart valve disorders from taking the drug.

## Other Diet Pills

Despite the negative publicity attached to fen-phen, the quest for a pharmaceutical fix for overweight continues. In 2003 Congress took notice of the herbal dietary supplement ephedra after the FDA received more than 16,000 complaints blaming the substance for the onset of heart attacks, strokes, and at least 100 deaths. A 1994 federal law allows the makers of dietary supplements to place their products on the market without testing their safety, but prohibits them from making misleading or false statements about the products. Ephedra has been promoted as a diet pill, an energy booster, and an enhancer of memory and sexual and athletic performance. Two measures regarding ephedra were pending in Congress in late 2003. One measure (H.CON.RES.52) expressed "the sense of Congress that all major sports organizations should ban the use of ephedra and dietary supplements containing ephedrine." The other measure (HR 1075 IH) sought to amend the Federal Food, Drug, and Cosmetic Act with respect to dietary supplements containing natural or synthetic ephedrine group alkaloids.

In 2003 the three most prescribed weight-loss drugs on the market were phentermine, Meridia, and Xenical. Xenical, whose generic name is orlistat, was approved by the FDA in April 1999 for use by patients whose BMI is 30 (considered obese), as well as for those who are overweight and suffer from high blood pressure, high cholesterol, or diabetes. Xenical does not suppress the appetite like other diet drugs. Instead, it prevents fat absorption by blocking the enzymes that normally break fat down into smaller molecules. In a four-year study conducted at the University of Texas Health Science Center at San Antonio, it was found that obese patients who combined Xenical with lifestyle and dietary changes were less likely to contract type 2 diabetes than patients who only changed their diet.

The diet drug Meridia was introduced in 1998. Its target subjects are similar to Xenical's. Meridia blocks the absorption of serotonin (a brain chemical) into the cells, thus curbing a person's appetite. Denise Grady, in "Quest for Weight-Loss Drug Takes an Unusual Turn" (*The New York Times,* April 15, 2003), wrote that Xenical, Meridia, and phentermine were only "moderately useful" when it came to weight loss. Obese individuals taking Meridia, for example, lost no more than 10–14 pounds over a six-month period. "The human body seems to guard its fat stores jealously, and attempts to outsmart the system often fail outright or backfire, causing dangerous side effects," Grady observed.

Zonisamide, a drug used to treat epilepsy, is being studied for possible use as a diet drug. Its common side effect is significant weight loss.

## WEIGHT-LOSS SURGERY

Some individuals do not respond to dieting, drugs, or lifestyle changes. Those who are 100 pounds or more overweight, or who have a BMI of 40 or greater, are deemed to suffer from clinically severe obesity. An increasing number of such individuals are turning to weight-loss (bariatric) surgery. According to the NIH, an estimated 40,000 bariatric surgical procedures were carried out in the United States in 2001, and an estimated 86,000 procedures were projected for 2002.

While surgery may produce complications or even death, a candidate for bariatric surgery may face a greater risk of death from not having the surgery because of the life-threatening conditions that often accompany severe obesity. The two most common types of bariatric surgery are vertical banded gastroplasty (a reversible procedure) and gastric bypass (an irreversible procedure). Both procedures involve isolating a small pouch of stomach with staples, which creates a smaller stomach that limits food intake.

Because of the growing number of cases of adolescent obesity, several children's hospitals have launched adolescent bariatric programs. Pediatric experts have proposed guidelines for the surgery, which are summarized in an article in *Medical Devices & Surgical Technology Week* (August 31, 2003). The teen candidate should have obesity-caused problems and weigh at least 30 pounds more than adult candidates for the surgery. It is recommended that the operation not be performed until the teen has nearly reached full height potential. A panel of experts should be convened at hospitals performing the surgery to evaluate a candidate's physical and psychological health.

## EATING DISORDERS

### Anorexia Nervosa

Many persons with a weight problem struggle to lose weight and control their overeating. However, some (mainly females, but also some males) are obsessed with the fear of gaining weight, and literally starve themselves. This condition, known as anorexia nervosa, often begins with a desire to take off a few pounds, and then, experts believe, becomes an obsession that rules the dieter's life.

Anorexia nervosa results in severe weight loss—to at least 15 percent below normal body weight. Anorexics become terrified of gaining weight, and continue to believe they are overweight even though they may be extremely thin. They experience depression and weakness, their nails and hair become brittle, and their skin dries. The medical complications of anorexia are similar to those of starvation. While the body attempts to protect its most vital organs, the heart and brain, it goes into "slow gear." Monthly menstruation stops in women, and breathing, pulse, and thyroid functions slow down. Anemia, swelling joints, and osteoporosis can result. Eventually, low blood pressure and an irregular heartbeat may lead to cardiac arrest.

Middle-class, white, teenage girls who strive for perfection, who think they are not "good enough," and who feel controlled by others (parents or peers) are most vulnerable to becoming anorexic. Women whose careers depend on their size—dancers, models, performers, gymnasts—are also at risk for anorexia. Anorexia peaks at age 14 or 15 and again at 18, significant times of stress among young American women. The National Institute of Mental Health (NIMH) reports that between 0.5 and 3.7 percent of women suffer from anorexia nervosa at some time in their lives, and approximately 0.56 percent of people with anorexia die each year, a death rate about 12 times higher than the annual death rate due to all causes of death among females ages 15–24 in the general population.

### Bulimia Nervosa

Also called binge-purge syndrome, bulimia nervosa sometimes, but not always, accompanies anorexia. A bulimic eats compulsively, ingesting huge amounts of high-calorie, high-fat food. Then, disgusted with this behavior, he or she purges through forced vomiting and/or abuse of laxatives.

Many bulimics have normal body weights or are overweight because of the large amounts of food they eat. Unlike persons with binge eating disorders, bulimics purge, fast, or perform vigorous exercises after episodes of binge eating. Bulimics who maintain normal weights can keep their eating disorders a secret for years. The binge-purge cycle can, however, result in heart failure because the body loses vital minerals. The acid in vomit can erode the teeth, glands in the neck can become swollen, and the esophagus can become chronically inflamed.

Some bulimics are addicted to certain foods in the same way alcoholics are addicted to liquor. Many are severely depressed and suicidal. Not all bulimics, however, have psychiatric illnesses. Some bulimic behavior is a "fad," especially on college campuses where overeating and purging are sometimes a part of dorm life. Bulimia peaks in young women between ages 18 and 26. The NIMH estimates that 1.1–4.2 percent of women have bulimia nervosa at some time in their lives.

The NIMH notes that anorexia and bulimia exist primarily in industrialized, economically advanced countries and that they are much less common among black women. These disorders are almost unheard of in developing or third-world countries. "Thinness," it seems, is not highly prized by people whose hunger is not a matter of choice.

### Binge Eating Disorder

Binge eating disorder is a condition that between 2 and 5 million Americans experience in any six-month period.

It is probably the most common eating disorder. A person with a binge eating disorder frequently eats an abnormally large quantity of food while feeling a loss of control over his or her eating.

Binge eating disorder is common among the obese. Obese persons with the disorder are very likely to have been overweight at younger ages than those without the disorder. They are also more likely to engage in frequent episodes of losing and regaining weight (yo-yo dieting), while also being at risk for the same health problems and diseases that accompany obesity. The disorder is slightly more common in women—three women are affected for every two men. Both whites and blacks are affected by this disorder, although the frequency of occurrence in other ethnic groups is unknown.

## EXERCISE

### The Exercise-Diet Approach

Some experts no longer recommend dieting for weight loss, but instead focus on achieving physical health through exercise. They encourage an appreciation of good food combined with regular exercise.

### How Much Exercise Do Americans Need?

Everyone agrees that exercise helps promote good health and weight control. Nonetheless, fitness experts differ as to how much exercise is needed. The CDC recommends a minimum cumulative 30 minutes of moderate exercise over the course 5 or more days of the week to achieve some of the health benefits of exercise. A person could accomplish this by walking for 10 minutes in the morning, gardening in the afternoon, and taking another 10-minute walk after dinner. To achieve even more health benefits, the CDC recommends vigorous-intensity physical activity for 20 minutes or more on 3 or more days of the week. For children and teens, the U.S. Department of Health and Human Services recommends 60 minutes of moderate exercise on most days of the week.

The NIH reports that physical inactivity is a risk factor for heart diseases. Studies have shown that inactive persons are twice as likely to develop heart disease as those who are more active. Even persons who have had heart attacks can improve their chances of survival if they start exercising.

Steven Blair, director of epidemiology and clinical applications at the Cooper Institute for Aerobics Reseach in Dallas, Texas, found that men who went from being moderately fit to being highly fit showed a 15 percent decline in mortality. Moreover, when men went from being unfit to moderately fit, there were even greater benefits—a 40 percent decline in deaths from all causes.

Experts stress the importance of exercise for everyone, including the elderly. Physical activity results in reduced risk of heart disease, disability, and death. Studies show that it is never too late to start exercising. Senior citizens who take up weight lifting build their strength, improve their balance, and strengthen their bones, decreasing their risk for osteoporosis. The American College of Sports Medicine suggests that senior citizens engage in aerobic activities for 20 minutes 3–5 times a week.

### What Kind of Exercise Is the Best?

While lightweight activities will help anyone to achieve some health benefits, many experts advocate an exercise routine that incorporates vigorous physical activities (aerobics). Dr. Kenneth H. Cooper, the head of the Cooper Institute for Aerobics Research, was the first to promote endurance-type exercise, coining the word "aerobics" in 1968 (from "aerobic," meaning "living in air" or "utilizing oxygen"). Examples of aerobic activities are walking, running, biking, and swimming. Experts also recommend adding flexibility and strength training to an exercise routine. The bottom line, say many experts, is that the best exercise includes activities that the participant enjoys and will return to again and again.

LIFESTYLE VERSUS STRUCTURED INTERVENTIONS. Andrea L. Dunn et al. noted that, although a strong link between physical inactivity and ill health has been established, about 60 percent of the U.S. population remains inadequately active or completely inactive. In "Comparison of Lifestyle and Structured Interventions to Increase Physical Activity and Cardiorespiratory Fitness: A Randomized Trial" (*The Journal of the American Medical Association,* vol. 281, no. 4, January 27, 1999), researchers recognized that many Americans do not exercise for various reasons. These include lack of time, lack of social support, bad weather, lack of access to fitness centers, disruptions of daily routine, and dislike for strenuous physical activity.

With the help of the Cooper Institute Institutional Review Board in Dallas, Texas, researchers compared the effects on sedentary adults of improving physical activity and cardiorespiratory fitness, using two intervention programs—a physical activity program geared toward a person's lifestyle, and a traditional fitness-center program. Participants in the lifestyle group were advised to perform at least 30 minutes of moderate-intensive physical activity on most or all days of the week in a manner suited to their lifestyle. During regular meetings, they learned cognitive and behavioral strategies to maintain their physical activity. Group meetings involved mall walking, volleyball, and other activities to reinforce their cognitive and behavioral skills. The study showed that at 24 months, participants of both the lifestyle group and the fitness center–based intervention improved their physical activity, cardiorespiratory fitness, and blood pressure, and achieved positive changes to their percentage of body fat.

FIGURE 9.9

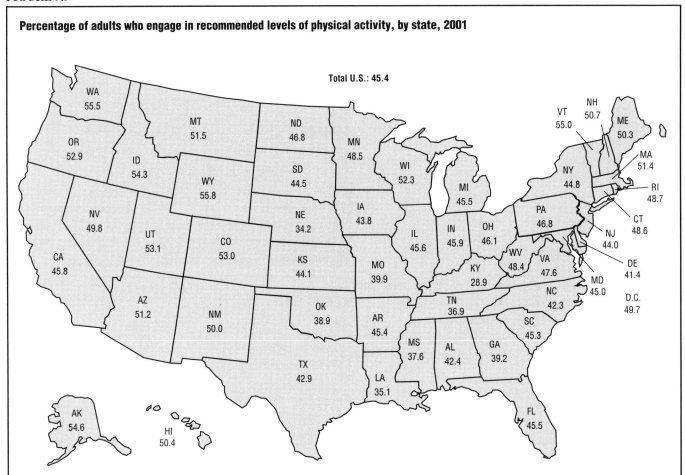

**Percentage of adults who engage in recommended levels of physical activity, by state, 2001**

Total U.S.: 45.4

Note: Respondents reported moderate-intensity activities (i.e., brisk walking, bicycling, vacuuming, gardening, or anything else that causes small increases in breathing or heart rate) for ≥ 30 minutes per day ≥ 5 days per week or vigorous-intensity activities (i.e., running, aerobics, heavy yard work, or anything else that causes large increases in breathing or heart rate) for ≥ 20 minutes per day, ≥ 3 days per week.

SOURCE: Adapted from "Table 2. Age-adjusted percentage of respondents aged ≥ 18 years who engaged in activities consistent with physical activity recommendations, by state/area—Behavioral Risk Factor Surveillance System (BRFSS), United States, 2000 and 2001," in *Morbidity and Mortality Weekly Report*, vol. 52, no. 32, August 15, 2003

## How Much Do Americans Exercise?

The CDC, in its *Morbidity and Mortality Weekly Report* (August 2003), found that most adults are not getting enough physical activity to promote health. In 2001 only 45.4 percent engaged in activities consistent with the CDC's physical activity recommendations. On a state-by-state basis, the percentage of adults who engaged in activities consistent with the CDC's recommendations ranged from a low of 28.9 percent (Kentucky) to a high of 55.8 percent (Wyoming). (See Figure 9.9.)

The CDC also studied physical activity among children. Its survey of children and their parents revealed that the majority (61.5 percent) of children ages 9–13 do not participate in any organized physical activity during their non-school hours, and more than one-fifth (22.6 percent) do not engage in any free-time physical activity. (See Table 9.7.)

**THE SURGEON GENERAL'S REPORT.** In 1996 the Surgeon General reported in *Physical Activity and Health* (CDC and the President's Council on Physical Fitness and Sports, Washington, DC) that only about 15 percent of adults participated in regular vigorous physical activity (defined as 3 times a week for at least 20 minutes). Approximately 22 percent of adults engaged in any level of physical activity for a sustained period of time (5 times a week for at least 30 minutes). About 25 percent did no physical exercise at all.

Inactivity was more prevalent among women than men, among blacks and Hispanics than whites, among older than younger adults, and among the less wealthy than the more wealthy. The most popular activities were walking and gardening, or yard work.

About half of young people ages 12–21 participated in regular vigorous activity; one-fourth were not active at all. Inactivity was more likely in young females than in young

**TABLE 9.7**

**Children's participation in organized and leisure-time activity, 2002**

(Percent)

| Characteristics | Participated in organized physical activity during preceding 7 days | Participated in free-time physical activity during preceding 7 days |
|---|---|---|
| **Sex** | | |
| Female | 38.6 | 74.1 |
| Male | 38.3 | 80.5 |
| **Age (years)** | | |
| 9 | 36.1 | 75.8 |
| 10 | 37.5 | 77.0 |
| 11 | 43.1 | 78.9 |
| 12 | 37.7 | 77.5 |
| 13 | 38.1 | 78.0 |
| **Race/ethnicity** | | |
| Black, non-Hispanic | 24.1 | 74.7 |
| Hispanic | 25.9 | 74.6 |
| White, non-Hispanic | 46.6 | 79.3 |
| **Parental education** | | |
| < High school | 19.4 | 75.3 |
| High school | 28.3 | 75.4 |
| > High school | 46.8 | 78.7 |
| **Parental income** | | |
| ≤ $25,000 | 23.5 | 74.1 |
| $25,001–$50,000 | 32.8 | 78.6 |
| > $50,000 | 49.1 | 78.3 |
| **Total** | **38.5** | **77.4** |

SOURCE: "Table 1. Percentage of children aged 9–13 years who reported participation in organized and free-time physical activity during the preceding 7 days, by selected characteristics—Youth Media Campaign Longitudinal Survey, United States, 2002," in *Morbidity and Mortality Weekly Report,* vol. 52, no. 33, August 22, 2003

males and in black young females than in white young females. Physical activity declined sharply as the school grade increased. Only 19 percent of high school students reported being physically active for 20 minutes or more in daily physical education classes.

# CHAPTER 10
# HUNGER AND PUBLIC ASSISTANCE PROGRAMS

In the early 1800s Thomas Robert Malthus, a British economist and mathematician, developed the theory that the food supply grows arithmetically, increasing by two, four, six, eight, ten, etc., but that population grows geometrically—two, four, eight, sixteen, thirty-two, etc. Based on this theory, Malthus believed the world would eventually run out of food, and people would face starvation and death.

Malthus could not have imagined the spectacular developments in the science of growing and preserving food. With modern technology, farmers have been able to produce more food per acre than ever before. Two hundred years ago fresh food could not be moved from one region to another without spoiling because there was no refrigeration and transportation was very slow. Today food can be shipped around the world and eaten almost as fresh as it was when first picked, caught, or prepared.

Medical knowledge and technology, however, are keeping people alive longer and longer, and this achievement, combined with the fact that the population of developing countries continues to increase, means that some observers again fear that food supplies will not be enough to feed everyone in the world.

Most Americans are well fed. In 1998 the U.S. Department of Agriculture (USDA) set the daily Recommended Energy Allowance for the United States at 2,247 calories (Judy Putnam et al., " U.S. Per Capita Food Supply Trends: More Calories, Refined Carbohydrates, and Fats," *FoodReview,* vol. 25, issue 3, Winter 2002). A person who consumes fewer than 2,100 calories per day is considered "hungry." The average American consumed just under 2,700 calories per day in 2000, a 24.5 percent increase (530 calories) since 1970, according to the USDA's *Agriculture Fact Book 2001–2002.* In terms of caloric intake, then, most Americans are well fed.

The Food and Agriculture Organization (FAO) of the United Nations uses a minimum requirement of about 1,800 calories on average per capita per day to define adequate nutrition. By that measure, the FAO used 1998–2000 data to calculate that 840 million people worldwide were malnourished.

## IS THERE HUNGER IN AMERICA?

### Hunger and Food Insecurity

Although the United States is one of the richest countries in the world, some Americans are still poor and hungry. According to the USDA, "'Hunger' is the uneasy or painful sensation caused by a lack of food. It can result from the recurrent and involuntary lack of access to food. 'Severe hunger' exists in households when children go hungry or adults experience prolonged or acute hunger. 'Food insecurity' is used to describe inadequate access to enough food at all times for a healthy, active life. It can be a warning sign for hunger."

The latest USDA survey of hunger and food insecurity, conducted in 2001, found that 89.3 percent of American households were food-secure, a 1.25 percent increase from 1998. (See Table 10.1.) Nevertheless, this signifies a decrease in food-secure households from 1999. About 10.7 percent of all U.S. households reported experiencing food insecurity in 2001, a 9.3 percent decrease from 1998.

### Characteristics of Low-Income, Food-Insecure Households

Approximately 32.3 percent of low-income U.S. households (those with incomes below 130 percent of the poverty level) reported being food-insecure in 2001, the same percentage as in 1999. (See Table 10.2.) Different kinds of households experienced hunger at different rates. About 11 percent of all households reported experiencing hunger in 2001; this figure was highest for female-head, no-spouse households (13.2 percent) and for men

TABLE 10.1

**Prevalence of food security, food insecurity, and hunger for households and persons, by year, 1998–2001**

| Unit | Total[1] | Food secure | | Food insecure | | | | | |
|---|---|---|---|---|---|---|---|---|---|
| | | | | All | | Without hunger | | With hunger | |
| | 1,000 | 1,000 | Percent | 1,000 | Percent | 1,000 | Percent | 1,000 | Percent |
| **Households** | | | | | | | | | |
| 1998 | 103,309 | 91,121 | 88.2 | 12,188 | 11.8 | 8,353 | 8.1 | 3,835 | 3.7 |
| 1999 | 104,684 | 94,154 | 89.9 | 10,529 | 10.1 | 7,420 | 7.1 | 3,109 | 3.0 |
| 2000 | 106,043 | 94,942 | 89.5 | 11,101 | 10.5 | 7,786 | 7.3 | 3,315 | 3.1 |
| 2001 | 107,824 | 96,303 | 89.3 | 11,521 | 10.7 | 8,010 | 7.4 | 3,511 | 3.3 |
| **All individuals (by food security status of household)[2]** | | | | | | | | | |
| 1998 | 268,366 | 232,219 | 86.5 | 36,147 | 13.5 | 26,290 | 9.8 | 9,857 | 3.7 |
| 1999 | 270,318 | 239,304 | 88.5 | 31,015 | 11.5 | 23,237 | 8.6 | 7,779 | 2.9 |
| 2000 | 273,685 | 240,454 | 87.9 | 33,231 | 12.1 | 24,708 | 9.0 | 8,523 | 3.1 |
| 2001 | 276,661 | 243,019 | 87.8 | 33,642 | 12.2 | 24,628 | 8.9 | 9,014 | 3.3 |
| **Adults (by food security status of household)[2]** | | | | | | | | | |
| 1998 | 197,084 | 174,964 | 88.8 | 22,120 | 11.2 | 15,632 | 7.9 | 6,488 | 3.3 |
| 1999 | 198,900 | 179,960 | 90.5 | 18,941 | 9.5 | 13,869 | 7.0 | 5,072 | 2.5 |
| 2000 | 201,922 | 181,586 | 89.9 | 20,336 | 10.1 | 14,763 | 7.3 | 5,573 | 2.8 |
| 2001 | 204,340 | 183,398 | 89.8 | 20,942 | 10.2 | 14,879 | 7.3 | 6,063 | 3.0 |

| Unit | Total[1] | Food secure | | Food insecure | | | | | |
|---|---|---|---|---|---|---|---|---|---|
| | | | | All | | Without hunger among children | | With hunger among children | |
| | 1,000 | 1,000 | Percent | 1,000 | Percent | 1,000 | Percent | 1,000 | Percent |
| **Households with children** | | | | | | | | | |
| 1998 | 38,036 | 31,335 | 82.4 | 6,701 | 17.6 | 6,370 | 16.7 | 331 | .9 |
| 1999 | 37,884 | 32,290 | 85.2 | 5,594 | 14.8 | 5,375 | 14.2 | 219 | .6 |
| 2000 | 38,113 | 31,942 | 83.8 | 6,171 | 16.2 | 5,916 | 15.5 | 255 | .7 |
| 2001 | 38,330 | 32,141 | 83.9 | 6,189 | 16.1 | 5,978 | 15.6 | 211 | .6 |
| **Children (by food security status of household)[2]** | | | | | | | | | |
| 1998 | 71,282 | 57,255 | 80.3 | 14,027 | 19.7 | 13,311 | 18.7 | 716 | 1.0 |
| 1999 | 71,418 | 59,344 | 83.1 | 12,074 | 16.9 | 11,563 | 16.2 | 511 | .7 |
| 2000 | 71,763 | 58,867 | 82.0 | 12,896 | 18.0 | 12,334 | 17.2 | 562 | .8 |
| 2001 | 72,321 | 59,620 | 82.4 | 12,701 | 17.6 | 12,234 | 16.9 | 467 | .6 |

[1] Totals exclude households whose food security status is unknown because they did not give a valid response to any of the questions in the food security scale. In 2001, these represented 353,000 households (0.3 percent of all households).

[2] The food security survey measures food security status at the household level. Not all individuals residing in food-insecure households are appropriately characterized as food insecure. Similarly, not all individuals in households classified as food insecure with hunger nor all children in households classified as food insecure with hunger among children were subject to reductions in food intake or experienced resource-constrained hunger.

SOURCE: Mark Nord, Margaret Andrews, and Steven Carlson, "Table 1—Prevalence of food security, food insecurity, and hunger by year," in *Measuring Food Security in the United States: Household Food Security in the United States, 2001,* Food Assistance and Nutrition Research Report Number 29, U.S. Department of Agriculture, Economic Research Service, Washington, DC, October 2002

living alone (14.2 percent). Black low-income households were more likely to experience hunger (13.3 percent) than Hispanic (10.2 percent) or white (10.3 percent) households.

## FEDERAL PROGRAMS THAT FEED THE HUNGRY

Food-assistance programs were begun during the Great Depression to help feed the poor and unemployed and to keep farm prices stable by giving the surplus to people who needed it. Surpluses occur when some of the agricultural product is not sold on the open market. Established in 1969, the USDA's Food and Nutrition Service (FNS) administers the nation's current food-assistance programs. The agency's goals are to provide needy people with access to a more nutritious diet, to improve the eating habits of the nation's children, and to help farmers by stabilizing farm prices through the purchase and distribution of surplus foods.

The FNS works in partnership with the states in all of its programs. States determine most administrative details regarding distribution of food benefits and eligibility of participants, while the FNS provides funding to cover most of the states' administrative costs. According to the U.S. Census Bureau's *Statistical Abstract of the United States* (December 2002), in fiscal year (FY) 2000 the federal government spent $32.1 billion in food-assistance programs.

In general, food-assistance expenditures follow macroeconomic conditions: when unemployment is high, food-assistance expenditures (such as those for food stamps) are relatively high, and vice versa. (See Figure 10.1.)

**TABLE 10.2**

## Prevalence of food security, food insecurity, and hunger in households with income below 130 percent of the poverty line, 2001

| Category | Total[1] | Food secure | | Food insecure | | | | | |
| | | | | All | | Without hunger | | With hunger | |
| | 1,000 | 1,000 | Percent | 1,000 | Percent | 1,000 | Percent | 1,000 | Percent |
|---|---|---|---|---|---|---|---|---|---|
| **All low-income households** | 16,904 | 11,450 | 67.7 | 5,454 | 32.3 | 3,609 | 21.3 | 1,845 | 10.9 |
| **Household composition** | | | | | | | | | |
| With children < 18 | 7,608 | 4,462 | 58.6 | 3,146 | 41.4 | 2,273 | 29.9 | 873 | 11.5 |
| With children < 6 | 4,037 | 2,422 | 60.0 | 1,615 | 40.0 | 1,235 | 30.6 | 380 | 9.4 |
| Married couple families | 3,080 | 1,879 | 61.0 | 1,201 | 39.0 | 901 | 29.3 | 300 | 9.7 |
| Female head, no spouse | 3,806 | 2,075 | 54.5 | 1,731 | 45.5 | 1,227 | 32.2 | 504 | 13.2 |
| Male head, no spouse | 523 | 367 | 70.2 | 156 | 29.8 | 109 | 20.8 | 47 | 9.0 |
| Other household with child[2] | 199 | 141 | 70.9 | 58 | 29.1 | 35 | 17.6 | 23 | 11.6 |
| With no children < 18 | 9,296 | 6,988 | 75.2 | 2,308 | 24.8 | 1,336 | 14.4 | 972 | 10.5 |
| More than one adult | 3,888 | 3,046 | 78.3 | 842 | 21.7 | 507 | 13.0 | 335 | 8.6 |
| Women living alone | 3,475 | 2,594 | 74.6 | 881 | 25.4 | 518 | 14.9 | 363 | 10.4 |
| Men living alone | 1,933 | 1,347 | 69.7 | 586 | 30.3 | 312 | 16.1 | 274 | 14.2 |
| With elderly | 4,223 | 3,454 | 81.8 | 769 | 18.2 | 557 | 13.2 | 212 | 5.0 |
| Elderly living alone | 2,206 | 1,822 | 82.6 | 384 | 17.4 | 264 | 12.0 | 120 | 5.4 |
| **Race/ethnicity of households** | | | | | | | | | |
| White non-Hispanic | 9,116 | 6,600 | 72.4 | 2,516 | 27.6 | 1,581 | 17.3 | 935 | 10.3 |
| Black non-Hispanic | 3,750 | 2,226 | 59.4 | 1,524 | 40.6 | 1,026 | 27.4 | 498 | 13.3 |
| Hispanic[3] | 3,214 | 2,031 | 63.2 | 1,183 | 36.8 | 856 | 26.6 | 327 | 10.2 |
| Other non-Hispanic | 825 | 594 | 72.0 | 231 | 28.0 | 146 | 17.7 | 85 | 10.3 |
| **Area of residence** | | | | | | | | | |
| Inside metropolitan area | 12,644 | 8,519 | 67.4 | 4,125 | 32.6 | 2,705 | 21.4 | 1,420 | 11.2 |
| In central city[4] | 5,413 | 3,572 | 66.0 | 1,841 | 34.0 | 1,174 | 21.7 | 667 | 12.3 |
| Not in central city | 4,548 | 3,102 | 68.2 | 1,446 | 31.8 | 953 | 21.0 | 493 | 10.8 |
| Outside metropolitan area | 4,260 | 2,931 | 68.8 | 1,329 | 31.2 | 904 | 21.2 | 425 | 10.0 |
| **Census geographic region** | | | | | | | | | |
| Northeast | 2,605 | 1,876 | 72.0 | 729 | 28.0 | 494 | 19.0 | 235 | 9.0 |
| Midwest | 3,519 | 2,476 | 70.4 | 1,043 | 29.6 | 658 | 18.7 | 385 | 10.9 |
| South | 6,909 | 4,556 | 65.9 | 2,353 | 34.1 | 1,580 | 22.9 | 773 | 11.2 |
| West | 3,871 | 2,541 | 65.6 | 1,330 | 34.4 | 877 | 22.7 | 453 | 11.7 |
| **Individuals in low-income households (by food security status of household)** | | | | | | | | | |
| All individuals in low-income households | 45,941 | 29,405 | 64.0 | 16,536 | 36.0 | 11,508 | 25.0 | 5,028 | 10.9 |
| Adults in low-income households | 29,577 | 20,042 | 67.8 | 9,535 | 32.2 | 6,391 | 21.6 | 3,144 | 10.6 |
| Children in low-income households | 16,364 | 9,363 | 57.2 | 7,001 | 42.8 | 5,117 | 31.3 | 1,884 | 11.5 |

[1] Totals exclude households whose income was not reported (about 17 percent of households), and those whose food security status is unknown because they did not give a valid response to any of the questions in the food security scale (0.7 percent of low-income households).

[2] Households with children in complex living arrangements, e.g., children of other relatives or unrelated roommate or boarder.

[3] Hispanics may be of any race.

[4] Metropolitan area subtotals do not add to metropolitan area totals because central-city residence is not identified for about 17 percent of households in metropolitan statistical areas.

SOURCE: Mark Nord, Margaret Andrews, and Steven Carlson, "Table 4—Prevalence of food security, food insecurity, and hunger in households with income below 130 percent of the poverty line by selected household characteristics, 2001," in *Measuring Food Security in the United States: Household Food Security in the United States, 2001,* Food Assistance and Nutrition Research Report Number 29, U.S. Department of Agriculture, Economic Research Service, Washington, DC, October 2002

## Food Stamp Program

The Food Stamp Program, the largest of the federal food-assistance programs, began as a pilot program in 1961. Congress established it as a permanent program through the Food Stamp Act of 1964 (PL 88-525). It is designed to increase the food-purchasing ability of low-income families to the point where they can afford nutritionally adequate low-cost diets. Paper coupons or electronic benefits transfers are used in place of money in food stores all over the country. Food stamps can only be used for foods to prepare at home and not for tobacco, alcohol, lunch-counter items, or foods to be eaten in the store. Data from the U.S. Department of Agriculture indicate that 54 percent of all food-assistance expenditures ($20.6 billion) supported the Food Stamp Program. Figure 10.2 shows the trend in USDA spending on all food-assistance programs, compared with that of the Food Stamp Program, from 1970 to 2002.

In order to be eligible for food stamps, individuals must meet income guidelines and certain work requirements. Benefits are based on household size, income, and certain non-food expenses (including housing costs, dependent-care expenses, and child-support payments) and are adjusted annually for inflation. Generally, the monthly income of the household must be at or below 130 percent of the federal poverty guidelines. In FY 2001 monthly

FIGURE 10.1

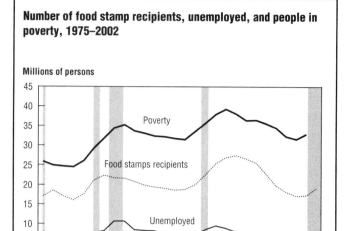

**Number of food stamp recipients, unemployed, and people in poverty, 1975–2002**

Note: Gray bars indicate recessions.

SOURCE: "Number of food stamp recipients, unemployed, and people in poverty, 1975–2002," in *The Food Assistance Landscape,* Food Assistance and Nutrition Research Report Number 28-2, U.S. Department of Agriculture, Economic Research Service, Washington, DC, March 2003

FIGURE 10.2

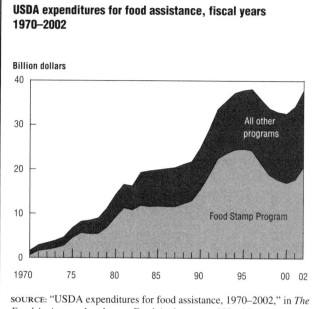

**USDA expenditures for food assistance, fiscal years 1970–2002**

SOURCE: "USDA expenditures for food assistance, 1970–2002," in *The Food Assistance Landscape,* Food Assistance and Nutrition Research Report Number 28-2, U.S. Department of Agriculture, Economic Research Service, Washington, DC, March 2003

**TABLE 10.3**

**Federal nutrition assistance at-a-glance, 2001–02**

| Program | | Fiscal year 2001 | Fiscal year 2002 | Change |
|---|---|---|---|---|
| Food stamp program | Average monthly participation (thousands) | 17,313 | 19,110 | 10.4% |
| | Average monthly benefit per person (dollars) | 74.83 | 79.55 | 6.3% |
| | Total annual expenditures (billions) | 17.8 | 20.6 | 15.5% |
| WIC | Average monthly participation (thousands) | 7,306 | 7,489 | 2.5% |
| | Total annual expenditures (billions) | 4.1 | 4.3 | 4.6% |
| National School Lunch Program | Average daily participation (thousands) | 27,506 | 27,909 | 1.5% |
| | Total annual expenditures (billions) | 6.5 | 6.8 | 5.3% |
| School Breakfast Program | Average daily participation (thousands) | 7,787 | 8,125 | 4.3% |
| | Total annual expenditures (billions) | 1.5 | 1.6 | 7.7% |
| Child and Adult care Food Program | Meals served in: | | | |
| | • child care centers (millions) | 923 | 987 | 6.8% |
| | • family day care homes (millions) | 717 | 709 | -1.1% |
| | • adult day care centers (millions) | 40 | 44 | 9.7% |
| | Total annual expenditures (billions) | 1.7 | 1.9 | 6.5% |
| Total program expenditures | Dollars (billions) | 34.2 | 37.8 | 10.6% |

Note: the figures are based on preliminary data provided by the Food and Nutrition Service as of November 2002 and are subject to change. Total program expenditures include figures from other programs not shown in table.

SOURCE: "Federal Nutrition Assistance At-A-Glance," in *The Food Assistance Landscape,* Food Assistance and Nutrition Research Report Number 28-2, U.S. Department of Agriculture, Economic Research Service, Washington, DC, March 2003

benefits averaged $75 per person. (See Table 10.3.) In FY 2002 the average monthly benefit per person grew to about $80. According to *Food Assistance Landscape,* the per person increase in benefits between FY 2001 and 2002 (6.3 percent) was the largest increase in these benefits since 1991 ("Food Stamp Program Expands," Economic Research Service, USDA, Washington, D.C., March 2003).

After an all-time peak monthly participation of 28 million people in the spring of 1994, Food Stamp Program participation declined steadily, due in part to the changes brought about by the 1996 Personal Responsibility and Work Opportunity Reconciliation Act (PL 104-193), a welfare reform law that eliminated benefits to most legal immigrants and able-bodied adults with no dependents. (In 1998 the Agricultural Research, Extension, and Education Reform Act [PL 105-185] restored food stamp benefits to legal immigrants who were receiving benefits or assistance for blindness or disability, who were younger than 18, or who were 65 or older as of August 22, 1996). The continuing strong economy and the accompanying decrease in unemployment also contributed to the decline. Participation rose again in 2001 and 2002, possibly because of high unemployment rates and a weaker economy. In fact, there was a 10.4 percent increase in participation from FY 2001 to FY 2002, when more than 19 million people participated in the program.

**PARTICIPATION IN THE FOOD STAMP PROGRAM.** In FY 2002 total federal expenditures on the Food Stamp Program were $20.6 billion. According to *Characteristics of Food Stamp Households: Fiscal Year 2002* (Advance

FIGURE 10.3

**Distribution of food stamp participants, 2002**

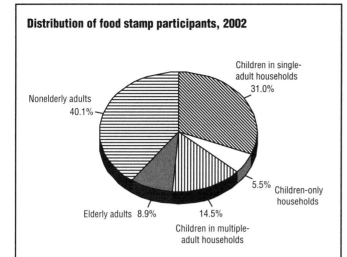

SOURCE: "Figure 2: Distribution of Food Stamp Participants, 2002," in *Characteristics of Food Stamp Households: Fiscal Year 2002 (Advance Report)*, U.S. Department of Agriculture, Food and Nutrition Service, Office of Analysis, Nutrition, and Evaluation, Washington, DC, July 2003

FIGURE 10.4

**Electronic Benefit Transfer issuances as percent of total food stamp program issuance, 1991–2003**

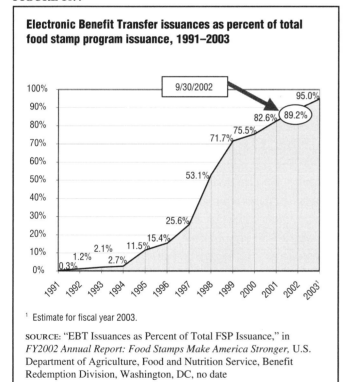

[1] Estimate for fiscal year 2003.

SOURCE: "EBT Issuances as Percent of Total FSP Issuance," in *FY2002 Annual Report: Food Stamps Make America Stronger*, U.S. Department of Agriculture, Food and Nutrition Service, Benefit Redemption Division, Washington, DC, no date

TABLE 10.4

**Race/ethnicity of food stamp participants, 2002**

| Race | Participants | |
| --- | --- | --- |
| | Number (thousands) | Percent |
| Total | 19,044 | 100.0 |
| White, non-Hispanic | 7,931 | 41.6 |
| African-American, non-Hispanic | 6,651 | 34.9 |
| Hispanic | 3,465 | 18.2 |
| Asian | 536 | 2.8 |
| Native American | 303 | 1.6 |
| Other | 159 | 0.8 |

SOURCE: "Table 6—Race/Ethnicity of Food Stamp Participants, 2002," in *Characteristics of Food Stamp Households: Fiscal Year 2002 (Advance Report)*, U.S. Department of Agriculture, Food and Nutrition Service, Office of Analysis, Nutrition, and Evaluation, Washington, DC, July 2003

**ELECTRONIC BENEFITS TRANSFER (EBT).** In the past, food stamp participants received their monthly benefits in the form of paper coupons to redeem for foods at authorized food stores. In an effort to eliminate illegal trafficking in food stamps, the government introduced electronic benefits transfers (EBTs), which operate like a bank card. When food purchases are made, the store uses the card to debit the recipient's food stamp account. As of September 30, 2002, 89.2 percent of food stamp benefits were delivered using EBTs. (See Figure 10.4.) That percentage was expected to increase to 95 percent for FY 2003.

## Child Nutrition Programs

The USDA operates four programs to provide meals and snacks to preschool- and school-age children. In FY 2001 expenditures for three of these programs—the National School Lunch Program, the School Breakfast Program, and the Child and Adult Care Food Program—amounted to $9.7 billion. During FY 2002 federal spending increased for each of these programs. The highest increase in spending was for the School Breakfast Program (7.7 percent), followed by the Child and Adult Care Food Program (6.5 percent) and the National School Lunch Program (5.3 percent). This is a continuation of the trend of steady increases in program costs.

**NATIONAL SCHOOL LUNCH PROGRAM.** The National School Lunch Program provides lunch to children in public and non-profit private schools and in residential child care institutions. The USDA provides cash and some commodities to these schools to offset food-service costs. In return, the schools must serve lunches that meet federal nutritional requirements. The program is available to virtually every child, and low-income students may qualify to receive their lunches free or at a reduced price.

The cost of the National School Lunch Program has been rising steadily for many years. It has the

Report, USDA, July 2003), half (51 percent) of food stamp recipients were children, 40 percent were non-elderly adults, and 9 percent were elderly. (See Figure 10.3.) Of the total recipients in 2002, whites (non-Hispanic) comprised 42 percent; African Americans (non-Hispanic), 35 percent; and Hispanics (of any race), 18 percent. (See Table 10.4.)

FIGURE 10.5

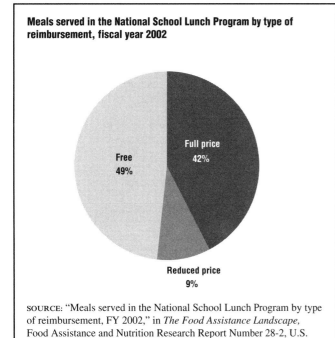

Meals served in the National School Lunch Program by type of reimbursement, fiscal year 2002

SOURCE: "Meals served in the National School Lunch Program by type of reimbursement, FY 2002," in *The Food Assistance Landscape,* Food Assistance and Nutrition Research Report Number 28-2, U.S. Department of Agriculture, Economic Research Service, Washington, DC, March 2003

FIGURE 10.6

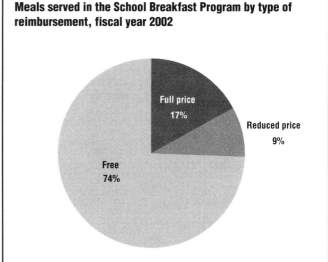

Meals served in the School Breakfast Program by type of reimbursement, fiscal year 2002

SOURCE: "Meals served in the School Breakfast Program by type of reimbursement, FY 2002," in *The Food Assistance Landscape,* Food Assistance and Nutrition Research Report Number 28-2, U.S. Department of Agriculture, Economic Research Service, Washington, DC, March 2003

second-largest monthly enrollment of the food-assistance programs. In FY 2002 over 28 million children (58 percent of all children attending a participating institution) received subsidized lunches, at a cost of $6.8 billion. Almost 50 percent of the children got free lunches, and another 9 percent received reduced-priced lunches. (See Figure 10.5.)

A 1992 *School Nutrition Dietary Assessment* found that although school lunches were nutritious, they provided 38 percent of calories from total fat and 15 percent of calories from saturated fat. This is more fat than specified by the USDA's *Dietary Guidelines for Americans,* which recommends that 30 percent or fewer calories come from total fat and less than 10 percent of calories come from saturated fat. The study also found that lunches provided an average of 1,479 milligrams of sodium—almost two-thirds the National Research Council's recommendation for daily intake.

Starting in the 1996–97 school year, schools had to meet USDA nutritional guidelines in promoting the health of children. School cafeterias have always had the difficult task of trying to serve nutritious meals to children, who often prefer high-fat, high-sodium meals such as pizza or macaroni and cheese. The USDA's Team Nutrition Program is helping school cafeterias make changes to their menus, reducing the fat content of foods and providing more healthy choices. How effective have these efforts been? A May 2003 report from the General Accounting Office (GAO; *School Lunch Program: Efforts Needed to Improve Nutrition and Encourage Healthy Eating*) found

that while schools were making progress, more improvements were needed. Students were still consuming too many calories from fat and schools were not providing enough encouragement toward healthy eating. The GAO recommended more nutrition education and reduced access to foods with little nutritional value.

**SCHOOL BREAKFAST PROGRAM.** Begun in 1966, the School Breakfast Program became permanent in 1975. Eligibility is the same as for the National School Lunch Program. Although participation in the program has grown steadily since 2000, the breakfast program is still smaller than the lunch program. In recent years, the USDA has encouraged schools that participate in the lunch program to offer the School Breakfast Program.

In FY 2002 the program served almost 1.4 billion breakfasts to low-income children at a cost of $1.6 billion. About three-quarters (74 percent) of the meals were served free, and another 9 percent were offered at reduced prices. (See Figure 10.6.)

**CHILD AND ADULT CARE FOOD PROGRAM.** The Child and Adult Care Food Program provides cash and food to child care centers, family day care homes, and adult day care centers. In FY 2002, 1.74 billion meals were served— 98 percent in child care centers and family day care homes, and 3 percent in adult day care centers. Expenditures increased 6.5 percent from FY 2001 to FY 2002. Nearly 75 percent of all meals were free; another 9 percent were at reduced prices.

FIGURE 10.7

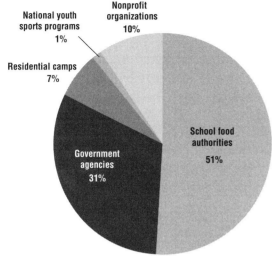

**Distribution of Summer Food Service Program meals, by provider, 2001**

SOURCE: "School districts served half of all SFSP meals," in *The Food Assistance Landscape,* Food Assistance and Nutrition Research Report Number 28-2, U.S. Department of Agriculture, Economic Research Service, Washington, DC, March 2003

FIGURE 10.8

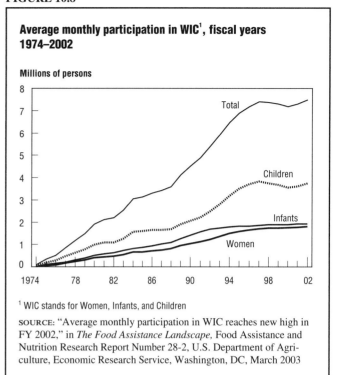

**Average monthly participation in WIC[1], fiscal years 1974–2002**

[1] WIC stands for Women, Infants, and Children

SOURCE: "Average monthly participation in WIC reaches new high in FY 2002," in *The Food Assistance Landscape,* Food Assistance and Nutrition Research Report Number 28-2, U.S. Department of Agriculture, Economic Research Service, Washington, DC, March 2003

**SUMMER FOOD SERVICE PROGRAM.** During school vacations, the Summer Food Service Program provides free meals and snacks to children 18 and younger, and to handicapped persons over age 18, in places where at least half of the children come from households with incomes at or below 185 percent of the federal income poverty guidelines. During the summer of 2001, more than 130 million meals and snacks were served. Figure 10.7 shows the distribution of Summer Food Service Program meals by type of provider.

**SPECIAL MILK PROGRAM.** Expansion of the National School Lunch and School Breakfast Programs, both of which include subsidized milk, has led to a substantial reduction in the Special Milk Program since its peak in the late 1960s. Participation is now limited to schools, summer camps, and child care institutions that have no federally assisted meal program, or to prekindergarten or kindergarten children who attend half-day sessions and have no access to milk programs. Milk is offered free or at reduced cost. In FY 1998 the program cost $17 million, a slight decrease over the previous year. In 2002, about 8,300 institutions (schools, child care centers, and summer camps) participated in the program. The program received $16.1 million in federal funds in FY 2002 (the latest year for which data were available)—a 3.9 percent increase over funds appropriated in FY 2001.

## Supplemental Food Programs

**SPECIAL SUPPLEMENTAL NUTRITION PROGRAM FOR WOMEN, INFANTS, AND CHILDREN (WIC).** The Special Supplemental Nutrition Program for Women, Infants, and Children (WIC) is the third-largest food-assistance program. It provides nutritious supplemental foods, nutrition education, and health care referrals at no cost to low-income pregnant women, women in the period after childbirth, infants, and children up to the age of five. To be eligible, income must be below 185 percent of the federal income poverty guidelines. States can, however, set lower income limits.

Although all food-assistance programs promote improved nutrition as an objective, only WIC requires that a health official or a nutritionist first determine a recipient's nutritional needs. Eligible mothers get monthly food vouchers from their local health clinics. They can redeem these vouchers for specific foods rich in nutrients, such as infant formula, eggs, fruit juice, milk, cheese, and cereal. In FY 2002 these monthly benefits averaged $34.87 per person.

Under the WIC Farmers' Market Nutrition Program, recipients receive coupons to buy fresh fruits and vegetables at participating farmers' markets. A study sponsored by the USDA's Food and Nutrition Service in 1990 showed that women who participated in the program during their pregnancies had lower Medicaid costs for themselves and their babies than women who did not participate. (Low-income people receive government-paid health care under Medicaid.)

FIGURE 10.9

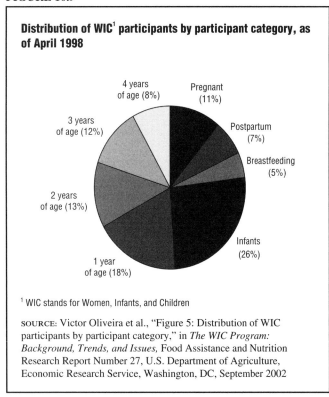

**Distribution of WIC¹ participants by participant category, as of April 1998**

4 years of age (8%)
Pregnant (11%)
3 years of age (12%)
Postpartum (7%)
Breastfeeding (5%)
2 years of age (13%)
Infants (26%)
1 year of age (18%)

¹ WIC stands for Women, Infants, and Children

SOURCE: Victor Oliveira et al., "Figure 5: Distribution of WIC participants by participant category," in *The WIC Program: Background, Trends, and Issues,* Food Assistance and Nutrition Research Report Number 27, U.S. Department of Agriculture, Economic Research Service, Washington, DC, September 2002

Participation in WIC continues to grow (see Figure 10.8), with expenditures totaling $4.3 billion in FY 2002, a 4.6 percent increase from FY 2001. In FY 2002, 7.5 million persons received WIC support. About half of WIC funding recipients are children, and one-quarter are infants. Figure 10.9 shows the distribution of WIC participants by category in 1998.

COMMODITY SUPPLEMENTAL FOOD PROGRAM. The Commodity Supplemental Food Program (CSFP) serves women and children up to six years of age, who are not WIC participants, as well as low-income people age 60 and over. While WIC uses vouchers, the CSFP distributes monthly food parcels. In FY 2002 the program provided monthly food parcels to about 410,000 people, an 11 percent increase from 1997. As more women and children switch to the WIC program, the CSFP serves an increasing proportion of the elderly. In FY 2002, 337,000 elderly people participated in the program each month, as did more than 73,000 women and children. Federal appropriation for the program in 2002 totaled $92.9 million.

**Food Donation Programs**

FOOD DISTRIBUTION PROGRAM ON INDIAN RESERVATIONS. The USDA provides food to families who live on or near Indian reservations. The program is an alternative to the Food Stamp Program for those whose remote location limits access to food stores. In FY 2002 (the latest year for which data were available), more than 110,000

Native Americans participated and the federal government spent $75.8 million on the program.

NUTRITION SERVICES INCENTIVE PROGRAM. Under an amendment to the Older Americans Act of 2000, the name of the Nutrition Program for the Elderly was changed to the Nutrition Services Incentive Program (NSIP). As provided for by public law (PL 108-7), the program was transferred to the Administration on Aging. The NSIP provides cash and food to the states for meals for senior citizens. Food is served in senior-citizen centers or delivered by Meals-on-Wheels programs. There is no income test for eligibility; all persons over 60 are eligible. Recipients can contribute as much as they wish to the cost of the meals, although the meals are free to those who cannot afford to pay. In FY 2001 the program provided 21 million meals each month, with a federal appropriation of $150 million.

THE EMERGENCY FOOD ASSISTANCE PROGRAM. The Emergency Food Assistance Program (TEFAP) was started in 1982 to help distribute government surpluses of butter, cheese, non-fat dry milk, honey, rice, cornmeal, and flour to needy families. Federal costs for TEFAP rapidly increased until the late 1980s, when surpluses were used up. As government stocks were depleted, food distribution had to be either discontinued or financed with federal funds.

The Federal Agriculture Improvement and Reform Act (PL 104-127; also known as the 1996 Farm Bill) made TEFAP a permanent program based on funding rather than purchases of surplus foods. In FY 1997 TEFAP and the Food Donation Programs to Soup Kitchens and Food Banks were combined into a single program, and in 1998 expenditures totaled nearly $235 million. For FY 2003 TEFAP was to receive $190 million in federal funding.

**2002 Farm Bill Food-Assistance Provisions**

The 2002 Farm Bill reauthorized the Food Stamp Program and related food-assistance programs through FY 2007. New provisions for these programs included the reinstatement of legal immigrants already receiving disability benefits to eligibility for the Food Stamp Program as of October 2002. As of April 2003 all legal immigrants who had lived continuously in the United States for five years could apply for food stamp benefits. In addition, all legal immigrant children, no matter how long they had lived in the United States, were eligible to apply for food stamp benefits as of October 2003.

The 2002 Farm Bill also reauthorized funding provisions of the Food Stamp Act. For FY 2003–2007 up to $5 million in annual funds may be awarded to competitive projects designed to improve access to the Food Stamp Program, including community outreach efforts.

# IMPORTANT NAMES AND ADDRESSES

**American Dietetic Association**
120 South Riverside Plaza
Suite 2000
Chicago, IL 60606-6995
(312) 899-0040
FAX: (312) 899-4899
URL: http://www.eatright.org

**Calorie Control Council**
5775 Peachtree-Dunwoody Rd.
Suite 500-G
Atlanta, GA 30342
(404) 252-3663
URL: http://www.caloriecontrol.org

**Council for Responsible Nutrition**
1828 L St. NW
Suite 900
Washington, DC 20036-5114
(202) 776-7929
FAX: (202) 204-7980
E-mail: webmaster@crnusa.org
URL: http://www.crnusa.org

**Food Marketing Institute**
655 15th St. NW
Suite 700
Washington, DC 20005
(202) 220-0730
FAX: (202) 220-0877
E-mail: fmi@fmi.org
URL: http://www.fmi.org

**National Center for Food and Agricultural Policy**
1616 P St. NW, 1st Floor
Washington, DC 20036
(202) 328-5048
FAX: (202) 328-5133
E-mail: ncfap@ncfap.org
URL: http://www.ncfap.org

**National Restaurant Association**
1200 17th St. NW
Washington, DC 20036-3097
(202) 331-5900

FAX: (202) 331-2429
E-mail: info@dineout.org
URL: http://www.restaurant.org

**Public Citizen**
**Health Research Group**
1600 20th St. NW
Washington, DC 20009
(202) 588-1000
FAX: (202) 588-7796
URL: http://www.citizen.org/hrg

**U.S. Department of Agriculture**
**Agricultural Research Service**
Room 1-2250
5601 Sunnyside Ave.
Beltsville, MD 20705-5128
(301) 504-1638
FAX: (301) 504-1648
E-mail: arsweb@nal.usda.gov
URL: http://www.ars.usda.gov

**U.S. Department of Agriculture**
**Center for Nutrition Policy and Promotion**
1120 20th St. NW
Suite 200 North Lobby
Washington, DC 20036
(202) 418-2312
E-mail: cnpp-web@www.usda.gov
URL: http://www.cnpp.usda.gov

**U.S. Department of Agriculture**
**Economic Research Service**
1800 M Street NW
Washington, DC 20036-5831
(202) 694-5100
FAX: (202) 694-5641
E-mail: service@ers.usda.gov
URL: http://www.ers.usda.gov

**U.S. Department of Agriculture**
**Food Safety and Inspection Service**
FSIS Food Safety Education and
Communications Staff
1400 Independence Ave. SW

Room 2932-South Bldg.
Washington, DC 20250-3700
(202) 720-7943
FAX: (202) 720-1843
E-mail: fsis.webmaster@usda.gov
URL: http://www.usda.gov/agency/fsis/
homepage/htm

**U.S. Department of Health and Human Services**
**Centers for Disease Control and Prevention**
1600 Clifton Rd. NE
Atlanta, GA 30333
(404) 639-3311
URL: http://www.cdc.gov

**U.S. Department of Health and Human Services**
**Food and Drug Administration**
**Center for Food Safety and Applied Nutrition**
5600 Fishers Lane
Rockville, MD 20857
(888) 463-6332
URL: http://www.cfsan.fda.gov

**Weight-control Information Network**
1 Win Way
Bethesda, MD 20892-3665
(202) 828-1025
(202) 828-1028
FAX: (301) 984-7196
E-mail: win@info.niddk.nih.gov
URL: http://www.niddk.nih.gov/health/
nutrit/nutrit.htm

**Wheat Foods Council**
10841 South Crossroads Dr., Suite 105
Parker, CO 80138
(303) 840- 8787
FAX: (303) 840-6877
E-mail: wfc@wheatfoods.org
URL: http://www.wheatfoods.org

# RESOURCES

The U.S. Department of Agriculture (USDA) is responsible for collecting and reporting information on food in the United States. The Economic Research Service (ERS) of the USDA organizes much of that information, producing a wide range of valuable publications on agriculture and food. Its journal *FoodReview,* renamed *Amber Waves* early in 2003, affords an excellent overview of domestic food consumption and expenditures, foreign aid, and food-assistance programs. *FoodReview's* Annual Spotlight on the U.S. Food System (1998) was an important resource in preparing this book. *Food Consumption, Prices, and Expenditures, 1970–1997* (1998) presents historical data on the per capita consumption of food and its cost. *Dietary Guidelines for Americans, 2000* was also an excellent resource.

The USDA National Agricultural Statistics Service conducted the *1997 Census of Agriculture* (1999), providing important data for this book. USDA's *Agricultural Baseline Projections to 2012* also provided useful information.

The USDA's *1994–96 Continuing Survey of Food Intakes by Individuals and Diet and Health Knowledge Survey* (1997), published by the Agricultural Research Service, is the government's main source of data on individual food intake. The *Agriculture Fact Book 2001–2002* (2003), produced by the Office of Communications, offers useful information about U.S. agriculture, rural America, nutrition, consumer issues, and trade.

In *Consumer Expenditures in 2001* (2003), the Bureau of Labor Statistics (BLS) of the Department of Labor examined how people spent their income. The *Public Health Reports,* published bimonthly by the U.S. Department of Health and Human Services (HHS) and the Association of Schools of Public Health, discussed "The Selling of Olestra" (1998). The *Morbidity and Mortality Weekly Report,* prepared by the Centers for Disease Control and Prevention (CDC) of the HHS, periodically provides health studies and reports concerning nutrition.

The Food and Drug Administration (FDA) publishes agricultural information bulletins that provide useful articles on food safety and nutrition. The FDA's Pesticide Program *Residue Monitoring 2001* (2003) examined food safety.

The Food Marketing Institute published *Trends in the United States: Consumer Attitudes & the Supermarket, 2003,* a survey of supermarket shopping patterns.

Nutrition is an important issue for many Americans, and many newsletters address these concerns. The Center for Science in the Public Interest publishes *Nutrition Action Health Letter;* Tufts University puts out *The Tufts University Diet and Nutrition Letter;* and the University of California's School of Public Health publishes the *University of California at Berkeley Wellness Letter.* All of them provide useful information and current research on nutrition. Oklahoma State University's Web site contains information on sources of fiber.

The National Restaurant Association surveyed consumers in *Nutrition and Restaurants: A Consumer Perspective* (1993) and in *Meal Consumption Behavior* (1996). The Wheat Foods Council's *Grains of Truth About Fad Diets & Obesity* (2003) was also very helpful.

# INDEX